AF691568

A PRACTICAL GUIDE TO ELECTRODIAGNOSIS IN DOGS AND CATS

First published in 2024 by Libri Publishing

Copyright © Libri Publishing

The right of Hélène Vandenberghe, Edward Ives and Nicolas Granger to be identified as the editors of this work has been asserted in accordance with the Copyright, Designs and Patents Act, 1988.

ISBN 978-1-911450-93-1

All rights reserved. No part of this publication may be reproduced, stored in any retrieval system or transmitted in any form or by any means, electronic, mechanical, photocopying, recording or otherwise, without the prior written permission of the copyright holder for which application should be addressed in the first instance to the publishers. No liability shall be attached to the author, the copyright holder or the publishers for loss or damage of any nature suffered as a result of reliance on the reproduction of any of the contents of this publication or any errors or omissions in its contents.

A CIP catalogue record for this book is available from
The British Library

Cover and design by Carnegie Book Production

Front cover image adapted with permission from Ivalalearn
(part of the Veterinary Information Network® family).

Libri Publishing
Brunel House
Volunteer Way
Faringdon
Oxfordshire
SN7 7YR

Tel: +44 (0)845 873 3837

www.libripublishing.co.uk

A PRACTICAL GUIDE TO ELECTRODIAGNOSIS IN DOGS AND CATS

Hélène Vandenberghe,
Edward Ives,
Nicolas Granger

Foreword

Veterinary neurology has been crying out for this book for ages!

Electrodiagnostic testing is clearly important as a means of detecting abnormalities and quantifying function of the nervous system but in recent years it has become relatively neglected in clinical veterinary neurology. This decline has occurred to such an extent that, currently, many private referral clinics in the USA do not even have the necessary equipment. Instead, veterinary neurology has become dominated by imaging. While the widespread availability of MRI initially led to rapid expansion of differential diagnosis lists in small animal neurology, there is now a growing appreciation of the limitations of imaging in diagnosis of many neurologic conditions.

For instance, there are many examples where the assessment of function is as important as imaging findings, if not more so. It is of course well established that electrodiagnostics are necessary for accurate categorisation of peripheral nerve diseases and, arguably, for junctionopathies and muscle diseases. Even so, the relative value of electrodiagnostic testing compared with imaging is easily underestimated, as illustrated by current methods for diagnosis of degenerative lumbosacral stenosis (DLSS). At present, DLSS is primarily diagnosed by imaging, even though it is recognised that the findings in normal and affected individuals greatly overlap. Conversely, electrodiagnostic testing can directly identify aberrant nerve function and so could be considered to provide more reliable recognition of nerve compression (albeit not the cause). However, such is the current dominance of veterinary neurology by imaging that the value of electrodiagnostic tests is usually assessed against the gold standard provided by imaging!

Recent increased recognition of the value of electrodiagnostics in modern veterinary neurology is most apparent in two specific areas. First, there have been many explorations of assessment of spinal cord 'long tract' function by evoked potentials, particularly after severe spinal cord injury. These methods will likely be key in providing evidence to refine the timing and need for surgical interventions or the introduction of novel therapies, such as cell transplants. Second, there is a rapidly burgeoning interest in applying EEG in dogs for more precise diagnosis of seizures and seizure-like disorders. An obvious application is for categorising paroxysmal events, but recent accumulated expertise has also led to increased recognition of non-convulsive status epilepticus, which has major implications for management. In some parts of the world there is now a strong drive to identify surgical targets in epileptic animals and EEG will be a central component of this exciting innovation in veterinary neurology. Both these increasingly important electrodiagnostic techniques are the subject of excellent chapters in this book.

Although electrodiagnostic tests are irreplaceable in evaluating the nervous system, the application and interpretation of the procedures can appear daunting, especially to trainees. This book provides the essential material to both allow novices to become confident with everyday tests and to also provide guidance to jaded old-timers on more recherche procedures. Key points at the beginning of each chapter provide a rapidly assimilated introduction to guide readers to appropriate pages, and a great merit of this text overall is its clear and logical organisation. As well as explanations of the physiological basis for the tests themselves, the book also contains highly practical sections detailing exactly HOW to do the procedures and more theoretical aspects that aid interpretation of the results and understanding of how various diseases are expressed. There are abundant illustrations that augment text explanations.

With its wide-ranging yet concise format, written by highly accomplished neurologists with decades of practical experience in applying electrodiagnostic tests, I thoroughly recommend this book to anyone with an interest in veterinary neurology, especially those training in this specialty. While I have pointed out some currently obvious areas where electrodiagnostics have become increasingly highly valued, perhaps future readers, like you, will develop new applications of these techniques or develop wholly new techniques!

Prof. Nick Jeffery
Department of Small Animal Clinical Sciences
Texas A&M University

July 5th 2024

Introduction

Electrophysiologic studies can be extremely valuable for the diagnosis and further characterisation of various neurological conditions in animals.

There has been a large number of publications that describe the recording techniques and expected results in normal animals and, less commonly, the results for various disease states. However, this field seems to have been rather effaced in the past couple of decades, perhaps with the increasing availability of advanced imaging techniques in companion animals, such as magnetic resonance imaging. This has, in turn, resulted in the potential for a lack of familiarity with electophysiologic studies. Some specialist centres around the world are highly proficient in these techniques and frequently perform such studies, whilst others perform them rarely, if at all, and lack both experience and confidence.

It is true that electrophysiology may not appear intuitive at a first glance and has two major limitations in companion animals: (i) animals need to be anaesthetised, which is a situation that does not marry well with some neuromuscular conditions in which respiratory weakness can be a feature; and (ii) acquiring the data can be time consuming and there can be challenges when it comes to interpreting the results. However, with basic understanding of the discipline, good methodology and practice, electrophysiology becomes very approachable and feasible for the clinician, and most examinations can be completed in 15 minutes (e.g., electromyography) to 45 minutes (e.g., when a full study is performed).

The importance of electrophysiology is clearly illustrated by the fact that some conditions, including those with severe clinical presentations (such as acute idiopathic polyradiculoneuritis), will have normal magnetic resonance imaging but very clear findings using electrophysiology. This immediately places the clinician in a situation where they can 'rule in' conditions rather than 'ruling them out', which is a major objective in clinical medicine. Of equal importance is that electrophysiology can be used to confirm a clinical suspicion of neuromuscular disease (versus an orthopaedic condition or myelopathy for instance), localise the problem, and guide decision-making regarding additional diagnostic tests, such as performing muscle/nerve biopsies or brachial plexus imaging for instance.

In this manual, we would like to reach veterinary colleagues practising neurology, in particular specialists in training who constitute the future of veterinary neurology, moving away from the current black-and-white vision that veterinary surgeons may have of electrophysiology: either 'I love it' or 'I hate it'. Hopefully adding the 'I now understand this' for others! We therefore hope that this manual will allow the reader to understand the basic principles behind electrophysiology (we do not intend to provide a long discussion around physics and electrical currents), and how to practically apply these techniques in the clinic to serve their diagnostic needs and improve their patients' outcomes. We also hope that this will help to spread the use of electrophysiology more widely and, by doing so and with a common methodology, help to establish electrophysiologic characteristics of numerous neuromuscular disorders in order to be able to diagnose them more efficiently in the future.

Table of contents

SECTION 1

Anatomy and physiology of the peripheral nervous system and principles of electrophysiology

Nicolas Granger, Hélène Vandenberghe,
Edward Ives, Benjamin Metcalfe

Key points:

- The membrane potential is the potential difference between the intracellular and extracellular space.
- The resting membrane potential arises from ion gradients across the cell membrane with more negative charges inside the cell compared to outside. It is typically -70mV to -90mV.
- When the depolarising potential reaches a threshold, a nerve action potential is triggered by opening of voltage-gated sodium channels and influx of sodium inside the cell, as an all-or-nothing mechanism.
- When the nerve action potential reaches the nerve terminal, it triggers an influx of calcium in the pre-synaptic area and acetylcholine release at the neuromuscular junction. This leads to a post-synaptic end-plate potential, triggering a muscle action potential if a threshold is reached.

- The nerve conduction velocity is higher in large diameter and myelinated axons because of saltatory conduction.
- The potentials recorded during electrodiagnosis are extracellular recordings of intracellular events originating from the muscles or nerves.
- Nerve stimulation uses a bipolar (cathode and anode) montage. Depolarisation of the nerve membrane occurs below the cathode and the nerve action potential propagates in both directions from its point of stimulation.
- Two types of potentials can be recorded: near-field potentials are recorded by a pair of electrodes located close to the source generating the potential, whilst far-field potentials are produced by neural generators located away from the recording electrodes.
- Recording in the nerve or muscle typically uses a 'differential' bipolar (cathode and anode) measurement. An amplifier measures the difference in voltage between two points: a cathode electrode and an anode electrode.

1. Anatomy of the peripheral nervous system

(i) Anatomic organisation of the peripheral nervous system

The peripheral nervous system is located outside the brain and spinal cord. It comprises the nerve roots of cranial and spinal nerves, the peripheral motor/sensory/mixed nerves, neuromuscular junctions and muscles. The cell bodies of the motor neurons are located in the ventral grey matter of the spinal cord (spinal nerves) or the brainstem (cranial nerves III – XII). The axons of these cell bodies exit the spinal cord as the ventral nerve roots, which leave the spinal canal via intervertebral foramina. These motor fibres contribute to the motor portion of the individual peripheral nerves that innervate the skeletal muscles via neuromuscular junctions.

The cell bodies of the sensory neurons reside within enlargements along the peripheral nerves called sensory ganglia. For the spinal nerves, these 'dorsal root ganglia' are located outside the spinal cord within each intervertebral foramen. Axons from the cell bodies within each ganglion form the sensory nerve roots that project proximally to the dorsal grey matter of the spinal cord, whilst dendrites project distally as the sensory nerve. The motor and sensory nerve roots unite at each intervertebral foramen, distal to the dorsal root ganglion, to form a mixed spinal nerve. The muscles innervated by axons originating from a single spinal cord segment (i.e., one motor nerve root) are called a myotome, and the cutaneous area supplied by one spinal cord segment (i.e., one sensory nerve root) is called a dermatome.

(ii) Anatomy of the peripheral nerves

Peripheral nerves contain nerve trunks, which are themselves composed of multiple axons. These axons are organised within fascicles embedded in connective tissue of collagen, elastic fibres and fat. Each axon is covered by the endoneurium, each fascicle is contained within a perineurium, and the entire nerve is surrounded by the epineurium (Kimura, 2013; Michell, 2013; Shapiro and Preston, 2013) (**Figure 1.1**).

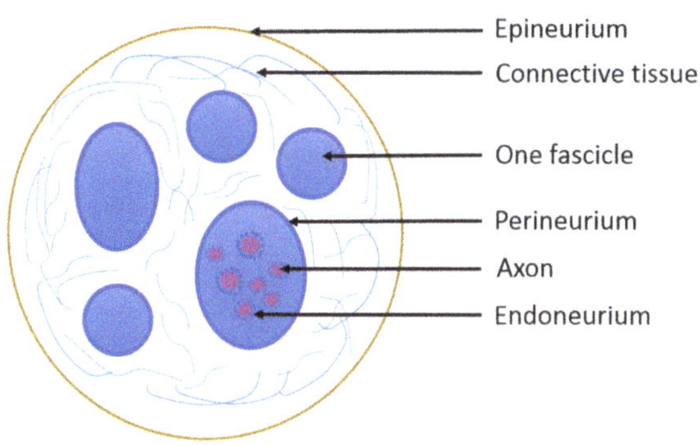

Figure 1.1. Microstructure of a nerve trunk.

(iii) Classification of the peripheral nerves

Peripheral nerves can be classified according to several parameters: (a) the information their axons convey; (b) the myelination or absence of myelination of the axons; and (c) the diameter of the axons.

The peripheral nervous system is broadly divided into the somatic and autonomic nervous system, with the latter being subdivided into sympathetic or parasympathetic fibres that regulate vital, involuntary physiological processes such as blood pressure, heart rate, gastrointestinal and glandular functions. The somatic nervous system is composed of motor and sensory fibres that innervate the muscles and skin. These fibres can be myelinated or unmyelinated, with myelinated axons covered by a myelin sheath formed by the surface membrane of Schwann cells (Kimura, 2013). The nodes of Ranvier are uninsulated gaps along the myelinated fibres between areas covered by adjacent Schwann cells (see **Figure 1.3** later in this chapter).

Peripheral nerve fibres can be further classified as follows:

- A-fibres are large-diameter myelinated axons that can be divided into four subtypes: (i) Aα (or Ia) fibres are the primary receptors of the muscle spindle and Golgi tendon organs, involved in transmitting proprioceptive information from the muscles and joints to the spinal cord; (ii) Aβ fibres are the secondary receptors of the muscle spindle (involved in proprioception) and part of the cutaneous mechanoreceptors; (iii) Aδ fibres are free nerve endings associated with somatic pain; and (iv) Aγ fibres are fibres from the motor neurons controlling the intrinsic activation of the muscle spindle.
- B-fibres are small-diameter myelinated fibres involved in transmission of autonomic information.
- C-fibres are small-diameter unmyelinated fibres that respond to thermal, mechanical, and chemical stimuli, or a combination of these stimuli.

The number, characteristics, and proportions of these axons within each fascicle varies (Michell, 2013; Shapiro and Preston, 2013), and this has direct consequences on electrodiagnostic recordings, as we will see later in 'Section 4 – Appendicular motor nerve conduction studies'.

2. Physiology of the peripheral nerves and useful electrophysiologic principles

Although peripheral nerve physiology and the physics of electrophysiology might initially appear daunting, it is worthwhile investing a small amount of time in understanding some basic electrical principles. This will allow you as a clinician to understand the basic concepts required to correctly perform, recognise, and interpret electrodiagnostic tests and their findings in animals.

(i) Membrane potential

Neurons are electrically active and excitable cells with specialised membranes. These membranes are made of impermeable bilayers of lipids and protein channels which allow the selective passage of specific ions. The membrane potential is the potential difference between the intracellular and extracellular space. Its value depends on which types of ion channel are open at any one time, and the relative concentrations of ions between the intracellular and extracellular spaces.

(ii) Resting membrane potential

During the resting state, there is more negative charge inside the cell than outside the neuronal cell membrane. This resting membrane potential is typically between -70 and -90mV for neurons. Potassium (K^+) and organic anions are found at higher concentrations in the intracellular space, whilst sodium (Na^+) and chloride (Cl^-) are found at higher concentrations in the extracellular space. This provides a gradient for ions to flow in or out of the cell when their respective channels are open. Concentration gradients are maintained by the Na^+/K^+ ATPase pump via active efflux of Na^+ into the extracellular space, maintaining the negative charge inside the cell – the energy of one ATP molecule is used to exchange 3 intracellular Na^+ ions for 2 extracellular K^+ ions. In the resting state, the cell membrane is mostly permeable to potassium, which moves freely across the membrane.

(iii) Action potential

The neuronal membrane potential can change depending on chemical signals called neurotransmitters that are released by nearby cells. Some neurotransmitters are excitatory, causing an influx of Na^+ and Ca^{2+}, thus reducing the negative charge within the cell and depolarising the cell membrane. Other neurotransmitters are inhibitory, causing an increase in the K^+ and Cl^- conductance, which increases the negative charge within the cell and hyperpolarises the cell membrane (i.e., making it less excitable). Neurotransmitters generate graded potentials in the dendrites, which influence the production of a 'generator potential' in the axon of the same cell. When this generator potential reaches a threshold of ~ -65mV, an action potential starts at the axon hillock on an all-or-nothing basis. The axon hillock is the conical part of the cell body where the axon departs, and synaptic inputs are summated.

The depolarisation/repolarisation process relies largely on voltage-gated sodium and potassium channels. These channels are controlled by voltage sensors and open/close when the membrane potential reaches a certain level, which is specific to each channel. First, there is opening of voltage-gated sodium channels, leading to an influx of sodium inside the cell. Once a threshold is reached (~ -65mV), any sodium channel that had remained closed opens, leading to a further and rapid depolarisation. Voltage-gated sodium channels are 'time locked' and close after a few milliseconds, hence the axon remains depolarised for a limited amount of time. At this stage, there is opening of voltage-gated potassium channels and potassium moves out of the cell. The cell membrane potential therefore becomes more negative again, goes through a short phase of hyperpolarisation, and eventually returns to its resting potential. Afterwards, the voltage-gated sodium channels remain closed for a period called the 'refractory period', during which a second stimulus cannot trigger an action potential. The refractory period is divided into: (i) the absolute refractory period, when the sodium channels are still closed after an action potential; and (ii) the relative refractory period, during which sodium channels come out of their inactivation and the neuron can be excited, but only with a stimulus stronger than the one normally needed to initiate an action potential (**Figure 1.2**).

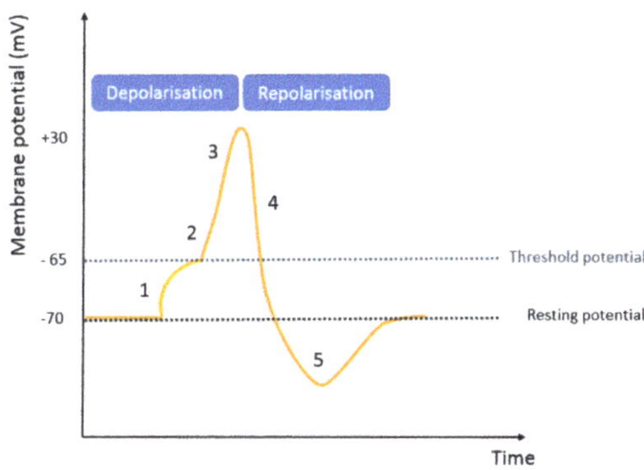

Figure 1.2. Nerve action potential, demonstrating the voltage measured across the cell membrane over time. 1. A stimulus causes opening of voltage-gated sodium channels; 2. A threshold is reached and more voltage-gated sodium channels open resulting in sodium rushing into the cell; 3. Voltage-gated sodium channels begin to close and voltage-gated potassium channels begin to open; 4. Voltage-gated sodium channels are closed and voltage-gated potassium channels are open: potassium rushes out of the cell; 5. Some voltage-gated potassium channels are still open, leading to a transient hyperpolarisation.

(iv) Electric current

An electric current corresponds to the flow of charges over time (e.g., electrons in a metallic wire or ions in an axon). This occurs from one point of a volume or conductor to another point when there is an electric potential difference (voltage, measured in volts [V]) between the two points.

Negative charges (like electrons) flow from the negative end to the positive end of a conductor (e.g., electron current), whilst positive charges move from the positive to the negative end. By convention, the current's direction is that of the positive charges. The current (in amperes [A]) is the voltage (difference in potential in volts [V]) divided by the resistance (in ohms [Ω]) of the material it travels through.

(v) Electrodes – cathode, anode and 'reference'

The anode is the positive terminal of an electric current source, and the cathode is the negative terminal. This concept applies for both electrical stimulation, where a pair of needle electrodes may be the sources stimulating a nerve, and for recording, where the nerve itself (or the muscle) is the source of the current that is detected by two recording electrodes, a cathode (E1) and an anode (E2).

Regarding the terminology used for recording electrodes, the cathode is the active 'recording' electrode (E1), which is attached to the black port of the amplifier, and the anode (E2) is attached to the red port of the amplifier. The potential difference between the electrical activity recorded at the cathode compared to that at the anode is used to generate the trace displayed on the screen of the electrodiagnostic unit (see below). A third electrode is also placed for recording, which is connected to the green-coloured socket of the amplifier. This is frequently termed the 'earth' or 'ground' electrode. However, this is a misnomer as its purpose is not to divert stray current from the patient into the ground in the event of an electrical malfunction (as the EMG machine itself may have via its power plug). This electrode is in fact a common reference point for the anode and active (cathode) recording electrodes. The amplifier of the EMG machine takes the voltage at the cathode compared to this reference point and subtracts the voltage at the anode compared to this common 'ground' (E0) to give a net voltage difference between cathode (E1) and anode (E2). Therefore, the 'ground electrode' does not have a role in patient safety and simply acts as a reference point representing background electrical activity in the surrounding environment that is common to all recording electrodes. As has been suggested in human medicine (Robinson *et al.*, 2016), the authors have therefore referred to this electrode as the 'reference electrode' throughout the text, rather than a ground or earth. This choice of nomenclature may initially appear confusing, particularly as in previous texts the anodal recording electrode has been commonly termed the 'reference' for the active cathode. However, our goal in using these terms is to promote the correct terminology that may be used in future publications and hope the explanation above is useful in supporting this.

(vi) Propagation of action potentials and saltatory conduction

Action potentials are generated at one end of the nerve (e.g., a sensory receptor or motor neuron cell body) and travel to the other end of the axon (e.g., a sensory potential ascending along axons of a mixed peripheral nerve to reach a dorsal root ganglion). In unmyelinated axons, this corresponds simply to a flow of charges along the axon. However, in myelinated axons this conduction is accelerated by a process called saltatory conduction. Peripheral nerves contain myelinated axons (e.g., A-fibres), with Schwann cells forming segments of myelin along the axon. These segments play an insulating role, with no charges exchanged across the insulated segments. A node of Ranvier is the non-insulated part of the axon in between two myelinated segments. Charges can be exchanged in and out of the axon at these nodes – the voltage difference at the level of a node of Ranvier is such that the positive charges are outside the axon in the extracellular space and the negative charges are within the axons underneath the cell membrane (**Figure 1.3**).

Action potentials can only occur at the nodes of Ranvier, where there are many sodium channels and only a few potassium channels. When an action potential is initiated, sodium ions rush into the axon at the nodes of Ranvier. This phenomenon is called a 'sinking current' and one that we will see again in

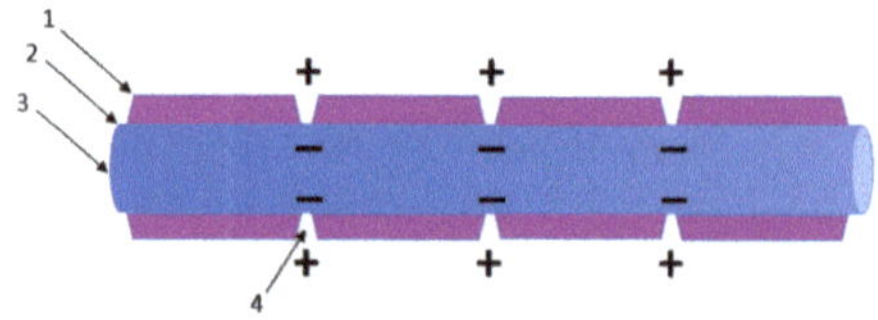

Figure 1.3. Resting membrane potential at the level of the node of Ranvier. There is more negative charge inside the axon than outside the axonal membrane, with the potential difference being around -70 mV in the resting state. 1. Myelin sheath; 2. Axonal membrane; 3. Axon; 4. Node of Ranvier.

the next sections (**Figure 1.4A**). The intracellular environment at that level becomes more positively charged than the intracellular environment at the next node(s) along the axon. This creates an electrical gradient between the depolarised section of the axon (at the node of Ranvier) and the more negative environment at the nodes around it. Consequently, the positive ions are pushed inside the axon towards the next node(s), which then in turn depolarises (**Figure 1.4B**). There is also a current source outside the axon flowing from the positive regions to the negative region of the extracellular space (**Figure 1.4B**).

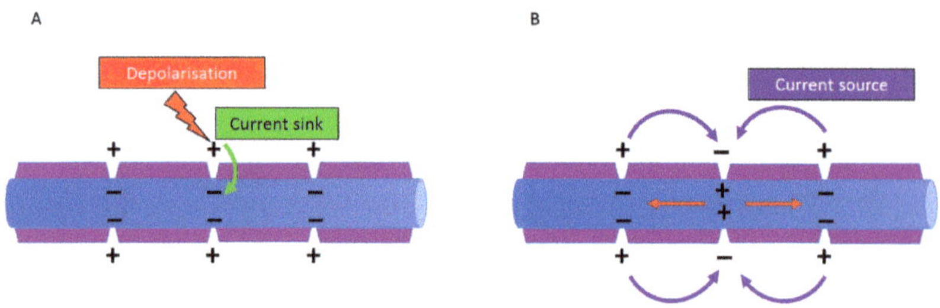

Figure 1.4. Depolarisation at the level of a node of Ranvier. **A.** When depolarisation occurs at a node of Ranvier, sodium ions rush into the axon, creating a current sink. The intracellular environment becomes more positively charged than the extracellular environment resulting in depolarisation. **B.** An electrical gradient is created between the depolarised node of Ranvier and the next nodes (more negative intracellular environment), and the positive ions are pushed inside the axon towards the next nodes (red arrows), leading to depolarisation of the next node and saltatory conduction of the impulse down the axon (in this instance in both directions). There is a current source outside the axon flowing from the positive regions to the negative region of the extracellular space.

The myelinated segments between nodes insulate the axon from passive loss of positive ions across the cell membrane, meaning that there is still sufficient charge by the time it reaches the next node to trigger another action potential. This results in rapid conduction along the axon as the electrical impulse skips from one node of Ranvier to the next. This process is termed saltatory conduction and significantly increases the conduction velocity along the axon (>50m/s in myelinated axons *versus* <10m/s in non-myelinated axons).

During electrodiagnostic testing, the action potential is generated where the clinician decides to stimulate the nerve with an electric current, which is not necessarily the location where a nerve would normally be depolarised. This means that, unlike in the natural situation when action potentials are generated at one end (e.g., at the sensory receptor or motor neuron cell body) and travel to the other, the action potential will propagate in both directions from its point of stimulation, as for the example shown in **Figure 1.4B.**

(vii) Factors influencing conduction velocity and amplitude of the action potential

There is a positive correlation between conduction velocity and both axon diameter and the presence of myelin. Myelinated axons will have faster conduction velocities than unmyelinated axons because of the insulation effect and the possibility of saltatory conduction. For axon diameter, there is less resistance along larger diameter axons meaning that more current will flow, leading to faster conduction and higher action potential amplitudes. In contrast, less current will flow along smaller diameter axons with more resistance, leading to slower conduction and smaller action potential amplitudes.

3. Recording of electrical potentials and their waveforms

(i) Peaks and troughs of waveforms and polarity in electrophysiology

Potentials recorded during electrodiagnostic testing are extracellular recordings of intracellular events that originate from muscles or nerves (intracellular recording is possible but difficult and not routinely done in a clinical setting).

Let's consider two recording electrodes, a cathode (E1) and an anode (E2), placed near a node of Ranvier along a peripheral nerve, or outside a muscle cell membrane (**Figure 1.5A**). The amplifier records the difference in potential between the anode and the cathode (active electrode): E2 minus E1. In the resting state, the difference between E2 and E1 is negligible, and the trace depicted on the monitor display is flat (**Figure 1.5A**). If depolarisation occurs closest to E1, the extracellular space becomes increasingly negatively charged relative to the electrode E2. This means that the resultant E2 minus E1 is a positive value increasing over the duration of the depolarisation and resulting in an upward deflection of the trace on the monitor display (**Figure 1.5B**).

This brings us to an important point regarding how these electrical events are displayed on the screen of the amplifier and

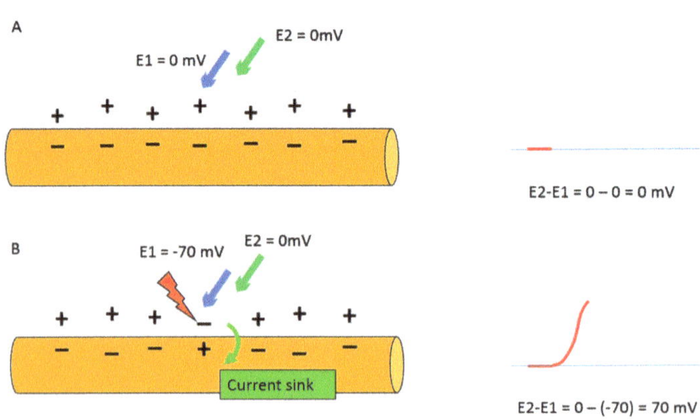

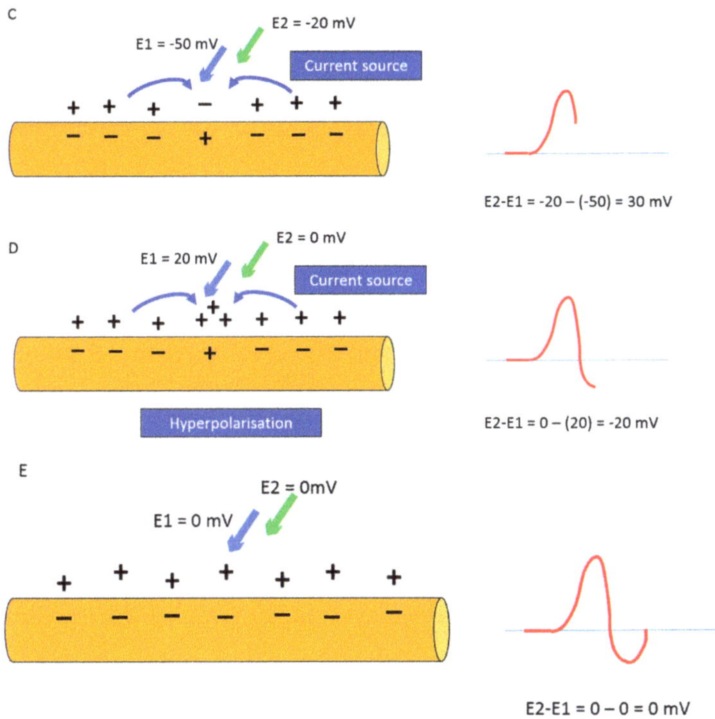

Figure 1.5. Example of recording outside a denervated muscle fibre (electromyography recording using two monopolar needles). The amplifier records the potential difference between two needle electrodes (E2 *minus* E1), where E2 is the anode electrode and E1 the cathode electrode. **A.** Before depolarisation, the difference in potential is negligible. **B.** After depolarisation (e.g., following irritation by needle placement) there is a current sink and the extracellular space in the region closest to E1 becomes increasingly negatively charged. The difference of potential therefore becomes increasingly positive (0mV minus -70mV = +70mV – these values are arbitrary), leading to an upward deflection of the trace on the monitor display. **C.** Positive charges in the extracellular space then move towards the increased negativity at the site of depolarisation as a current source. This appears as a progressive *downwards* deflection of the trace because there is now increasing positivity in the extracellular space under E1 (e.g., a change from -70mV to -50mV) and E2 may also have become slightly more negative, being nearby the depolarisation site. **D.** This phenomenon continues up to a state of hyperpolarisation, where E1 becomes positively charged and the resultant potential difference between E2 and E1 is negative. **E.** Finally, the cell membrane returns to its resting potential, E2 and E1 become equal, and the trace returns to baseline.

the nomenclature used to describe the individual 'peaks' and 'troughs' of the waveform. As the monitor displays the potential difference between the anode and cathode electrodes, rather than the actual extracellular charge *per se*, an increase in positive charge adjacent to the recording needle will be displayed as downward deflection of the trace (a 'trough' below the baseline), whilst increased negativity in the extracellular space will result in an upward deflection of the trace (a 'peak' above the baseline). This principle is important when interpreting traces, for understanding the terms used to describe individual waveforms, and how this relates to the cellular events that underlie them. For example, a positive sharp wave in electromyography is a large downward (positive) deflection of the trace; other waveforms such as evoked potentials may have subpeaks that are named accordingly (e.g., P1, N1 and P2 of a cortical somatosensory evoked potential will correspond to the first downward – positive – deflection, the first upward – negative – deflection and the second downward – positive – deflection).

(ii) Biphasic and triphasic waveforms

In the following section, we will consider how biphasic and triphasic waves are formed (Barry, 2015; Dumitru, 2000). We can broadly consider two situations: (i) the waveform of potentials during electromyography (EMG) recordings; and (ii) the waveform of potentials during nerve conduction studies. The primary difference between these two situations is that the waveforms recorded during EMG are mostly spontaneous, with the recording needle being near to or at the source of the spontaneous muscle membrane depolarisation, or at a region that depolarises due to placement of the needle itself. In contrast, during nerve conduction studies (sensory nerve conduction studies for example), the clinician places recording needles along a peripheral nerve and the recordings correspond to potentials moving towards and then past the recording needles following direct stimulation of the nerve or its receptor endings.

We will consider a pair of recording electrodes (a cathode and an anode) placed above either a muscle fibre or a myelinated axon of a peripheral nerve: one is the active electrode (E1 – cathode) and one is the anode electrode (E2), as defined above. We will consider the difference in potential E2 minus E1 throughout these examples.

a. Biphasic waveform from potentials recorded above a muscle fibre during electromyography

In this example, the clinician inserts a concentric needle into the muscle. This type of needle contains both a cathode and an anode within the same shaft (see 'Section 2 – Equipment and set up'). Therefore, in this instance, E1 and E2 are close together, in fact part of the same needle, but at the microscopic level E1 and E2 will still be considered distant. The needle is positioned in the extracellular space and physically irritates a muscle fibre end-plate. This leads to depolarisation of the muscle membrane and a current sink, resulting in increased negative charge in the extracellular space under E1 and an upwards deflection of the trace (as described in **Figure 1.5B**): the intracellular space has become positive whereas the extracellular space has become negative. Next, positive charges in the extracellular space will move towards the site of depolarisation (current source) leading to a progressive increase in positivity in the extracellular space and a downward deflection of the trace (i.e., E1 is now becoming gradually more positive with regards to E2 – see **Figure 1.5C**) up to a state of hyperpolarisation (**Figure 1.5D**). Finally, the cell membrane returns to its resting potential and there is no longer a difference in potential between the cathode and the anode, so the trace returns to baseline (**Figure 1.5E**).

b. Triphasic waveform from potentials recorded above a myelinated axon

Let's now consider an action potential flowing along a myelinated axon and the pair of recording electrodes (E1 and E2) placed

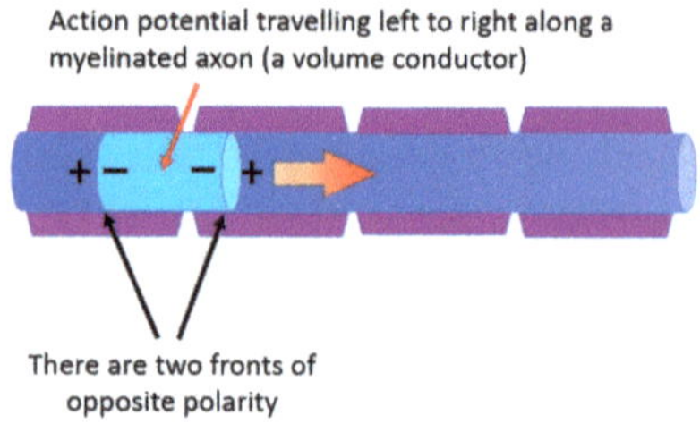

Figure 1.6. An action potential travels in a volume conductor along the axon and is composed of a pair of wave fronts of opposite polarity.

above the nerve. In this instance, the clinician typically uses two monopolar needles macroscopically distant from each other (~1 to 2cm) so that one acts as the anode under which the polarity varies little. The action potential is travelling along the nerve towards these recording electrodes by saltatory conduction (Barry, 2015). The action potential travels in a volume conductor and is composed of a pair of wave fronts of opposite polarity (**Figure 1.6**). For simplification, we will consider through the example below the 'positivity' or 'negativity' resultant from these two wave fronts.

Initially, there is no difference in potential between E2 and E1 when the action potential is far away from the recording electrodes (**Figure 1.7A**). Note that E2 will remain away from the travelling potential and therefore null throughout this example, and the values for E1 are arbitrary. As nearby nodes of Ranvier are sequentially depolarised, a current source will appear that corresponds to movement of positive charges towards the node of Ranvier being depolarised; this results in a short phase of hyperpolarisation at the level of E1 (an initial extracellular positivity) and leads to downward deflection of the trace (**Figure 1.7B**). As the action potential continues to travel to reach the node of Ranvier close to E1 and the current source has further propagated, the resultant change is a reduced positivity/progressive negativity perceived by E1 relative to E2 which leads to an upward deflection of the trace (**Figure 1.7C**). Depolarisation then occurs at the node of Ranvier closest to E1 and the sink current leads to movement of positive charges inside the axon and a further upward deflection of the

Figure 1.7. Example of depolarisation along a myelinated axon: triphasic wave. **A.** When the action potential is distant to the recording electrodes, there is no difference in potential between E2 and E1. **B.** Nearby nodes of Ranvier are depolarised resulting in a current source and movement of positive charges towards the node of Ranvier being depolarised. The movement of positive charges initially leads to downwards deflection of the trace (hyperpolarisation at E1) and then **(C)** an upwards deflection of the trace as the current source terminates**. D.** Depolarisation occurs at the node of Ranvier closest to E1 and the sink current leads to movement of positive (Na^+) charges into the axon and a further upward deflection of the trace as the extracellular space becomes negatively charged. **E.** The potential moves away from the node of Ranvier where the recording needles are placed, and another current source appears. This corresponds to movement of positive charges towards the node of Ranvier where the recording needles are placed, leading to a downward deflection of the trace. **F.** As this current source finishes, E1 will become progressively less positive relative to E2 and there is an upward deflection of the trace, before E2 and E1 return to the same polarity.

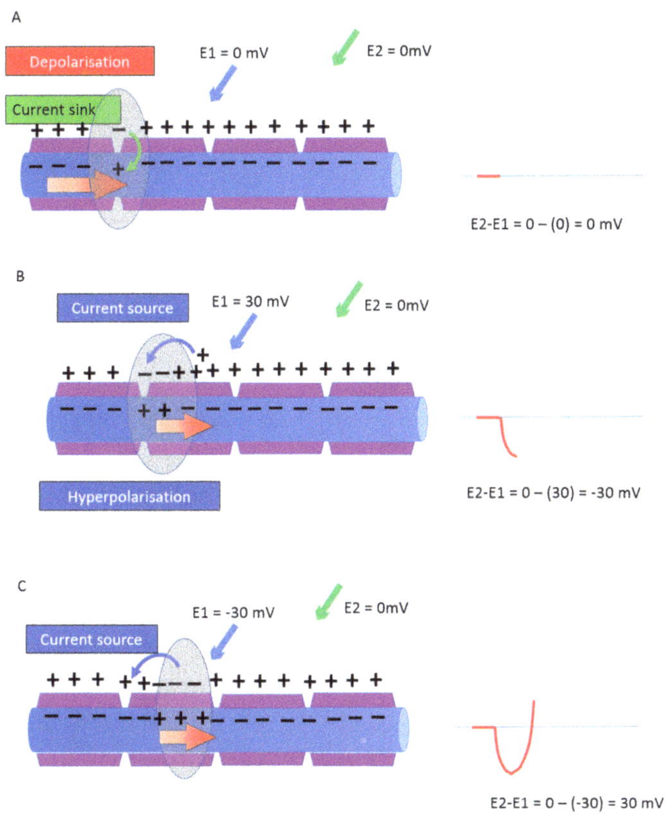

Figure 1.7. continued

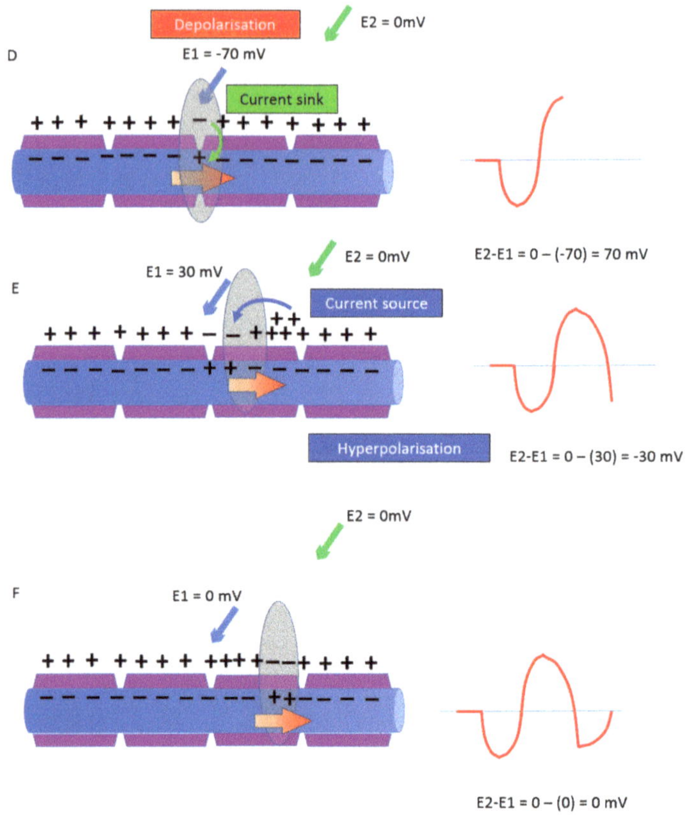

trace (the extracellular space becomes more negatively charged under E1 compared to E2) (**Figure 1.7D**). As the potential then moves away from the recording needles, another current source will appear corresponding to movement of positive charges towards the node of Ranvier where the recording needles are located; this increasing positivity at E1 leads to a downwards deflection of the trace (**Figure 1.7E**). Finally, as the action potential continues to move towards distant nodes of Ranvier and the current source finishes, the membrane potential at E1 returns to its resting state and there is an upward deflection of the trace returning back to the baseline (**Figure 1.7F**).

(iii) Variation in wave morphology

From the explanations above, one can now perceive how the location of the recording needles relative to the site of depolarisation can significantly affect the shape of the recorded waveforms. Fibrillation potentials in EMG frequently arise slightly away from the concentric recording needle and travel along the muscle fibre membrane towards it, as for an action potential travelling along an axon in the example above. They can therefore have an initial positive spike (downward deflection) and be triphasic, as described above. However, they may also be biphasic if the needle deforms the muscle fibre, blocking the propagation of the depolarisation away from the needle. If the needle records a fibrillation potential generated at its tip, the morphology will be initially negative and cannot be differentiated from an end-plate spike (see 'Section 3 – Electromyography' for further discussion regarding the different types of waveforms that can be seen and their individual morphologies).

(iv) Moving potentials and field potentials

Electrical potentials can be described based on the location of the recording electrodes relative to the source of the potential (that is 'near' the source or 'far' from the source). Furthermore, some potentials are moving potentials (e.g., travelling along an axon), whereas other potentials are static field potentials created by a group of neurons or muscle fibres.

Following stimulation of a peripheral nerve, potentials will travel along the nerve and can be detected by recording needles placed adjacent to the nerve as this axonal volley passes by. This is called a near field potential. An example of a moving near field potential is a sensory compound action potential. Another example of a moving near field potential would be that recorded by needles placed above the spinal cord following stimulation of a peripheral sensory or mixed nerve (i.e., ascending evoked spinal cord potentials [see 'Section 9 – Somatosensory evoked potentials']).

The recording needles placed in the muscle during a motor nerve conduction study will detect a 'near field' compound muscle action potential following stimulation of the peripheral motor fibres innervating that muscle.

Recording needles may also pick up non-propagating discharges from a distant, static source, such as a group of neurons. These are called far field potentials. In companion animals, these field potentials are typically studied by placing needles directly above them and they are therefore effectively recorded as 'near field' potentials, rather than placing needles at a distance from the source. A good example of this recording is the cord dorsum potential obtained following distal stimulation of the sciatic nerve. In this case, recording needles are placed above the lumbosacral spinal cord intumescence and pick up the field generated by depolarisation of interneurons in the dorsal aspect of the spinal cord grey matter. Other examples of static field potentials are the brainstem auditory evoked potentials, where recording needles are close to the generators (cochlea, vestibulocochlear nerve, brainstem), or potentials recorded during electroencephalography (EEG).

References

Barry JM. Axonal activity in vivo: technical considerations and implications for the exploration of neural circuits in freely moving animals. Front Neurosci. 2015 May 6;9:153. doi: 10.3389/fnins.2015.00153. PMID: 25999806; PMCID: PMC4422007.

Dumitru D. Physiologic basis of potentials recorded in electromyography. Muscle Nerve. 2000 Nov;23(11):1667-85. doi: 10.1002/1097-4598(200011)23:11<1667::aid-mus2>3.0.co;2-h. PMID: 11054745.

Kimura J. Electrodiagnosis in Diseases of Nerve and Muscle: Principles and Practice – 4th ed. Oxford University Press, 2013.

Michell AW. Understanding EMG. Oxford University Press, 2013.

Robinson LR, Christie M, Nandedkar, S. A message from the ground electrode. Muscle Nerve. 2016 Dec;54(6):1010-1011. doi: 10.1002/mus.25419.

Shapiro BE and Preston DC. Electromyography and Neuromuscular Disorders: Clinical-Electrophysiologic Correlations – 3rd ed. Elsevier Inc, 2013.

SECTION 2

Equipment and set up

Hélène Vandenberghe, Edward Ives, Nicolas Granger, Benjamin Metcalfe

Key points

- EMG machines comprise a hardware unit controlling an amplifier, stimulator, laptop software and loudspeakers; cables and electrodes are then connected to the stimulator and the amplifier to generate electrophysiologic data.
- The electrical signal and noise are recorded by electrodes. There are many different types of electrodes, and their use depends on the application (stimulation, recording) and structure being explored.
- Standard electrophysiologic recordings require the use of a minimum of two electrodes since all such recordings are differential. The cathode is the active electrode (negative, corresponding to the black port on the amplifier) and the recording is done by comparison to the anode electrode (positive, corresponding to the red port on the amplifier). A reference/'ground' electrode is required for each investigation, connected to the green port of the amplifier.
- Stimulation devices can deliver electrical, visual or auditory stimuli. Pairs of electrodes (cathode and anode) may be used for nerve or skin stimulation.

- The signal is carried to the amplifier using one or more leads dependent on the test.
- The signal and noise are magnified by the amplifier while the unwanted noise is attenuated by filters and algorithms. The monitor displays the voltage difference between the cathode and the anode recording electrodes.

Introduction

The equipment required to conduct electrodiagnostic investigations includes electrodes, an amplifier, cables to attach these electrodes to/from the amplifier and stimulator, visual and auditory displays (laptop and loudspeakers), a base unit and a stimulator (**Figure 2.1**). A portable electrodiagnostic unit is usually preferable in modern veterinary referral hospitals, because it can be placed on a trolley and wheeled easily from one room to another where the animal is maintained under general anaesthesia. This also reduces the need to move the animal if other ancillary tests are planned at that time. The screen of the laptop allows a visual representation of the electrical activity at the level of the electrodes to be displayed as a function of time, and adjustments to specific parameters or measurements made using inbuilt software.

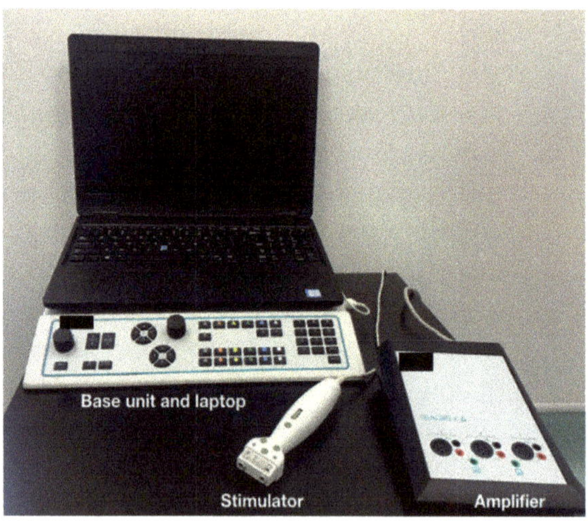

Figure 2.1. Portable electrodiagnostic device with the base unit and laptop, stimulator and amplifier.

Electrodiagnostic procedures were historically performed in a specifically designed room that was shielded from outside sources of electrical interference in order to optimise recording by reducing artefacts. The introduction of more advanced amplifiers, together with modern insulation of electrical cables and regular checks of a building's electrical installations and its electrical appliances, means that portable electrodiagnostic units do not necessarily need to be used in a shielded room. However, whilst modern equipment records fewer artefacts from appliances that generate electrostatic or electromagnetic fields (e.g., heat mats, radio, mobile phones), artefacts remain possible and are described later (see 'Section 3 – Electromyography').

1. Amplifier

The signals recorded during electrodiagnostic tests range from a few microvolts (µV) to a few millivolts (mV). In order to amplify the signals of interest across that range, amplifiers have a high input impedance, a high gain, a low noise level, and a large dynamic range.

Amplifiers have an 'inverting terminal' which is often black and corresponds to the cathode or negative port and a 'non-inverting terminal' which is often red and corresponds to the anode or positive port (**Figure 2.2**). If the signal enters at the cathode (as for EMG or nerve conduction studies), the amplifier is in an 'inverting' configuration and the output signal is inverted relative to the input signal.

For electromyography (EMG) recording, differential amplifiers will magnify the voltage difference between the anode electrode and the cathode electrode, and will also monitor and exclude electrical activity that is simultaneously recorded by both the recording electrodes and a reference electrode (see 'Section 1 – Anatomy and physiology of the peripheral nervous system and principles of electrophysiology) (**Figure 2.2**). This allows effective rejection of potentials from both local electrical equipment (e.g., power sources) and distant muscle potentials. Furthermore, the use of well-shielded electrode cables is important, as well as insulated cables from other equipment in the room.

It is important to understand how electrical events occurring at a cellular level are visually displayed on the screen of the unit (e.g., laptop) as this also relates to the nomenclature used to describe the polarity of individual 'peaks' and 'troughs' of the waveform. This is to avoid confusion, particularly as certain terms may initially appear counterintuitive. As the monitor displays the voltage difference between the recording electrodes, rather than simply the actual charge around the active electrode in the extracellular space, for an inverting configuration, an increase in positive charge adjacent to the active needle will be displayed as downward deflection of the trace, or a 'trough' below the baseline. Vice versa, an increase in negative charge in the extracellular space will result in an upward deflection of the trace, or a 'peak' above the baseline (see 'Section 1 – Anatomy and Physiology' for further discussion). This principle is important when interpreting traces, understanding the terms used to describe individual waveforms, and how this relates to the cellular events that underlie them. For example, a 'positive sharp wave' in electromyography is a type of waveform that appears as a large downward (positive) deflection of the trace.

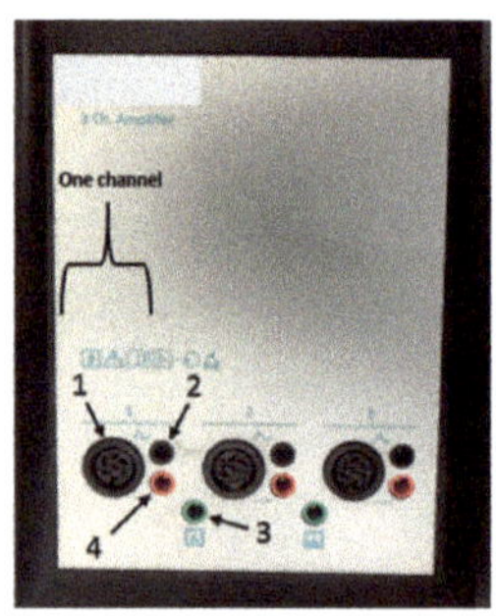

Figure 2.2. Three channel amplifier. 1. Amplifier input connector for the concentric needle electrode; 2. Amplifier input connector for the active electrode/cathode (monopolar needle electrode or surface electrode); 3. Amplifier input connector for the reference electrode; 4. Amplifier input connector for the anode electrode. NB: EMG is typically performed using connectors 1 and 3, and action potential recording requires the use of connectors 2, 3 and 4 (see later).

An exception to this is when the amplifier is in a 'non-inverting' configuration, where the signal enters at the anode (the 'non-inverting terminal'), which results in an output that is in phase with the input signal. This is used for BAER, EEG, ERG, or SEP recording for example. This explains why these techniques display positivity as an upwards trace and negativity as a downward deflection of the trace.

Amplifiers also have a rejection mode that allows them, for example, to discard two waves that are identical other than having inverted polarities: one being positive and the other negative. This is because such waves usually occur as random artefacts and means that only unique (positive or negative) waves will be amplified. It is also possible to set high- and low-bandpass filters. The frequency of muscle action potentials ranges from 2-20kHz, but in the presence of artefact this can be narrowed to 20Hz-10kHz. Once the equipment is set up, it is good practice to always use the same settings, as changing the high- and low-bandpass can affect the amplitude and latency of recorded potentials.

2. Loudspeakers

Electrophysiology units will play the recorded sound through loudspeakers, either via the laptop or from the base unit sitting under the laptop. This is particularly important for electromyography, in which specific waveforms are associated with distinctive sounds via the loudspeakers. Some systems are only formed of one machine, without a separate base unit, and hearing the recordings correctly can sometimes be challenging with these machines. The quality of the amplifier can also be less with these systems compared to those with a specific base unit and separate amplifier, all connected to a laptop.

3. Stimulator

The stimulating unit should ideally be separate from the main electrophysiology base unit and laptop (**Figure 2.3**). This is for safety reasons and to reduce artefacts, as it ensures that the stimulation circuit has no conductive paths to other parts of the system, other than through the patient's body (i.e., the current delivered by the two stimulating electrodes will only flow between these two electrodes and is not able to reach the rest of the equipment, accidentally stimulate other unintended sites, or lead to artefacts such as amplifier overload).

In an ideal world, each hospital would define its own reference values (current intensity, pulse width) for a given electrophysiological set-up as this might vary from one clinic to another and potentially influence interpretation of results.

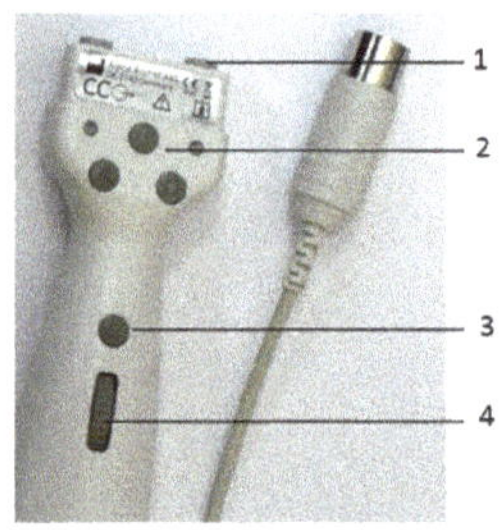

Figure 2.3. Stimulating unit. 1. Output electrode sockets; 2. Polarity and stimulation indicators; 3. Stimulation button; 4. Stimulation intensity control wheel.

4. Electrodes

There are many different types of electrodes available and their individual use is dependent on the application and the structures being explored (e.g., electromyography versus motor nerve conduction studies versus sensory nerve conduction studies). The further away the recording electrodes are from the source of the signal, the more they will record electrical activity from multiple sources. For example, surface electrodes placed on the skin overlying a muscle will pick up the signal from a relatively large portion of the muscle (several motor units). This is in comparison to needle electrodes within a muscle, that will pick up the signal from only one motor unit, or even single myofibres dependent on the type of needle.

It is good practice to either use new needles for each study, or to sterilise needles after each use. Cold chemical sterilisation with ethylene oxide is preferred for needles with integral cables to preserve the plastic coating of the electrode cable. Electrodes should be inspected regularly as the tips can become blunt and the insulating plastic coating of monopolar needles will deteriorate over time/with use, which is a common area of fault. It is always useful to have two sets of electrodes available, and to repeat the measurements with a second set when difficulties in recording or uncertainties are encountered; this is to ensure that any artefacts or abnormal waveforms are not originating from the needles/cables themselves.

(i) Surface electrodes

Surface recording electrodes are commonly used for electromyography in humans, particularly to record volitional electrical muscle activity (over a surface area of ~2cm). They are not practical in animals unless the fur is clipped over the recording area. However, more importantly, the impedance of the skin in dogs and cats is too high to allow good recording of spontaneous activity using surface electrodes. Therefore, there is generally a need to record using needle electrodes under the skin with an animal under general anaesthesia. There are some metal cup surface electrodes that reduce the skin impedance and can be used together with a contact electrode paste (such as that used for electroencephalography recordings) (**Figure 2.4**). These are practical, applicable to animals and allow good recordings, particularly to record tremor activity in awake animals and to assess the frequency of tremors. Surface electrodes can also work well when used as the reference electrode.

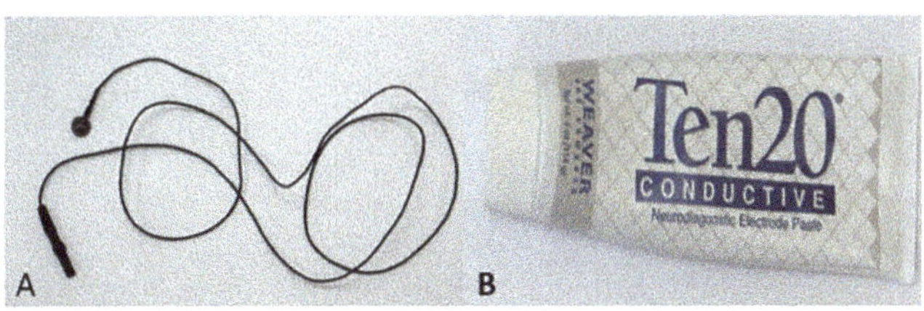

Figure 2.4. A. Metal cup surface electrode; B. Contact electrode paste.

(ii) Needle electrodes

a. Standard concentric needles (also known as coaxial needles)

Electromyography is classically performed in animals using a concentric needle to record muscle fibre activity. This type of electrode is made using two different metals, one contained within

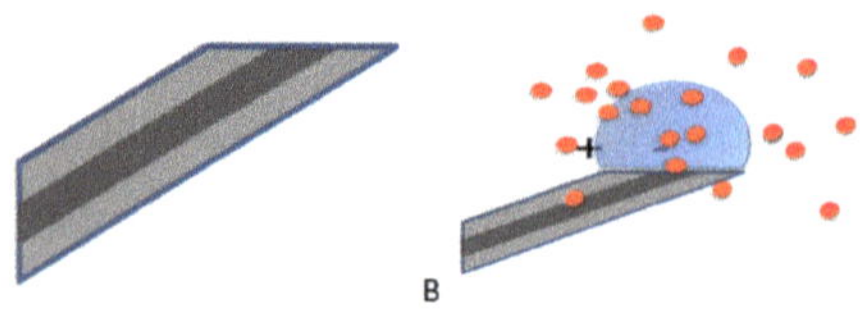

Figure 2.5. A. Drawing of a concentric needle electrode with a stainless-steel cannula (light grey) and wire contained within it (dark grey); B. The concentric needle records electrical potentials in myofibres (red) located within a hemisphere at its tip with a radius of ~0.5 – 2.5mm from its recording surface.

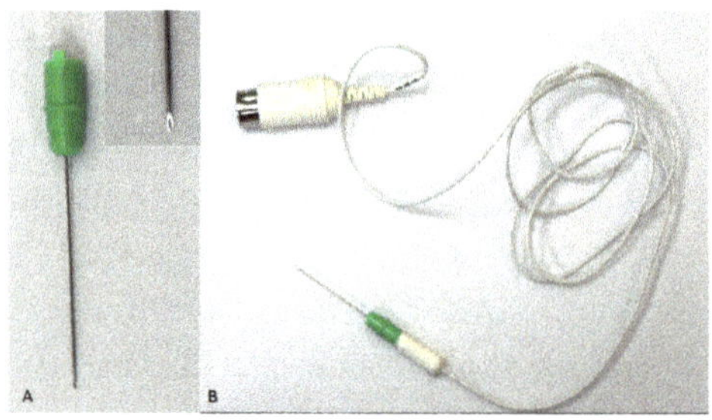

Figure 2.6. A. Disposable concentric needle electrode, 37mm length, with a needle diameter of 0.46mm (26G). Inset: magnification of the needle tip; B. Concentric needle electrode and its cable.

the other: a stainless-steel cannula of ~0.46mm that is similar to a hypodermic needle used in the clinic (the same size as a 26-gauge (G) needle), and a second solid 'wire' of metal within the cannula, made of nichrome, silver or platinum (recording surface of $0.07mm^2$) (**Figures 2.5A and 2.6**). This arrangement offers a hemispherical recording territory, with the needle measuring the potential difference between the two metals at the tip of the needle, usually within a ~0.5 – 2.5mm radius. This will allow recording of a small portion of a motor unit territory which extends over ~1cm (**Figure 2.5B**).

Concentric needles are less prone to recording background noise compared to monopolar needles. They also cause more tissue damage on insertion compared to monopolar needles, but this means that they can trigger more spontaneous myofibre activity in diseased or denervated muscle, which can be useful when detecting mild EMG changes.

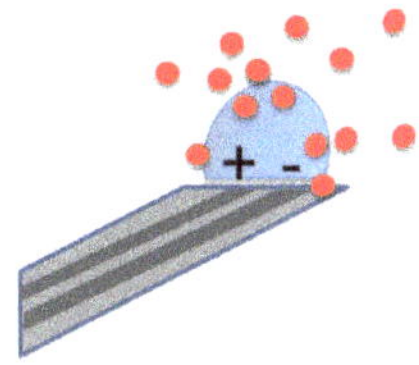

Figure 2.7. Drawing of a bipolar concentric needle with its cannula (light grey) and two wires contained within it (dark grey – anode / cathode), recording electrical potentials in myofibres (red) in a small nearby volume (blue hemisphere).

b. Bipolar concentric needles

Bipolar concentric needles are composed of a cannula containing two wires and they measure the potential difference between these two wires, with the cannula acting as the reference/'ground' (**Figure 2.7**). Therefore, the waveforms recorded using these needles are different to those classically observed with standard concentric needles. These needles are overall bigger (similar to a 23G hypodermic needle), but as the recording occurs between the two closely arranged (0.2mm) wires, they actually have a smaller recording area compared to a standard concentric needle. Bipolar concentric needles are rarely used in companion animals but can be useful to study a small number of muscle fibres.

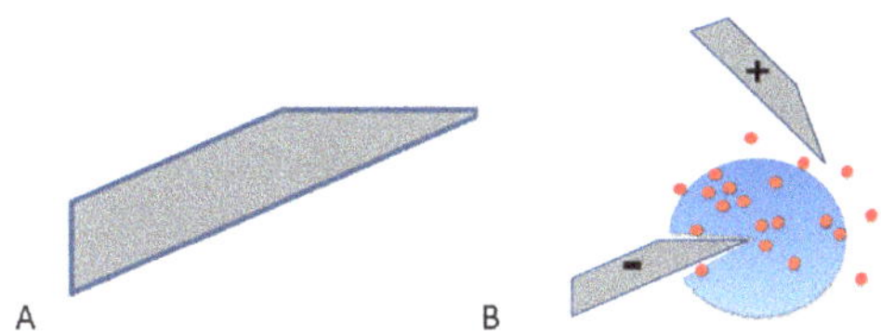

Figure 2.8. Drawings of: A. A monopolar needle electrode; B. Recording EMG with monopolar needles: (-) active recording electrode and (+) anode electrode. Recording from myofibres (red) located within a spherical volume of a few millimetres around the tip of the active electrode.

c. Monopolar needles

These needles are generally ~0.36mm (28G) in diameter and are composed of a single type of metal, usually stainless-steel. They can be either non-insulated (e.g., for nerve conduction studies) or insulated with a Teflon sleeve except for a ~0.2 – 0.4mm section

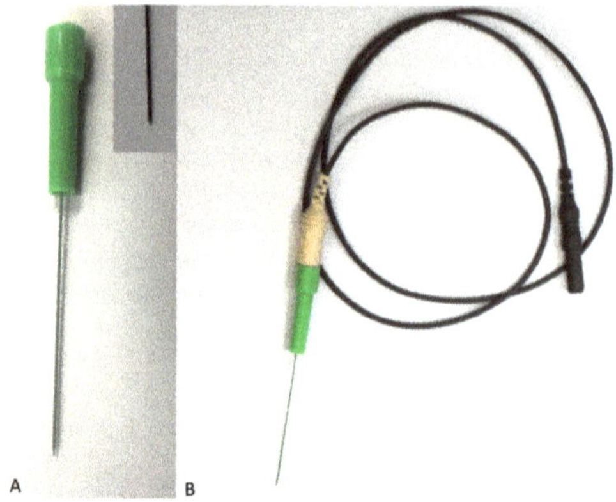

Figure 2.9. A. Insulated (Teflon-coated) monopolar needle electrode, 37mm in length, with a needle diameter of 0.46mm (26G). Inset: magnification of the needle tip; B. Monopolar needle electrode with its detachable cable.

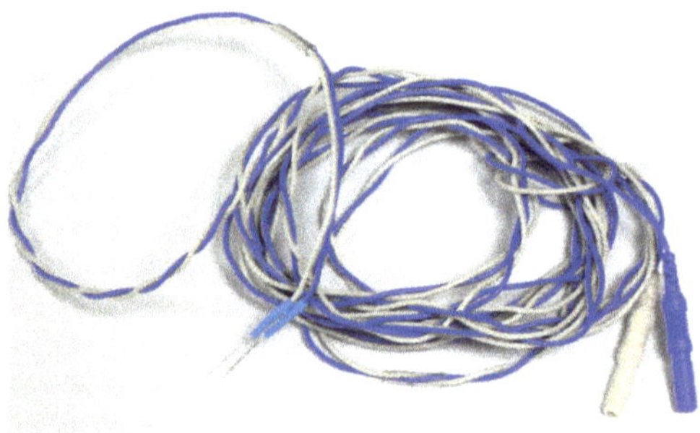

Figure 2.10. Non-insulated, platinium iridium subdermal needle electrodes with integrated twisted cables.

at the tip (e.g., for EMG recording) (**Figures 2.8, 2.9 and 2.10**). If a concentric needle is not used, two monopolar needles are required to perform EMG, placed 1 to 2cm apart, with one needle serving as the active recording electrode (cathode), connected to the black port of the amplifier, and the second acting as the anode, connected to the red port of the amplifier; the potential difference between the two needles is measured and recording is made from a spherical volume of muscle within a few millimetres of the tip of the active electrode (**Figure 2.8**). These needles will pick-up more background noise than concentric needles but record over a greater distance/volume of muscle. Therefore, they may be used in large animals (e.g., horses) and the waveforms will be different to those acquired with standard concentric needles.

In companion animals, pairs of monopolar needles are most frequently used for nerve conduction studies. They can be used to stimulate either a nerve (e.g., motor or sensory nerve conduction studies) or the skin (e.g., sensory nerve conduction studies), and are also used to record from various sites dependent on the test being performed:

- Within a muscle (compound muscle action potential for a motor nerve conduction study);
- Around a nerve (compound sensory action potential for a sensory nerve conduction study);
- Over the vertebral column/spinal cord (cord dorsum potential, ascending/descending spinal evoked potentials);
- Or over the skull/brain (somatosensory evoked potentials).

d. Single fibre needles

In order to measure potentials from individual muscle fibres, this type of needle has a much smaller leading edge compared to other needles. They typically contain a wire of 25μm in diameter that terminates in a bend towards the side of the needle around 3mm from its tip. The shaft serves as the reference electrode (**Figure 2.11**). These needles are not suited to recording compound muscle action potentials, which represent the combined electrical activity from multiple muscle fibres.

A high pass filter of 500Hz is used for single fibre EMG. When performing this test, >50 single muscle fibre action potentials are recorded after stimulation of intramuscular nerve bundles at the level of the motor point, and at least 20 individual muscle fibres are tested per muscle. Therefore, there is first a need to determine the motor point of the tested muscle (see 'Section 6 – Repetitive nerve stimulation'). Once the motor point has been identified, the lowest electrical current is applied through the cathode (active

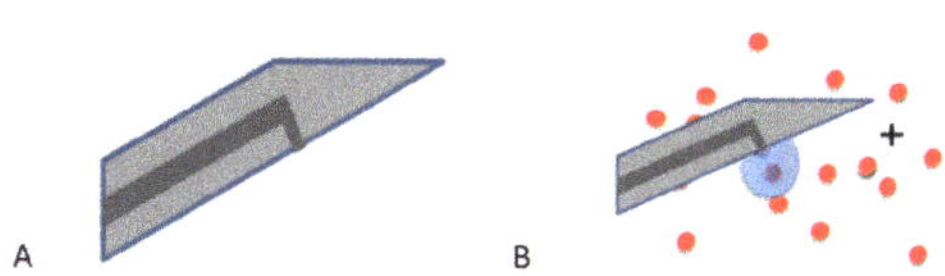

Figure 2.11. Drawings of: A. A single fibre needle electrode comprising a wire (dark grey) and shaft (light grey), with the latter acting as a reference; B. Recording of potentials from single muscle fibres within a very small radius of the wire's side port.

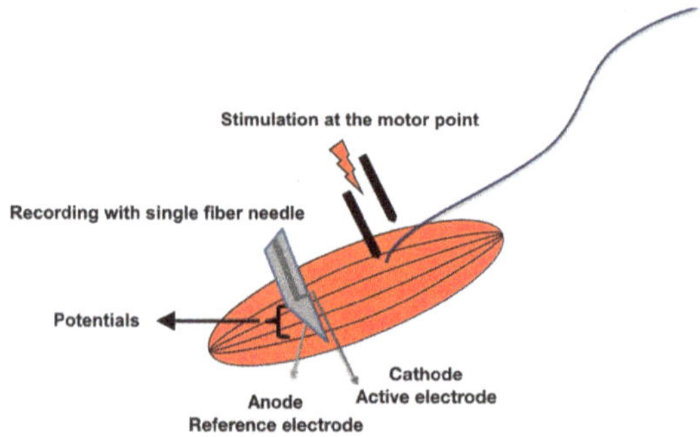

Figure 2.12. Drawing of the electrode set-up for single fibre electromyography.

electrode) and anode of a bipolar montage, and a single fibre EMG needle is used in various sites within the muscle for measurement of the action potentials from single muscle fibres (**Figure 2.12**).

Single fibre needles are designed to study diseases of the neuromuscular junction and can detect variations in the time of transmission through the neuromuscular junction between the different fibres forming a motor unit: this is termed the 'neuromuscular jitter' and is a measure of synaptic delay that can help diagnose diseases that affect neuromuscular transmission, such as *myasthenia gravis* (See 'Section 6: Repetitive nerve stimulation'). The jitter, however, can also be increased in other situations, such as those causing denervation (e.g., motor neuropathies) or during reinnervation where it reflects a state of variability of the neuromuscular transmission time. However, it should remain normal for purely myopathic disorders. Single fibre needles can also be used to measure the density of fibres around the needle, which varies in different disease states. Currently, the clinical use and experience with single fibre electromyography in companion animals is limited.

References and Further Reading

Kimura J. Electrodiagnosis in Diseases of Nerve and Muscle: Principles and Practice – 4th ed. Oxford University Press, 2013.

Michell AW. Understanding EMG. Oxford University Press, 2013.

Shapiro BE and Preston DC. Electromyography and Neuromuscular Disorders: Clinical-Electrophysiologic Correlations – 3rd ed. Elsevier Inc, 2013.

SECTION 3

Electromyography

Hélène Vandenberghe, Edward Ives,
Francesca Samarani, Nicolas Granger

Key points

- Electromyography (EMG) is a technique evaluating the electrical activity produced by skeletal muscles with a concentric needle electrode inserted into the muscle. It does not require nerve stimulation.
- In companion animals, EMG is performed under general anaesthesia and is usually the first step of an electrophysiologic evaluation.
- Under general anaesthesia, EMG should not identify any spontaneous electrical activity within a normal muscle, apart from electrical activity recorded during insertion of the needle (insertional activity) or next to the end-plate due to physiologic leakage of acetylcholine (miniature end-plate potentials, end-plate spikes). End-plate activity disappears with slight needle movement.
- Electromyography in animals with nerve (motor axonal neuropathy) or muscle (especially inflammatory or dystrophic) diseases often identifies spontaneous electrical activity, which is abnormal. There are several different types

of abnormal electrical activity which may be identified by studying the morphology and sound of the waveform.

- The type of abnormal electrical activity is often non-specific to the underlying disease.
- An abnormal EMG confirms the presence of a motor neuropathy or myopathy, and the distribution of abnormalities provides a map of the disease. Electromyography cannot distinguish between a neuropathy and a myopathy and nerve conduction studies are necessary for this.
- A normal EMG does not rule out a neuromuscular disorder. Many myopathies and junctionopathies, and some neuropathies (e.g., demyelinating), are silent on EMG.

Introduction

Electromyography (EMG) is the recording and evaluation of electrical activity produced by skeletal muscles using electrodes inserted into the muscle of interest. It measures spontaneous (or voluntary) muscle activity and therefore does not involve nerve stimulation. In companion animals, this is typically done under general anaesthesia during which muscle relaxation and reflex suppression means that there is no muscle activity that could lead to the recording of motor unit action potentials (MUAPs) (Van Nes, 1986; Cuddon, 2002). This aids in the recording of spontaneous myofibre activity alone, without overlying voluntary muscle activity that could complicate interpretation of the results. However, unlike nerve conduction studies, deep sedation may be used for EMG in some cases. This difference between veterinary patients and the conscious EMG studies performed in humans, means that voluntary recruitment of motor units cannot be studied in companion animals.

1. Recording technique

The recording parameters are as follows (**Table 3.1**). These can be increased or decreased as needed during examination.

Recording parameter	Value
Gain (i.e., amplitude, vertical axis)	50 to 100μV/cm
Sweep speed (horizontal axis)	2 to 10ms/cm
High frequency filter	10kHz
Low frequency filter	20Hz

Table 3.1. Recording parameters used for electromyography.

In order to perform an EMG evaluation, the following points should be considered:

- The reference electrode should be placed over a connective tissue/bony prominence (e.g., calcaneus, olecranon) and is connected to the green 'earth' socket of the amplifier.
- A concentric needle is most commonly used to record the electrical activity in EMG but monopolar needles may also be used (see 'Section 2 – Equipment and set up'). The plastic base of the recording needle is held firmly in the fingers like a pen. It is inserted through the skin and subcutaneous tissue into the muscle belly of interest. The hand holding the needle is rested on the skin so that the needle movement is precise, and the needle held immobile once inserted. If the needle is not supported, particularly for small muscles or shallow recording sites, it can lean or fall, which will result in muscle stimulation and induced electrical activity that can be hard to distinguish from true spontaneous myofibre activity.
- To increase the chances of identifying any significant abnormalities, five to ten regions should be tested for each muscle (unless significant amounts of spontaneous activity have already been observed for the first sampling sites). This is because abnormal electrical activity can be patchy within and between muscles. The needle is inserted into one part of the muscle belly and moved along a straight line from shallow to deeper, before being pulled back in short steps (Shapiro and Preston, 2013; Menkes and Pierce, 2019). Each muscle is then mapped in this way in 3 to 10 places, dependent on the size of the muscle.

- The clinician should look at the recording trace on the screen of the computer, whilst also listening to the sounds produced by the loudspeakers of the base unit. A brief pause, with the needle held immobile, is needed between each testing site to watch and listen for spontaneous myofibre activity. The display should be left to run continuously (free running mode). In general, sounds originating close to the recording needle are crisp, whilst sounds that are from distant sources tend to be duller. Some machines and software will allow storage of waveforms that appear repeatedly, and then display these in a specific part of the screen for analysis. It is also useful to be familiar with the way the software records the live EMG so that this can be replayed later. Most machines will automatically record the last 20 to 60 seconds of an assessment so that it is not redundant, but not the initial part when the needle is inserted.

Performing needle EMG leads to minor muscle injury and this needs to be considered if muscle biopsies are subsequently taken. For symmetrical diseases, one side of the animal can be used for EMG studies and the other side used for muscle biopsies. If a muscle that has been tested with needle EMG is sampled, then a comment should be made for the attention of the pathologist reading the biopsy. A study looking at the creatine kinase (CK) values at 4 hours, 24 hours and 48 hours after EMG in dogs and horses found that, although increased, it remained within the normal range (Steiss and Forsyth, 1984).

2. Muscular anatomy for electromyography

The muscles selected for examination are typically superficial and readily identified. A good knowledge of neuromuscular anatomy (skeletal muscles and their nerve supply) is essential for both performing and interpreting the electromyographic examination (Menkes and Pierce, 2019).

(i) Thoracic limb muscles

The thoracic limb muscles that may be screened using EMG are summarised in **Figure 3.1** and **Table 3.2** (Evans and de Lahunta, 2012).

Muscle	Nerve supply
Trapezius	(C5)C6-C7 nerve roots Suprascapular nerve
Supraspinatus	(C5)C6-C7 nerve roots Suprascapular nerve
Infraspinatus	(C5)C6-C7 nerve roots Suprascapular nerve
Deltoideus	(C6)C7-C8 nerve roots Axillary nerve
Triceps brachii	C7-C8-T1 nerve roots Radial nerve
Brachialis	C6-C7-C8 nerve roots Musculocutaneous nerve
Biceps brachii	C6-C7-C8 nerve roots Musculocutaneous nerve
Extensor digitorum communis	C7-C8-T1 nerve roots Radial nerve
Extensor digitorum lateralis	C7-C8-T1 nerve roots Radial nerve
Extensor carpi radialis	C7-C8-T1 nerve roots Radial nerve
Ulnaris lateralis	C7-C8-T1 nerve roots Radial nerve
Flexor carpi ulnaris	C8-T1(T2) nerve roots Ulnar nerve
Interossei palmare	C8-T1(T2) nerve roots Ulnar nerve

Table 3.2. Thoracic limb muscles and their innervation.

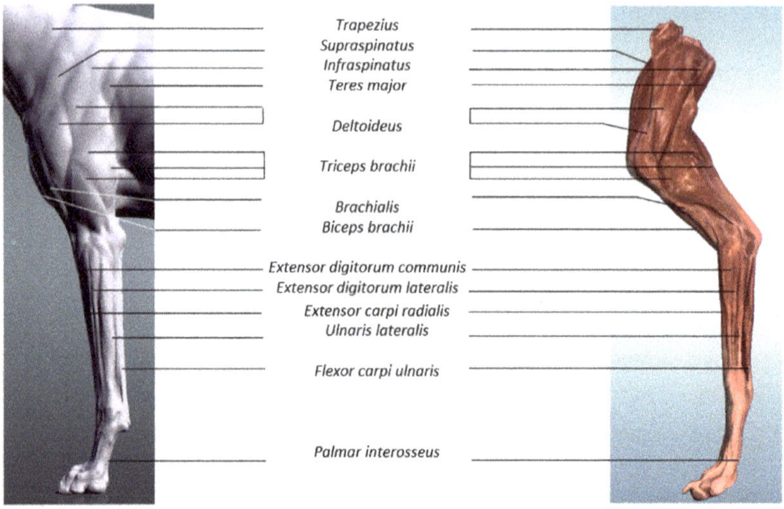

Figure 3.1. Representation of thoracic limb muscle locations for needle electromyography. Left thoracic limb of a dog, lateral aspect. *Adapted with permission from Ivalalearn (part of the Veterinary Information Network® family).*

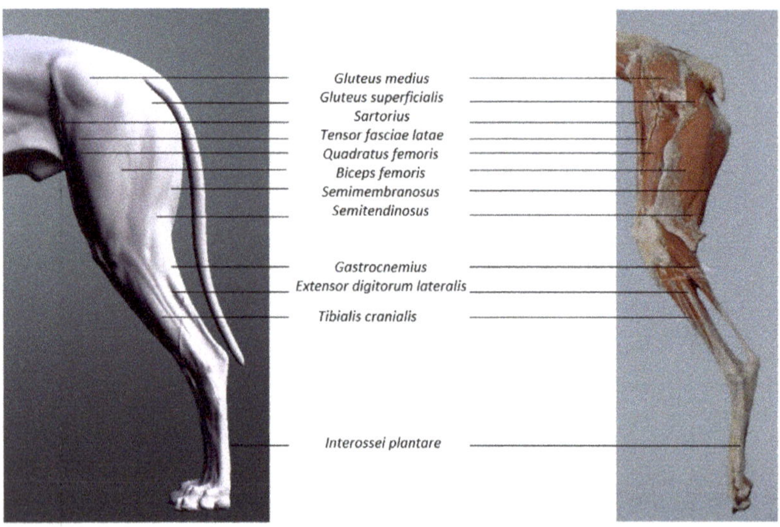

Figure 3.2. Representation of pelvic limb muscle locations for needle electromyography. Left pelvic limb of a dog, lateral aspect. *Adapted with permission from Ivalalearn (part of the Veterinary Information Network® family).*

(ii) Pelvic limb muscles

The pelvic limb muscles that may be screened using EMG are summarised in **Figure 3.2** and **Table 3.3** (Evans and de Lahunta, 2012).

Muscle	Innervation
Gluteus medius	L6-L7-S1 nerve roots Cranial gluteal nerve
Gluteus superficialis	L7(S1-2) nerve roots Caudal gluteal nerve
Sartorius	L4-5-6 nerve roots Femoral nerve
Quadratus femoris	L4-5-6 nerve roots Femoral nerve
Tensor fasciae latae	L6-L7-S1 nerve roots Cranial gluteal nerve
Biceps femoris	L6-L7-S1(S2) nerve roots Sciatic nerve
Semitendinosus	L6-L7-S1(S2) nerve roots Sciatic nerve
Semimembranosus	L6-L7-S1(S2) nerve roots Sciatic nerve
Gastrocnemius	L7-S1 nerve roots Tibial nerve
Flexor digitorum lateralis	L7-S1 nerve roots Tibial nerve
Tibialis cranialis	L6-L7 nerve roots Peroneal nerve
Interossei plantares	L7-S1 nerve roots Tibial nerve

Table 3.3. Pelvic limb muscles and their innervation.

(iii) Head muscles

The muscles of the head that may be screened using EMG are summarised in **Figure 3.3** and **Table 3.4** (Evans and de Lahunta, 2012).

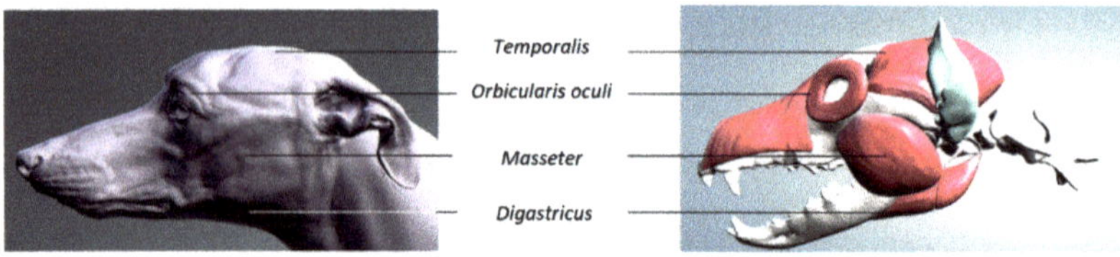

Figure 3.3. Representation of the muscles of the head for needle electromyography. Head of a dog left lateral view. *Adapted with permission from Ivalalearn (part of the Veterinary Information Network® family).*

Muscle	**Innervation**
Genioglossus (tongue)	Hypoglossal nerve (XII), caudal medulla oblongata
Temporalis	Mandibular nerve (V), pons
Masseter	Mandibular nerve (V), pons
Orbicularis oculi	Facial nerve (VII), cranial medulla oblongata
Digastricus	Cranial belly: Mandibular nerve (V), pons Caudal belly: Facial nerve (VII), cranial medulla oblongata

Table 3.4. Head muscles and their innervation.

(iv) Neck and trunk muscles

The most common neck and trunk muscles that may be used in needle EMG are summarised in **Figure 3.4** and **Table 3.5** (Evans and de Lahunta, 2012).

Muscle	**Innervation**
Sternocephalicus	Ventral branches of cervical nerves and accessory nerve
Cleidocephalicus	Accessory nerve
Trapezius	Accessory nerve
Latissimus dorsi	Caudal pectoral nerve, thoracodorsal nerve
Obliquus externus abdominis	Intercostal nerve, costoabdominal nerve, iliohypogastricus nerve, ilioinguinalis nerve

Table 3.5. Neck and trunk muscles and their innervation.

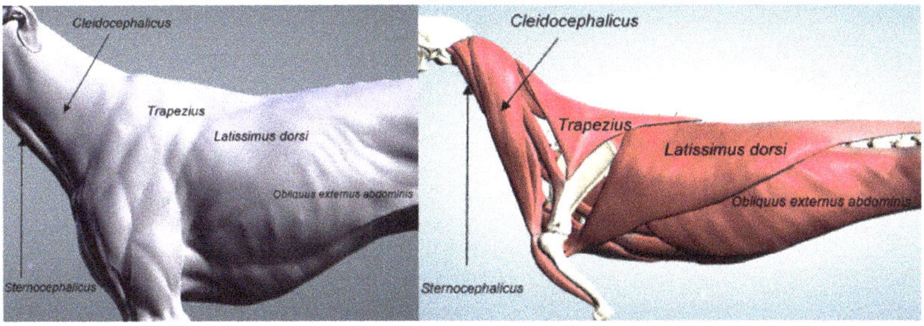

Figure 3.4. The most common muscles of the neck and trunk that may be screened using needle electromyography. Left lateral view of a dog. *Adapted with permission from Ivalalearn (part of the Veterinary Information Network® family).*

3. Normal electromyographic findings

If an animal is under general anaesthesia, normal skeletal muscles should be relaxed and electrically silent away from the end-plate zones, unless they are directly irritated by insertion of a needle electrode. Inserting the needle will induce a short period of insertional electrical activity, after which a silent (flat line) recording should be obtained. Normal spontaneous myofibre activity, without needle movement, can sometimes be noted if the tip of the recording needle is lying very close to a neuronal end-plate (neuromuscular junction). This is characterised by miniature end-plate potentials and/or end-plate spikes (Van Nes, 1986; Cuddon, 2002; Kimura, 2013; Shapiro and Preston, 2013).

(i) Insertional activity

For each muscle, the electromyographic examination starts with the assessment of insertional activity. This is the electrical activity seen when the needle electrode is passed through the myocytes, disrupting the sarcolemma and causing transient myofibre depolarisation. Insertional activity is also evoked by any quick movement of the needle electrode when inside the muscle (Cuddon, 2002; Daube and Rubin, 2009; Kimura, 2013; Shapiro and Preston, 2013).

The muscle fibre depolarisation causes a brief burst of positive or negative, high-frequency, high-amplitude spikes lasting a few hundred milliseconds (typically less than 230ms in humans), producing a crisp static sound. The amplitude depends on the speed and magnitude of electrode movement. In normal muscle, this is followed by a very quick return to electrical silence once the action potentials have propagated down the muscle fibres (**Figure 3.5**). This insertional activity confirms that the needle is within the muscle rather than in fibrous tissue, subcutaneous tissue or fat (Cuddon, 2002; Daube and Rubin, 2009; Kimura, 2013; Shapiro and Preston, 2013).

Increased/prolonged insertional activity is defined as any electrical activity (other than normal end-plate potentials) that lasts longer than 300ms after cessation of needle movement. It indicates instability or irritability of the muscle fibre membrane and can be noted in both neuropathic and myopathic conditions (Shapiro

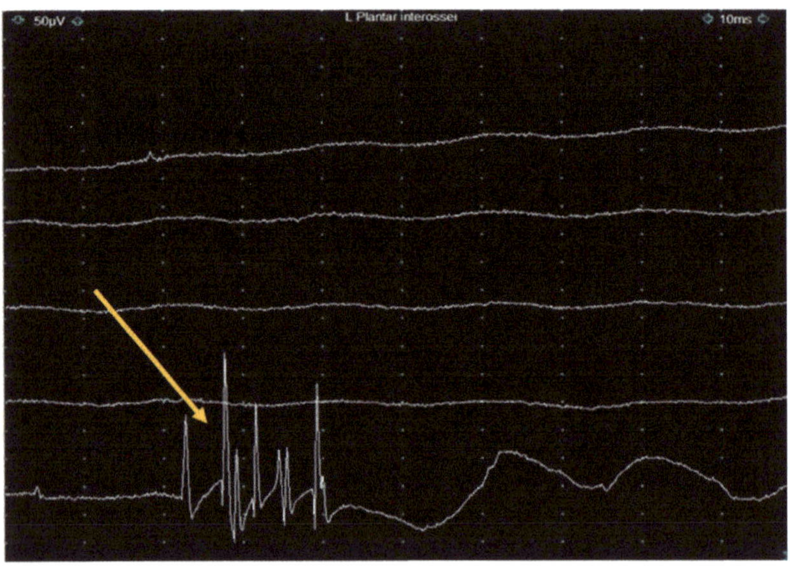

Figure 3.5. A normal, short burst of insertional electrical activity after needle movement in the left *plantar interosseous* muscle of an anaesthetised dog (yellow arrow). Note the normal electrically silent recording of the traces above, before needle movement. Horizontal scale = 10ms/division, vertical scale = 50μV/division.

and Preston, 2013). This can be the only abnormality observed in the early stages of peripheral motor neuropathies, before other abnormal forms of spontaneous myofibre activity develop, and can be recorded from 4 to 5 days after the onset of muscle denervation (Daube and Rubin, 2009; Kimura, 2013).

Decreased insertional activity can be seen in cases of chronic denervation or an advanced myopathy, when the muscle is replaced by fat or fibrous tissue. In these cases, needle movement through the replacement tissue does not trigger action potentials and few or no spikes are generated (Cuddon, 2002; Kimura, 2013; Shapiro and Preston, 2013).

(ii) Motor unit action potentials

The motor unit represents the cluster of 15-20 myofibres that are innervated by a single motor axon, with the axonal cell body residing in the ventral horn of the spinal cord. Spontaneous or, more commonly, voluntary firing of a motor neuron will therefore result in a potential with a large amplitude (100 to 3000µV) and long duration (1 to 12ms) as it represents the summation of activity from multiple myofibres. These motor unit action potentials are usually biphasic or triphasic, with an initial small positive (downward) deflection followed by a major negative deflection (**Figure 3.6**) (Cuddon, 2002; Kimura, 2013; Shapiro and Preston, 2013). They can also involve the depolarisation of several motor units and be even larger in amplitude if so.

If electromyography is performed under general anaesthesia in a normal animal, then there should be no motor unit action potentials (MUAPs) as the muscles are relaxed and there is no voluntary firing of the motor neuron cell bodies. However, if EMG is performed without general anaesthesia, for example in humans using surface electrodes, then MUAPs can be recorded in a resting state or recruited during voluntary movement (volitional EMG). When performing EMG of the laryngeal muscles in anaesthetised and spontaneously breathing companion animals, there will

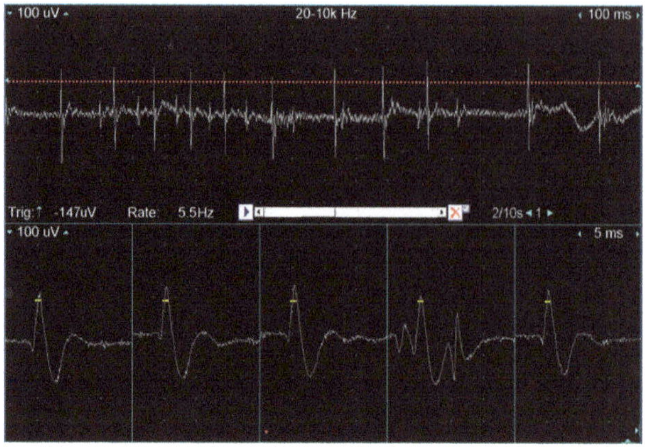

Figure 3.6. Motor unit action potentials in a standing, awake horse. Upper part: potentials of high amplitude (400μV). Horizontal scale = 100ms/division, vertical scale = 100μV/division. Lower part (magnification): large triphasic potentials (amplitude of 400μV) of long duration (10ms), with a small positive (downward) deflection followed by a larger negative deflection. Horizontal scale = 5ms/division, vertical scale = 100μV/division.

be the presence of MUAPs during the inspiratory phase, which is a normal finding. Motor unit action potentials can also be recorded in animals if they are sedated (or under a light plane of anaesthesia) and they react to needle placement, resulting in voluntary contraction of the muscle being tested.

The frequency of MUAPs depends on the state of the muscle (i.e., resting, in tension, or actively contracting). During voluntary contraction, it is possible to see the increase in MUAP frequency that comes with motor unit recruitment. This is called 'activation' and is regulated by the central nervous system, with small motor units being recruited first. When the muscle contraction is maximal, there is simultaneous discharge of numerous motor units, and it becomes impossible to recognise individual MUAPs. This is called an 'interference pattern' and provides valuable diagnostic information in humans, but is not applicable in animals (Kimura, 2013; Michell, 2013; Shapiro and Preston, 2013).

In humans, changes seen during conscious electromyography include (Kimura, 2013; Michell, 2013; Shapiro and Preston, 2013):

- Decreased amplitude of the MUAP, suggestive of myopathy, distal neuropathy with abnormal intramuscular nerve branches, or junctionopathy. This is because there are either fewer functional muscles fibres in the motor unit available for activation (myopathy), or because there is less transmission of the signal through the terminal axon branches (neuropathy) or the neuromuscular junctions (junctionopathy), resulting in stimulation of fewer muscle fibres to contribute to the compound potential;
- Giant MUAPs, characterised by an increased duration and amplitude. This is suggestive of reinnervation of denervated muscle fibres by axonal sprouting from surviving axons, with a resultant increase in the number of myofibres in the new motor units. These giant MUAPs are often polyphasic because new nerve branches have thinner myelin sheaths and therefore slower motor nerve conduction velocities. This means that the impulses to reinnervated muscle fibres arrive slightly later than those to others within the same motor unit, producing a compound potential with multiple phases;
- Decreased recruitment and an incomplete interference pattern during voluntary muscle contraction, suggesting axonal loss or conduction block;
- A normal number (normal recruitment) of low amplitude, short duration MUAPs in cases of myopathy;
- Decreased activation with fewer MUAPs in some central nervous system disorders.

(iii) Normal spontaneous electrical activity: miniature end-plate potentials and end-plate spikes

a. Miniature end-plate potentials

If a concentric needle is inserted into a normal muscle and happens to lie immobile close to an end-plate region (neuromuscular junction), it is possible to record small mono- or biphasic potentials (10 to 50μV of amplitude, 1 to 2ms in duration) that have an initial negative (upwards) deflection. These potentials correspond to depolarisation of the post-synaptic muscle fibre membrane following the normal release of small quanta of acetylcholine (typically from one synapse) into the synaptic cleft of the end-plate region (**Figure 3.7**). This depolarisation is insufficient to result in a visible muscle contraction (non-propagated sub-threshold end-plate potentials) but can be recorded during EMG if the needle lies in close proximity to a neuromuscular junction. These potentials are typically irregular, do not require needle insertion to occur and are frequently associated with end-plate spikes (see below). The sound associated with these miniature end-plate potentials is like a seashell held to the ear or waves on a shore. Small movements of the needle away from the end-plate zone will lead to their disappearance, which can sometimes help to distinguish miniature end-plate potentials from other forms of (abnormal) spontaneous activity (e.g., fibrillation potentials) (van Nes, 1986; Cuddon, 2002; Kimura, 2013; Shapiro and Preston, 2013).

There are descriptions of the absence of miniature end-plate potentials following denervation, reduction in their amplitude with *myasthenia gravis,* or reduction in their frequency with botulism. However, in small animals, these potentials have not been extensively investigated in disease states and they remain of little clinical significance in humans (Cuddon, 2002; Kimura, 2013).

b. End-plate spikes

End-plate spikes are commonly associated with miniature end-plate potentials. When the needle irritates a nerve terminal at the level of the end-plate region, it induces release of multiple quanta of acetylcholine into the synaptic cleft. This is sufficient to result in firing of a single muscle fibre (similar to a nerve action potential depolarising the fibre), typically at a high frequency, generating the end-plate spikes. They are therefore of higher amplitude (100 to 200µV) and longer in duration (3 to 4ms) than miniature end-plate potentials, irregular in frequency (5 to 50Hz) and are associated with a sound like fat spitting in a frying pan

(Shapiro and Preston, 2013). The waveform is biphasic, like that of a fibrillation potential (see later), but with an initial negative (upwards) deflection (**Figure 3.7**) (van Nes, 1986; Cuddon, 2002; Kimura, 2013; Shapiro and Preston, 2013). This is because end-plate spikes are detected when the tip of the recording needle is lying immediately next to an end-plate terminal, where the spike is generated. Fibrillation potentials that are recorded when the tip of the needle is next to their site of generation may also have an initial negative deflection (Kimura 2013). However, fibrillation potentials are more commonly generated away from the needle tip and will therefore have an initial positive deflection that precedes the negative phase, which is never a feature of end-plate spikes.

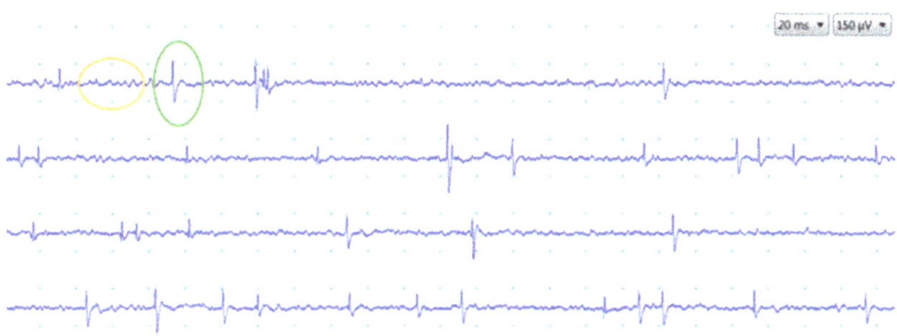

Figure 3.7. End-plate activity showing miniature end-plate potentials (orange circle) and end-plate spikes (green circle). Note the small and monophasic negative potentials for the miniature end-plate potentials, and the initial negative (upwards) deflection, biphasic morphology and irregular firing pattern for the end-plate spikes. Horizontal scale = 20ms/division, vertical scale = 150µV/division.

4. Abnormal electromyographic findings

(i) Generators of abnormal spontaneous electrical activity

In a case with disease affecting either the muscle fibres (myopathy) or the peripheral motor axons innervating the skeletal muscle (denervation), abnormal electrical activity can persist after normal insertional activity ('prolonged insertional activity', usually in the form of positive sharp waves), or appear as spontaneous firing of individual muscle fibres in the absence of neural stimulation (e.g., as fibrillation potentials in a relaxed muscle under general anaesthesia). This is because the post-synaptic muscle fibre membrane will recruit more acetylcholine receptors when it is isolated from axon terminals secondary to either axonal loss (denervation) or damage to the muscle membrane itself (myopathy). This process takes several days and dramatically increases the sensitivity of muscle fibres to any stimulation or to acetylcholine in the local environment, eventually resulting in spontaneous depolarisation of the post-synaptic membrane, even in the absence of neuronal firing.

Dependent on the cause, the primary generator site of abnormal spontaneous electrical activity can be the peripheral motor nerve or the muscle fibres themselves (**Table 3.6**) (Kimura, 2013; Michell, 2013; Shapiro and Preston, 2013).

Generator site	Type(s) of spontaneous electrical activity
Motor neuron/axon	Fasciculation, myokymia, neuromyotonia
Individual muscle fibre	Fibrillation potential, positive sharp wave, myotonia
Multiple muscle fibres	Complex repetitive discharges

Table 3.6. Generator sites of spontaneous electrical activity and types of electrical activity.

Spontaneous waveforms are characterised by:

- Their morphology: amplitude, phase direction (positive, negative, biphasic, triphasic);
- Their firing pattern (interspike interval change);
- The direction of the initial deflection of the potential from the baseline (Kimura, 2013; Shapiro and Preston, 2013).

Discharges from a single muscle fibre are of short duration, simple morphology (usually biphasic) and of lower amplitude (Michell, 2013).

(ii) Types of abnormal spontaneous electrical activity

Recognition of abnormal spontaneous activity is one of the most important parts of needle electromyography (EMG).

a. Fibrillation potentials

Fibrillation potentials are the consequence of spontaneous depolarisation of a single muscle fibre. They represent a potential travelling along the muscle fibre membrane and are recorded extracellularly. They are the most common form of abnormal spontaneous discharge recorded during needle EMG.

When a motor neuron is injured, the terminal portions of the axon degenerate back from the end-plate regions. The muscle(s) innervated by its branches are therefore disconnected from the nervous system and the chemosensitive area of the sarcolemma at the level of the motor end-plate spreads to involve the whole surface of the muscle fibre. This recruitment of increased numbers of nicotinic acetylcholine receptors along the muscle membrane eventually results in spontaneous electrical activity in response to only background levels of acetylcholine. Hypersensitivity of the post-synaptic acetylcholine receptors to this molecule following denervation also contributes to spontaneous activity (Kimura, 2013).

During the course of a disease, fibrillation potentials develop after a period of time dependent on the species: 5 to 8 days after onset of denervation in dogs and cats, 12 to 16 days in large animals, and approximately 16 days in humans (Cuddon, 2002; Kimura, 2013; Shapiro and Preston, 2013).

Fibrillation potentials are brief spikes (1 to 5ms in duration) of low amplitude (20-500µV). They are usually triphasic (when recorded at a distance along the muscle fibre from the site of discharge initiation), with an initial positive (downwards) deflection followed by a negative (upwards) spike and a final (usually small) positive phase (**Figures 3.8 and 3.9**) (Cuddon, 2002; Daube, 2009; Kimura,

2013). If the needle deforms the muscle fibre, therefore blocking the propagation of the depolarisation away from the needle, the morphology may only be biphasic (i.e., comprising the initial positive phase followed by a negative phase but without the third positive phase). If the needle records a fibrillation potential generated at its tip, the morphology will be initially negative and cannot be differentiated from an end-plate spike (see above). However, unlike fibrillation potentials, end-plate spikes are usually associated with miniature end-plate potentials and disappear if the electrode is moved away from the end-plate region. Fibrillation potentials have a regular firing pattern, with linear changes in the inter-spike interval, and sound like rain on a metal roof, frying eggs or wrinkling paper (Cuddon, 2002; Kimura, 2013; Shapiro and Preston, 2013).

Fibrillation potentials are the marker of active denervation. However, they can also be recorded in some myopathies in which damage to the muscle membrane causes instability and/or isolation of the muscle membrane from the end-plate regions (e.g., inflammatory myopathies, muscular dystrophies), and rarely in junctionopathies (e.g., botulism). Fibrillation potentials can sometimes be recorded in normal muscles without evidence of a lower motor neuron or muscle disorder. These changes are frequently mild and are thought to be associated with normal ageing in people, and/or some degree of external trauma to the nerves and muscles in distal parts of the foot (Falck and Alaranta, 1983).

Fibrillation potentials can be graded on a four-grade scale ranging from 1+ to 4+ based on their density on the screen and spread across a muscle, as follows (Michell, 2013; Kimura, 2013; Shapiro and Preston, 2013):

Grade 1+: one to a few potentials in more than one area;
Grade 2+: moderate number of potentials in 3 or more areas;
Grade 3+: large number of potentials in 3 or more areas;
Grade 4+: potentials completely filling the screen.

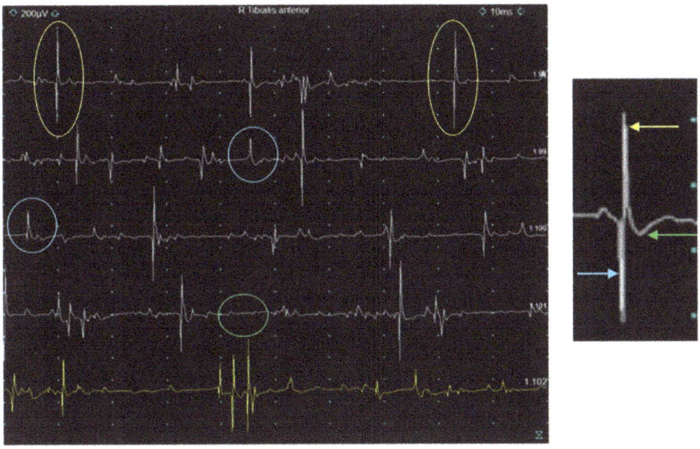

Figure 3.8. Fibrillation potentials in the right *tibialis cranialis* of a dog with degenerative polyneuropathy under general anaesthesia, grade 2+. Note some fibrillation potentials (yellow circles) with a triphasic morphology (inset), in which there is an initial positive phase (blue arrow), followed by a negative spike (yellow arrow) and a small positive phase (green arrow); other fibrillation potentials (blue circles) are biphasic, with an initial small positive phase and only a larger negative spike; note the presence of miniature end-plate potentials (green circle). Horizontal scale = 10ms/division, vertical scale = 200µV/division.

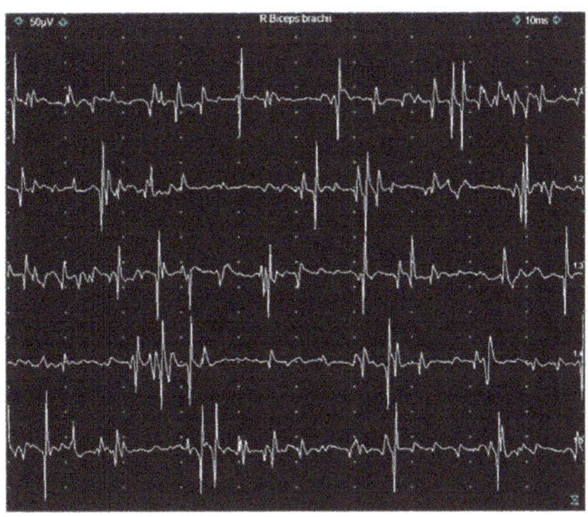

Figure 3.9. Fibrillation potentials, grade 3+, in the right *biceps brachii* of a dog with a traumatic brachial plexus injury (axonotmesis) under general anaesthesia. Horizontal scale = 10ms/division, vertical scale = 50µV/division.

In most cases, the grade reflects the severity of the disease. However, the grade can decrease in severity over time with either reinnervation or fibrosis (requiring correlation to the history and clinical findings).

b. Positive sharp waves

Positive sharp waves also represent spontaneous depolarisations of a single muscle fibre. They therefore represent the same pathophysiologic process as fibrillation potentials but differ in their morphology due to a difference in the position of the recording electrode in relation to where the travelling action potential terminates along the muscle membrane. If the muscle fibre is damaged by the needle insertion or by disease (denervation or myopathy), and the recording needle electrode is located where the action potential terminates along the muscle fibre, there will be no propagation of a potential past and away from the needle electrode (membrane inexcitability); this results in a biphasic potential comprised of an initial large, positive deflection, followed by a small, slower negative potential before the waveform returns to baseline (**Figure 3.10**) (Kimura, 2013). Positive sharp waves are typically less than 5ms in duration, with a variable amplitude of 50μV to 4mV (**Figure 3.10**), and sound like a racing car passing by.

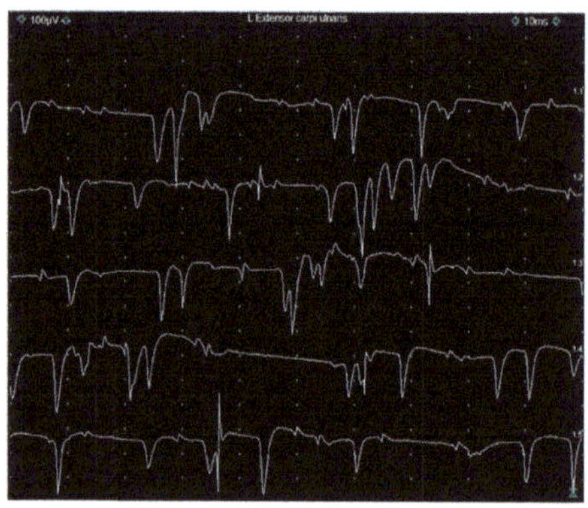

Figure 3.10. Positive sharp waves in the left *extensor carpi ulnaris* of a dog with traumatic brachial plexus injury (axonotmesis) under general anaesthesia. Note the initial sharp positive (downward) deflection followed by a slow and small negative phase. Horizontal scale = 10ms/division, vertical scale = 100μV/division.

c. Myotonic discharges

Myotonic discharges represent spontaneous repetitive firings of an individual muscle fibre and are generated because of instability or dysfunction of the muscle fibre membrane, or of the membrane ion channels (e.g., myotonic muscular dystrophies,

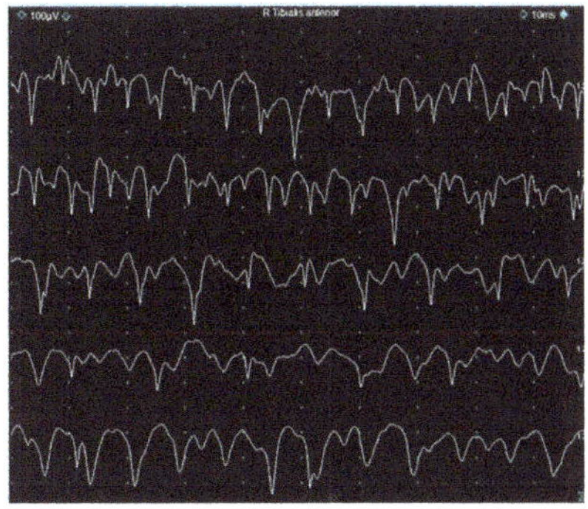

Figure 3.11. Myotonic discharges in the *tibialis cranialis* muscle of a dog with *myotonia congenita*. Note the waning and waxing of both the amplitude and frequency. Horizontal scale = 10ms/division, vertical scale = 100µV/division.

myotonia congenita, paramyotonia congenita, other myopathies). They are triggered by needle movement, persist after injection of a neuromuscular blocker and rarely occur with denervation (Kimura, 2013; Shapiro and Preston, 2013).

The discharges may be positive or negative potentials, which fire at a regular but exponentially increasing or decreasing frequency. This waxing and waning nature is characteristic of this type of potential, with firing rates usually between 20 and 150Hz (**Figure 3.11**). Their amplitudes may also decrease or increase over time (10µV-1mV). Myotonic discharges sound like a chainsaw or a dive bomber, and frequently lack the sudden 'start and stop' seen with complex repetitive discharges (see below)(Cuddon, 2002).

d. Complex repetitive discharges

Complex repetitive discharges were formerly referred to as 'pseudomyotonic discharges'. Unlike fibrillation potentials, positive sharp waves and myotonic discharges, they reflect the spontaneous activity of multiple muscle fibres. This results from the initial depolarisation of a single fibre that spreads directly to the muscle membranes of adjacent fibres. This means that they are 'time-locked', with all the fibres depolarising sequentially and in near synchrony. They typically have a regular firing rate, an amplitude ranging from 50µV to 1mV, and a duration of 50-100ms. If the depolarisation spreads in a circular movement, with the original pacemaker muscle fibre being reactivated, recurrent discharges are noted. Their morphology is very similar to waveforms originating from individual myofibres but represents a compound potential of multiple spikes. They fire consecutively with a high frequency, have an abrupt termination, and do not wax and wane like myotonic discharges (**Figures 3.12 and 3.13**). They typically sound like a machine gun via the loudspeaker (Kimura, 2013). They are generally identical from one discharge to the next but may change in appearance if extra paths are recruited (Daube and Rubin, 2009; Kimura, 2013; Shapiro and Preston, 2013).

Complex repetitive discharges are usually found in chronic neuropathies or myopathies (e.g., associated with hyperadreno-corticism). This is because they rely on the presence of adjacent

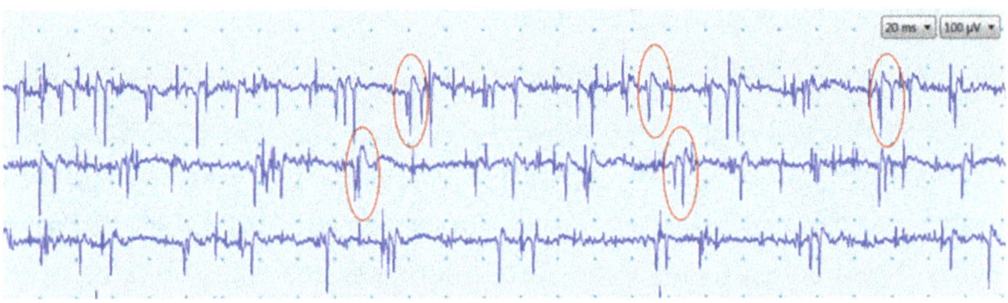

Figure 3.12. Complex repetitive discharges (red circles) in the *triceps brachii* muscle of a dog with a peripheral nerve sheath tumour of the radial nerve. Note the multiple spikes within a complex and the repetition of identical complexes. Horizontal scale = 20ms/division, vertical scale = 100µV/division.

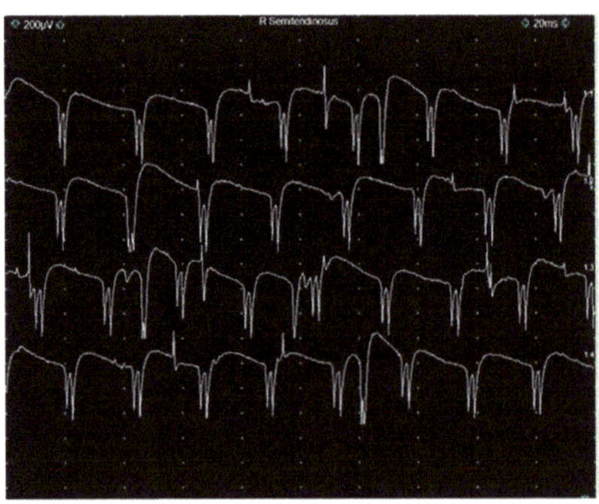

Figure 3.13. Complex repetitive discharges. Note the multiple spikes within a complex and the repetition of identical complexes. Horizontal scale = 20ms/division, vertical scale = 200µV/division.

denervated fibres for depolarisation to spread, which may not be present in acute disorders, in which denervated fibres may be next to normal fibres.

e. Abnormal spontaneous electrical activity from motor units: peripheral nerve hyperexcitability

Peripheral nerve hyperexcitability clinically manifests as muscle fasciculations, myokymia, neuromyotonia, cramps, or tetany. It can be focal or generalised, and each of these clinical features is associated with a specific EMG pattern (Vanhaesebrouck *et al.,* 2013). As the origin of the spontaneous myofibre activity is peripheral nerve hyperexcitability, and not from the brain or spinal cord, these electrical discharges will persist during general anaesthesia but disappear with neuromuscular blockade (e.g., curare) (Kimura, 2013). Electromyographic descriptions are available for myokymia and neuromyotonia in companion animals (Vanhaesebrouck *et al.,* 2013).

- Fasciculation potentials

Clinically, fasciculations are brief, random contractions/twitches of a portion of muscle that may (when located near the surface of a muscle) be visible at the skin surface (Lowrie and Garosi, 2016).

Fasciculation potentials result from a single, spontaneous, occasional discharge from one hyperactive motor neuron cell body or axon, leading to spontaneous firing of one individual motor unit. They represent depolarisation of more than one muscle fibre and are therefore polyphasic and larger than fibrillation potentials (**Figure 3.14**). They have a slow (less than 1-2Hz), irregular firing pattern on EMG (Kimura, 2013; Shapiro and Preston, 2013). To identify a fasciculation potential, it is recommended to remove one's hand from the recording needle and wait 30 seconds or longer to see if it occurs. When found, they sound like 'corn popping'. They can be observed in normal or diseased muscles (in which case they will be accompanied by spontaneous denervation activity).

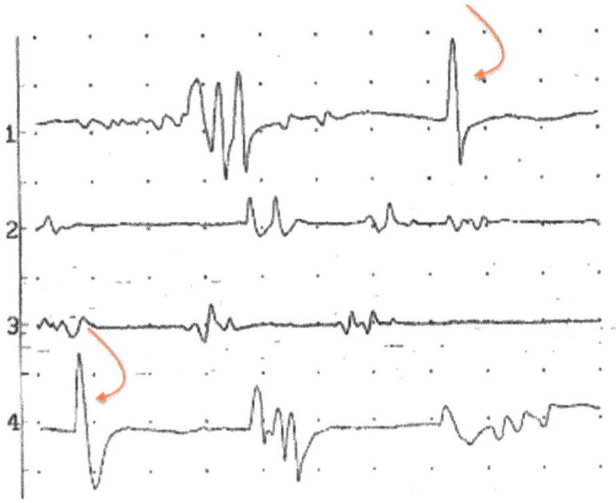

Figure 3.14. Fasciculation potentials (red arrows) in a Jack Russell Terrier with myokymia (Courtesy of Dr. An Vanhaesebrouck).

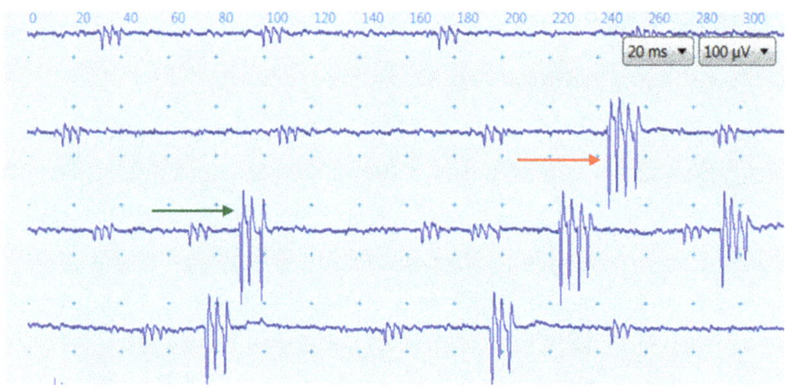

Figure 3.15. Myokymia. Bursts of potentials (some being triplets [green arrow], some quadruplets [red arrow]) with a high frequency (5-150Hz) within the burst, and a slow frequency between bursts. Horizontal scale = 20ms/division, vertical scale = 100µV/division.

• Myokymia

Myokymia manifests clinically as involuntary muscle contractions that result in rippling movements of the overlying skin (Lowrie and Garosi, 2016).

It represents rhythmic and spontaneous repetitive discharges of the same motor unit resulting from motor neuron or axonal hyperexcitability – in other words, these are grouped, repetitive fasciculations. This results in recurrent, brief (<1s), rhythmic bursts of motor unit potentials. The number of potentials in a burst may vary from one or two (doublet), to several (multiplet). The intra-burst frequency is between 5 and 150Hz (**Figure 3.15**) and they typically sound like soldiers marching (Vanhaesebrouck *et al.*, 2013; Lowrie and Garosi, 2016).

• Neuromyotonia

Clinically, neuromyotonia is characterised by muscle stiffness and delayed relaxation after contraction because of sustained firing of the muscle membrane and is more severe than myokymia (Lowrie and Garosi, 2016). Neuromyotonia and myokymia reflect a spectrum of the same pathophysiology and result from disorders leading to peripheral nerve hyperactivity. This includes autoimmune channelopathies affecting the voltage-gated potassium channel, which reduce the potassium conductance at the level of the nerve terminal and result in increased nerve terminal excitability.

Neuromyotonic discharges represent spontaneous electrical activities generated along the peripheral motor axons and differ from myokymia by their higher intra-burst frequency (150-300Hz). These bursts last for up to a few seconds and begin and end abruptly. The firing rate can also increase or decrease. The amplitude of the spikes (a compound muscle potential) often decreases over time due to muscle fatigue (Vanhaesebrouck *et al.*, 2013). They can fire continuously or in short bursts and have a 'pinging' sound via the loudspeaker (Vanhaesebrouck *et al.*, 2010; Lowrie and Garosi, 2016).

• Cramps

Cramps are involuntary and painful muscle contractions with an acute onset and short (seconds to minutes) duration. They are caused by peripheral nerve hyperexcitability and often lead to immobility of the affected muscle (e.g., sustained limb flexion)

(Lowrie and Garosi, 2016). Cramp has been described in dogs and is most commonly associated with hypocalcaemia (Gagliardo *et al.,* 2021). On EMG, cramps are characterised by repetitive and overlapping motor unit action potentials at high rates (up to 150Hz), resulting from activation of multiple motor units. They have an abrupt onset and rapid cessation. Discharge frequency initially gradually increases and subsequently decreases as the cramp subsides (Daube and Rubin, 2009; Vanhaesebrouck *et al.,* 2013; Lowrie and Garosi, 2016).

- Tetany/tetanus

Tetany is a prolonged, sustained muscle contraction without relaxation. On electromyography, doublets, triplets or multiplets of motor unit action potentials and simultaneous activity in both agonist and antagonist muscles are usually seen (de Risio *et al.*, 2006; Vanhaesebrouck *et al.*, 2013). The term *tetanus* is typically reserved for the sustained muscle contractions observed following infection by the anaerobic, spore-forming bacteria *Clostridium tetani* and resultant disinhibition of motor neuron firing following binding by the neurotoxin tetanospasmin to inhibitory interneurons (Renshaw cells) at the level of the spinal cord.

Discharge type *Origin*	Morphology	Amplitude and duration	Firing rate	Sound on loudspeaker	Picture
Insertional activity (normal activity) *Single muscle fibre*	Positive or negative spikes	200µV to 1mV A few hundred ms	High frequency	Crisp static sound	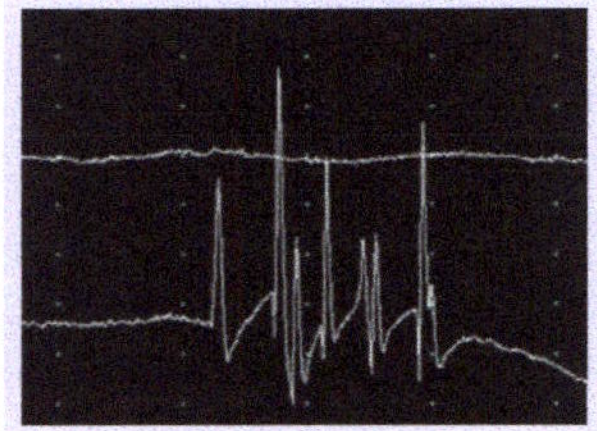
End-plate spike (normal activity) *Single muscle fibre*	Biphasic Initial negative deflection	100-200µV 3-4ms	Irregular frequency: 5-50Hz	Fat in a frying pan	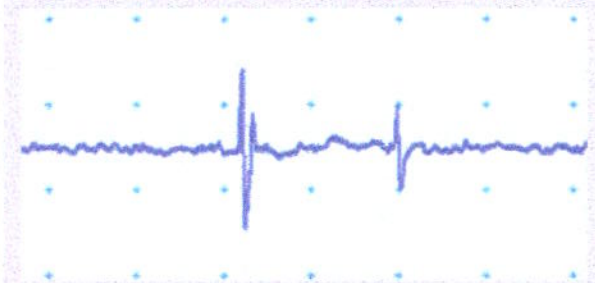
Fibrillation potential *Single muscle fibre*	Biphasic or triphasic, usually initial positive deflection	20-500µV 1-5ms	Regular 1-30Hz	Frying eggs, Rain on a metal roof	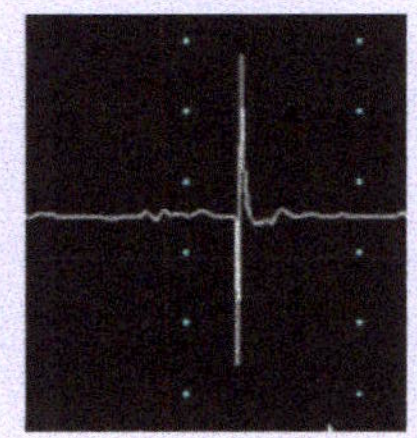

Discharge type ***Origin***	**Morphology**	**Amplitude and duration**	**Firing rate**	**Sound on loudspeaker**	**Picture**
Positive sharp wave *Single muscle fibre*	Initial short positive deflection then low amplitude slow negativity	50µV to 4mV 1-5ms	Regular 2-50Hz	Racing car	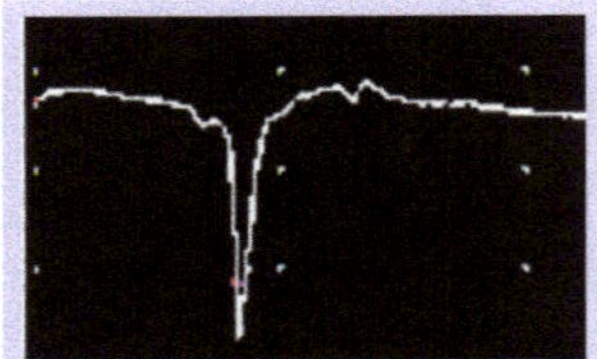
Myotonic discharge *Single muscle fibre*	Individual potentials that look like fibril-lation potentials or positive sharp waves	10µV to 1mV (waxing and waning)	Waxing and waning frequency (20-150Hz)	Chainsaw, Dive bomber, Accelerating and decelerating motorcycle engine	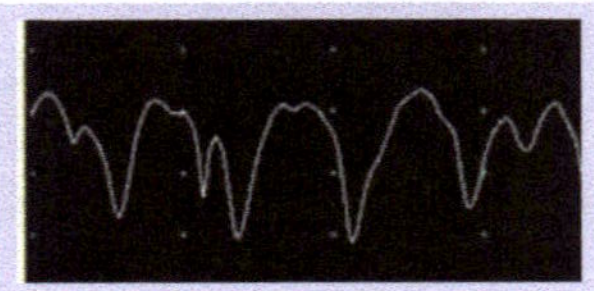
Complex repetitive discharge *Multiple muscle fibres*	Polyphasic with each discharge looking like a cluster of fibril-lation potentials or positive sharp waves of different sizes; each discharge is identical to the previous	50µV to 1mV 50-100ms	~30-40Hz Abrupt onset and cessation	Firing machine gun	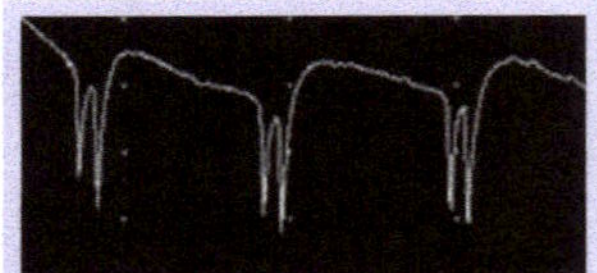

Table 3.7. Types of EMG recording originating from muscle fibres.

Spontaneous electrical activity	Morphology	Amplitude and duration	Firing rate	Sound on loudspeaker	Picture
Fasciculation	Polyphasic, with an initial small positive deflection. Similar to a fibrillation potential but larger amplitude and longer duration.	>1mV >5ms	Irregular Slow <1-2Hz	Corn popping	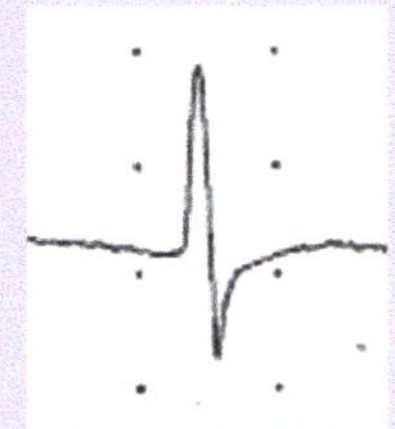
Myokymia	2-10 individual units that look like fasciculations	Brief (<1s), rhythmic bursts of motor unit potentials	Sudden onset and cessation, no waning and waxing. Regular firing rate; 5-150Hz intra-burst frequency	Marching soldiers	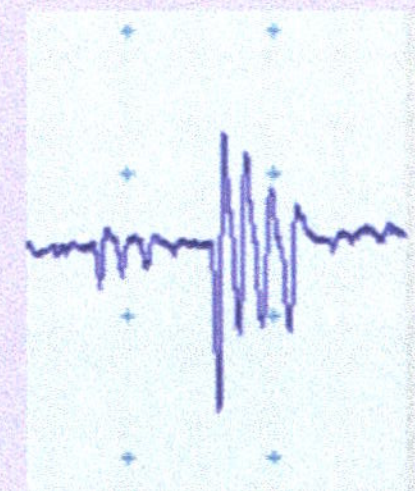
Neuromyotonia	Group of individual units that look like fasciculations	Amplitude often decreases over time Bursts can last up to a few seconds	Sudden onset and cessation 150-300Hz intra-burst frequency (can increase or decrease)	Pinging sound	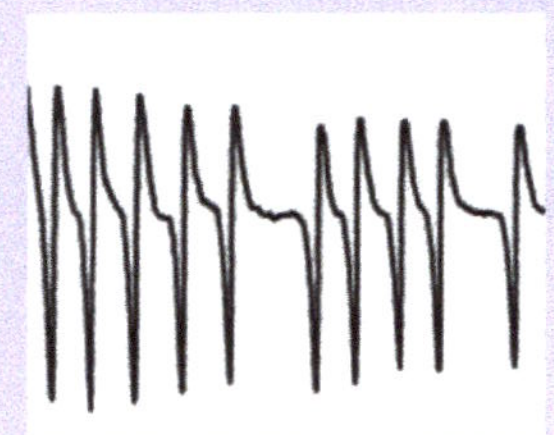

Table 3.8. Types of spontaneous EMG recording originating from motor axons (in order of increasing hyperexcitability) leading to activation of motor units.

Discharge type ***Origin***	**Morphology**	**Amplitude and duration**	**Firing rate**	**Sound on loudspeaker**	**Picture**
Miniature end-plate potential (normal) *Neuromuscular junction*	Small, rounded fluctuations of the baseline Disappear when needle moved away from the end-plate region	10-50μV 1-2ms	Irregular frequency: 5-50Hz	Seashell held to the ear Waves on a shore	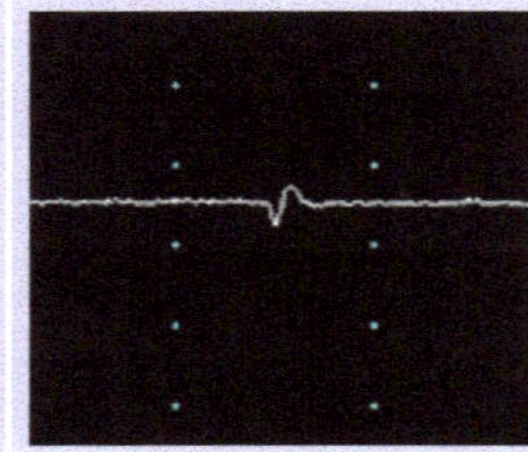

Table 3.9. Spontaneous electrical activity originating from the neuromuscular junction.

5. Artefacts

(i) Interferences during signal recording

The recording electrode(s) and amplifier can detect electrical currents in addition to those originating from muscles and nerves. If so, this will also appear on the computer display and be heard by the operator via the loudspeaker.

Some interferences are easily detected because of their unique discharge pattern and characteristic sound (e.g., high frequency audio interference from radio broadcasts), whilst others might mimic biological activity (e.g., mobile phones can mimic high-frequency complex repetitive discharges).

Electrostatic and electromagnetic sources from electrical apparatus used around the animal generate currents typically of 50-60Hz frequency. In particular, heating systems (e.g., a heat pad placed under the animal) can cause 60Hz oscillations on the computer display (**Figure 3.16**). Diathermy units in surgery can cause 120Hz oscillations. Unused power cords plugged into wall sockets, especially if these are multiple socket plugs into which the electrodiagnostic unit is also plugged, can generate artefacts. Light dimmers can also be a source of 60Hz oscillations (e.g., if one performs the study in an ultrasound room that is equipped with a light dimmer). Metal tables increase the likelihood to record artefacts.

Electrodes are a common source of artefacts. Needles with a small tip have a high impedance and can generate spikes when moved

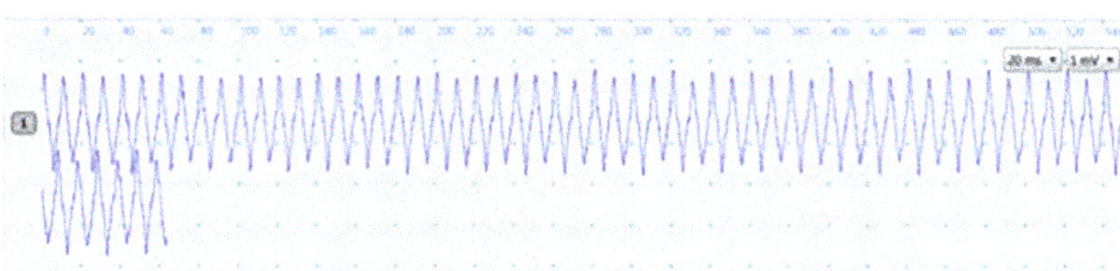

Figure 3.16. 60Hz artefact easily recognisable by the repetitive sinusoidal pattern. Horizontal scale = 20ms/division, vertical scale = 1mV/division.

in the muscle, with a similar appearance to fibrillation potentials (**Figure 3.17**). This is because the potential between the tissue fluid and the metal of the electrode (at the tip of the needle) does not necessarily remain constant over time resulting in changing potentials. A good way of making sure that the potentials are not artefacts is to ensure that abnormal EMG findings are repeatable.

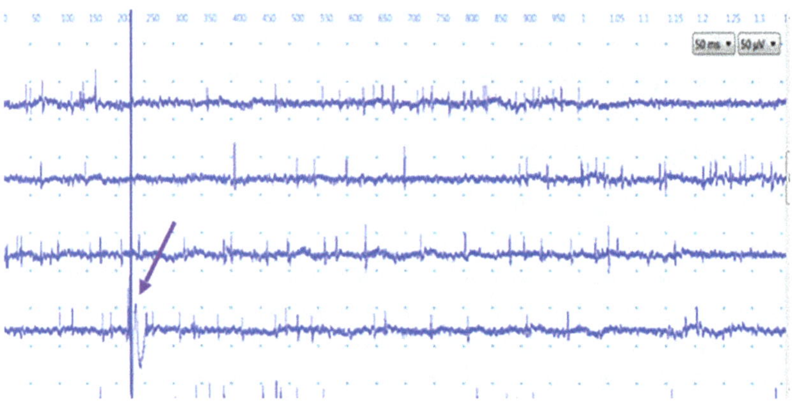

Figure 3.17. Spike generated by movement of a needle of high impedance. Horizontal scale = 50ms/division, vertical scale = 50μV/division.

There can also be a short-circuit at the tip of a concentric needle, especially if it has been re-used, and this can result in artefacts. A loose connection within the recording circuit, particularly affecting the cable(s) between the needle and amplifier, can also be a common source of artefacts. This can result from: (i) damage to the plastic insulation of a cable; (ii) damage to the wire within the plastic sleeve (even if the plastic appears intact), which can cause electrical potentials mimicking muscle action potentials; and (iii) damage at the base of the touch-proof connector, where the cable is regularly bent (common in the authors' experience) (**Figure 3.18**).

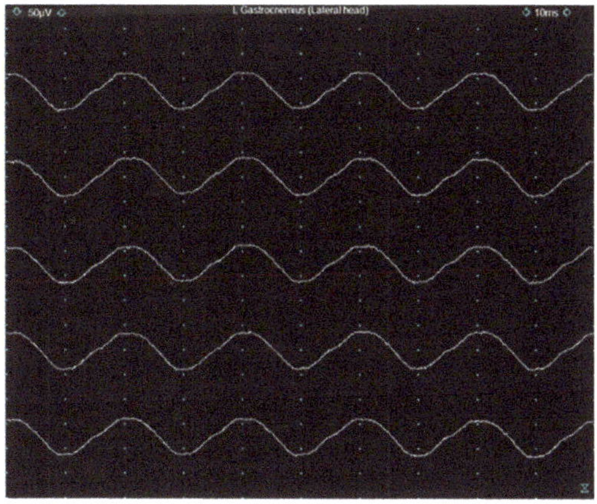

Figure 3.18. Recording artefact originating from poor connection between the needle and the amplifier. Horizontal scale = 10ms/division, vertical scale = 50µV/division.

Interference from the animal, rather than the equipment, can be caused by voluntary movement, in particular during the first few minutes after induction of anaesthesia and/or when the animal is moved or under a light plane of anaesthesia. This will appear as voluntary motor unit action potentials. An overlying electrocardiogram (ECG) from myocardial depolarisation can also be recorded when performing EMG on muscles close to the chest.

Finally, the presence of fat between the muscle and the recording needle can obscure the recording (**Figure 3.19**).

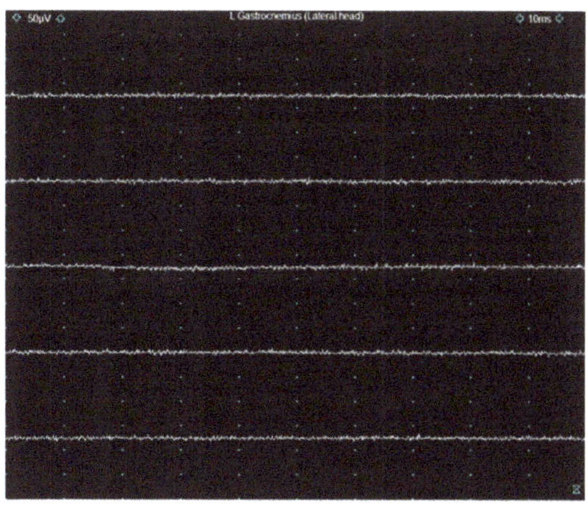

Figure 3.19. Electrical interference signal generated by the presence of fat between the muscle and the recording needle. Horizontal scale = 10ms/division, vertical scale = 50µV/division.

(ii) Solutions to reduce interference/artefacts

To reduce artefacts caused by needles and cables, it is best to use stainless steel or platinum electrodes and replace needles/cables regularly. During an examination, changing electrodes one at a time for a new one might be needed to test the possibility of a damaged cable or loose connection. It is also good practice to check the impedance of both the stimulating and recording needles. This can be done with an impedance meter designed to receive touch proof connections or by using in-built modalities offered by modern electrophysiology units.

Once both needles (including their impedance) and cables have been checked for faults, in the presence of unexplained interferences, it can be useful to:

- Unplug as many electrical appliances as possible within the room that is being used to conduct the examination;
- Check that a reference ('ground') electrode has been placed on the animal;
- Check the depth of anaesthesia or ask the anaesthetist to deepen the anaesthetic and assess if this resolves the problem, particularly if there is a high suspicion of voluntary muscle contraction and MUAPs overlying the trace.

One important tip when trying to identify the source of interference or artefact is to assess whether the recording is affected by needle position. If the interference persists when the recording needle is moved to a different location, then it is likely that the artefact is caused by a distant source, i.e. outside the patient. A good way to then eliminate these persistent artefacts, is to re-organise the position of the patient and the recording equipment in the room. The recording equipment can be placed in a different place around the animal or the table supporting the animal can be moved away from other electrical appliances or wall sockets. The heat pad should be disconnected.

6. Electromyography in neuromuscular disorders

The distribution of abnormal spontaneous electrical activity gives the 'EMG map' of the disease; this can support the neurological examination findings and assist in defining the neuroanatomic localisation. For example, in the case of a motor mononeuropathy, denervation potentials may be found in muscles belonging to the same myotome (innervated by the same motor nerve), with electromyographic changes first noted 5 to 8 days after initial axonal injury, supporting which nerve(s) are affected by the lesion. This can also help to differentiate orthopaedic from neurologic causes of lameness, in which EMG would be expected to be normal in the former and could be abnormal for the latter if there is muscle denervation.

Certain types of abnormal spontaneous electrical activity can be associated with specific neuromuscular disorders (myotonic discharges, for instance) (Cuddon, 2002). However, this is uncommon and, when taken in isolation, the recording of abnormal spontaneous muscle activity in an anaesthetised animal does not allow the distinction between a neuropathy and a myopathy (Cuddon, 2002). This is a limitation in animals but still gives important information to support the clinical findings and provides complementary information to that acquired from motor nerve conduction studies (see 'Section 4 – Appendicular motor nerve conduction studies'). Another consideration is that EMG recordings only correspond to the assessment of the function of the muscle and peripheral motor axons. Therefore, diseases causing lesions to other nerve fibres (e.g., sensory or autonomic), pure demyelination without axonal loss, or lesions affecting interstitial tissue within a muscle can escape detection with EMG alone. This all means that whilst an abnormal EMG is highly suggestive of denervation or a primary myopathy, a normal EMG examination does not rule out the possible presence of a neuromuscular disease.

The electrophysiological examination can also give some guidance regarding possible sites for muscle biopsies. The biopsies should ideally be performed in an affected muscle that is not at the end stage of the disease and (assuming the condition is generalised/bilateral/symmetrical) in the contralateral limb to the site that has been evaluated with the EMG.

(i) Motor/sensorimotor neuropathies

a. Acute neuropathy with axonal loss

In cases of acute axonal loss, Wallerian degeneration distal to the site of injury occurs within ~5 to 8 days. This is followed by denervation of the muscle(s) innervated by the affected motor unit distal to the lesion and subsequent detection of abnormal spontaneous electrical activity (e.g., fibrillation potentials, positive sharp waves). Consequently, the clinical signs of muscle weakness can be readily visible but if the electromyography is performed in the acute phase (<4-5 days) there may be no abnormal spontaneous electrical activity in the distal muscles tested (Cuddon, 2002; Kimura, 2013; Shapiro and Preston, 2013).

b. Chronic neuropathy with axonal loss

After the acute phase, there will be abnormal spontaneous electrical activity in the muscles distal to the affected nerve(s). The insertional activity is often increased but can be decreased in very chronic cases due to fibrous replacement. Fibrillation potentials and positive sharp waves are often noted, along with complex repetitive discharges in more chronic cases. The distribution of the abnormal spontaneous electrical activity indicates the 'neuroanatomic localisation' of the lesion(s) and a map of the affected nerves can be inferred from the muscles affected. The main limitation to precisely localising the site of a focal axonal injury is that many nerves travel a long distance before branching off to innervate a particular muscle. If only some fascicles of the nerve are affected, then some muscles distal to the lesion may still have a normal EMG examination (Cuddon, 2002; Kimura, 2013; Shapiro and Preston, 2013).

c. Purely demyelinating neuropathy, acute or chronic

There are usually no abnormalities found on EMG in cases with a purely demyelinating neuropathy without concurrent axonal loss (Shapiro and Preston, 2013). This is because the axon terminal remains intact at the motor end-plate and there is no stimulus for increased recruitment of nicotinic acetylcholine receptors by the muscle membrane. Affected animals can show significant weakness in spite of this, but motor nerve conduction velocities would be typically reduced (see 'Section 4 – Appendicular motor nerve conduction studies'). The EMG will also be normal in pure sensory neuropathies, with no involvement of the motor fibres to the muscles being tested.

d. Peripheral nerve hyperexcitability

Peripheral nerve hyperexcitability can result in fasciculations, myokymia, neuromyotonia, cramps and tetany, with generalised myokymia and neuromyotonia most commonly observed. This has been predominantly described in Jack Russell Terriers (Vanhaesebrouck *et al.,* 2010b), but has also been reported in other breeds (Van Ham *et al.*, 2004; Vanhaesebrouck *et al.,* 2011), and is frequently associated with hereditary spinocerebellar ataxia. Focal myokymia/neuromyotonia of the head has also been rarely described in dogs with structural brain lesions, including a puppy with idiopathic inflammatory brain disease (Walmsley *et al.*, 2006), an adult dog with an intracranial meningioma involving the facial nucleus and nerve (Holland *et al.,* 2010), and an adult dog with palatolingual myokymia associated with a pituitary tumour (Vanhaesebrouck *et al.,* 2010a). In these cases, neuromyotonic discharges were reported based on their high intra-burst frequency (150–300Hz).

(ii) Myopathies

It is important to note that EMG can be normal in some myopathies, with only minimal EMG changes found in others. However, electromyographic abnormalities are frequently encountered in the more common myopathies, including:

- Fibrillation potentials and positive sharp waves in cases with muscle inflammation or necrosis (e.g., polymyositis, muscular dystrophy, etc.);
- Myotonic discharges in case of myotonia congenita, myotonic muscular dystrophy and muscle channelopathies (e.g., paramyotonia congenita, hyperkalaemic periodic paralysis).

(iii) Junctionopathies

Most junctionopathies are associated with a normal EMG because the peripheral motor nerves and muscle fibres are unaffected. However, in cases of botulism, the EMG may show some spontaneous electrical activity around 2 weeks after the onset of clinical signs (van Nes and van der Most van Spij, 1986). Spontaneous electrical activity can also be seen in cases with *myasthenia gravis* and concurrent polymyositis (Shapiro and Preston, 2013; Mayousse *et al.*, 2017).

(iv) Orthostatic tremors

Orthostatic tremor is usually diagnosed in young large and giant breed dogs (e.g., Great Danes), or later in life in retriever breeds (Liatis *et al.,* 2022). It is characterised clinically by high frequency limb tremors while standing, that disappear when the animal is non-weight-bearing (Benito-León and Domingo-Santos, 2016). The diagnosis of this condition can be confirmed by awake electromyography using surface electrodes, which reveals recurrent motor unit action potentials of 13-18Hz and a distinctive 'helicopter' sound (**Figure 3.20**) (Liatis *et al.,* 2022).

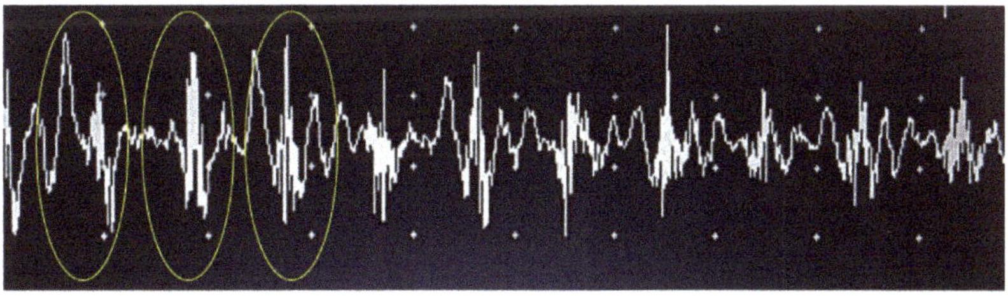

Figure 3.20. Surface EMG recordings in a standing 5-month-old Great Dane with primary orthostatic tremors, showing a high frequency of motor unit action potentials (yellow circles). Horizontal scale = 75ms/division (duration of the whole recording is 750ms, i.e. 0.75 s, hence frequency is 10/0.75=13.3Hz); vertical scale = 200μV/division.

References

Benito-León J, Domingo-Santos Á. Orthostatic Tremor: An Update on a Rare Entity. Tremor Other Hyperkinet Mov (N Y). 2016 Sep 22;6:411. doi: 10.7916/D81N81BT. PMID: 27713855; PMCID: PMC5039949.

Cuddon PA. Electrophysiology in neuromuscular disease. Vet Clin North Am Small Anim Pract. 2002 Jan;32(1):31-62. doi: 10.1016/s0195-5616(03)00079-2. PMID: 11785734.

Daube JR, Rubin DI. Needle electromyography. Muscle Nerve. 2009 Feb;39(2):244-70. doi: 10.1002/mus.21180. PMID: 19145648.

De Risio L, Zavattiero S, Venzi C, Del Bue M, Poncelet L. Focal canine tetanus: diagnostic value of electromyography. J Small Anim Pract. 2006 May;47(5):278-80. doi: 10.1111/j.1748-5827.2006.00046.x. PMID: 16674723.

Evans HE and de Lahunta A. Miller's Anatomy of the Dog – 4th Edition. Saunders/Elsevier, St. Louis, Missouri, USA, 2013.

Falck B, Alaranta H. Fibrillation potentials, positive sharp waves and fasciculation in the intrinsic muscles of the foot in healthy subjects. J Neurol Neurosurg Psychiatry. 1983 Jul;46(7):681-3. doi: 10.1136/jnnp.46.7.681. PMID: 6886709; PMCID: PMC1027494.

Gagliardo T, Ruggeri R, Di Paola A, Baroni M, Cherubini GB, Gallucci A, Falzone C, Trimboli S, Albul A, Gandini G. Clinical features of muscle cramp in 14 dogs. J Vet Intern Med. 2021 Jan;35(1):372-377. doi: 10.1111/jvim.15965. Epub 2020 Nov 28. PMID: 33247617; PMCID: PMC7848340.

Holland CT, Holland JT, Rozmanec M. Unilateral facial myokymia in a dog with an intracranial meningioma. Aust Vet J. 2010 Sep;88(9):357-61. doi: 10.1111/j.1751-0813.2010.00598.x. PMID: 20726972.

Kimura J. Electrodiagnosis in Diseases of Nerve and Muscle: Principles and Practice – 4th ed. Oxford University Press, 2013.

Liatis T, Gutierrez-Quintana R, Mari L, Czopowicz M, Polidoro D, Bhatti SFM, Cozzi F, Tirrito F, Brocal J, José-López R, Kaczmarska A, Cappello R, Harris G, Alves L, Rusbridge C, Rossmeisl JH. Primary orthostatic tremor and orthostatic tremor-plus in dogs: 60 cases (2003-2020). J Vet Intern Med. 2022 Jan;36(1):179-189. doi: 10.1111/jvim.16328. Epub 2021 Dec 12. PMID: 34897811; PMCID: PMC8783359.

Lowrie M, Garosi L. Classification of involuntary movements in dogs: Tremors and twitches. Vet J. 2016 Aug;214:109-16. doi: 10.1016/j.tvjl.2016.05.011. Epub 2016 May 19. PMID: 27387736.

Mayousse V, Jeandel A, Blanchard-Gutton N, Escriou C, Gnirs K, Shelton GD, Blot S. Evaluation of coexisting polymyositis in feline myasthenia gravis: A case series. Neuromuscul Disord. 2017 Sep;27(9):804-815. doi: 10.1016/j.nmd.2017.06.006. Epub 2017 Jun 16. PMID: 28687435.

Menkes DL, Pierce R. Needle EMG muscle identification: A systematic approach to needle EMG examination. Clin Neurophysiol Pract. 2019 Oct 21;4:199-211. doi: 10.1016/j.cnp.2019.08.003. PMID: 31886446; PMCID: PMC6921208.

Michell AW. Understanding EMG. Oxford University Press, 2013.

Shapiro BE and Preston DC. Electromyography and Neuromuscular Disorders: Clinical-Electrophysiologic Correlations – 3rd ed. Elsevier Inc, 2013.

Steiss JE, Forsyth G. Effect of electromyography on serum creatine kinase values in clinically normal dogs and horses. Am J Vet Res. 1984 Jun;45(6):1199-200. PMID: 6742582.

Vanhaesebrouck AE, Bhatti SF, Bavegems V, Gielen IM, Van Soens I, Vercauteren G, Polis I, Van Ham LM. Inspiratory stridor secondary to palatolingual myokymia in a Maltese dog. J Small Anim Pract. 2010 Mar;51(3):173-5. doi: 10.1111/j.1748-5827.2009.00865.x. Epub 2010 Jan 11. PMID: 20070491.

Vanhaesebrouck AE, Van Soens I, Poncelet L, Duchateau L, Bhatti S, Polis I, Diels S, Van Ham L. Clinical and electrophysiological characterization of myokymia and neuromyotonia in Jack Russell Terriers. J Vet Intern Med. 2010 Jul-Aug;24(4):882-9. doi: 10.1111/j.1939-1676.2010.0525.x. Epub 2010 May 11. PMID: 20492485.

Vanhaesebrouck AE, Bhatti SF, Polis IE, Plessas IN, Van Ham LM. Neuromyotonia in a dachshund with clinical and electrophysiological signs of spinocerebellar ataxia. J Small Anim Pract. 2011 Oct;52(10):547-50. doi: 10.1111/j.1748-5827.2011.01123.x. PMID: 21967102.

Vanhaesebrouck AE, Bhatti SF, Franklin RJ, Van Ham L. Myokymia and neuromyotonia in veterinary medicine: a comparison with peripheral nerve hyperexcitability syndrome in humans. Vet J. 2013 Aug;197(2):153-62. doi: 10.1016/j.tvjl.2013.03.002. Epub 2013 Apr 11. PMID: 23583699.

Van Ham L, Bhatti S, Polis I, Fatzer R, Braund K, Thoonen H. 'Continuous muscle fibre activity' in six dogs with episodic myokymia, stiffness and collapse. Vet Rec. 2004 Dec 11;155(24):769-74. PMID: 15638001.

van Nes JJ, van der Most van Spijk D. Electrophysiological evidence of peripheral nerve dysfunction in six dogs with botulism type C. Res Vet Sci. 1986 May;40(3):372-6. PMID: 3016850.

van Nes JJ. Clinical application of neuromuscular electrophysiology in the dog: a review. Vet Q. 1986 Jul;8(3):240-50. doi: 10.1080/01652176.1986.9694048. PMID: 3018992.

Walmsley GL, Smith PM, Herrtage ME, Jeffery ND. Facial myokymia in a puppy. Vet Rec. 2006 Mar 25;158(12):411-2. doi: 10.1136/vr.158.12.411. PMID: 16565340.

SECTION 4

Appendicular motor nerve conduction studies

Hélène Vandenberghe, Edward Ives, Nicolas Granger

Key points

- Motor nerve conduction studies involve the supramaximal stimulation of a motor nerve and recording of a compound muscle action potential (CMAP or M-wave), which is the summation of many muscle fibre action potentials.
- In practice, these studies provide information regarding fast-conducting, large-diameter axons. Therefore, small-diameter axons, which make up to majority of fibres in a peripheral nerve, are not assessed by routine nerve conduction studies.
- Motor nerve conduction studies allow assessment of the amplitude and area of the CMAP (reflecting the number of axons and functional myofibres) and calculation of the motor nerve conduction velocity (reflecting predominantly myelination).
- Following proximal nerve stimulation, the amplitude of the CMAP is of slightly lower amplitude and slightly longer duration than following distal nerve stimulation. This is called physiologic temporal dispersion.

- A conduction block happens when there is a dysfunction of the myelin preventing propagation of the action potential. This leads to a decrease in the amplitude of the proximal CMAP of more than 50 percent in comparison with the distal CMAP, without temporal dispersion.
- Demyelination can cause temporal dispersion and/or conduction block, with both reducing the amplitude of the CMAP. In the case of temporal dispersion, the duration of the CMAP also increases.
- Causes of a low amplitude CMAP include motor axonal loss, conduction block, temporal dispersion, abnormal neuromuscular transmission, and myopathies. A decrease in CMAP amplitude without temporal dispersion is consistent with an axonal disease, a severe myopathy or an abnormal neuromuscular transmission (e.g., botulism).
- Slowing of nerve conduction is predominantly caused by demyelination. However, conduction velocity may also decrease by up to 30 percent because of severe axonal loss without demyelination. A conduction slowing of more than 30 percent implies demyelination.
- In case of a nerve injury, electrophysiology performed in the first 7 to 10 days (before Wallerian degeneration of the distal axon) doesn't accurately assess the severity of nerve damage.

Introduction

Appendicular motor nerve conduction studies involve electrical stimulation of peripheral nerve motor fibres and recording of a compound muscle action potential (CMAP or M-wave) from the muscle(s) supplied by that nerve. It is a test that is frequently performed following electromyography (EMG), as the results are complementary, help to differentiate a myopathy from a motor neuropathy (or junctionopathy) and allow further refinement of the origin of the disease.

1. Technique

(i) Stimulation

Stimulating a nerve requires two monopolar needle electrodes (bipolar montage). In companion animals, nerve stimulation is performed using needle electrodes under general anaesthesia rather than the cutaneous surface electrodes that are frequently used in humans. Needle electrodes are more invasive but, as they can be inserted close to the nerve, they allow the use of a much lower intensity of stimulation (a few volts).

During stimulation, negative charges accumulate under the cathode (negative/active electrode connected to the black port of the stimulator) making the intra-axonal charge relatively more positive, which leads to depolarisation. The current flows from the cathode to the anode electrode (connected to the red port of the stimulator) where the nerve is hyperpolarised, leading to 'anodal conduction block' (local block of nerve conduction) at that level (Kimura, 2013).

For motor nerve conduction studies, the nerve should be stimulated in at least two sites; a proximal and a distal stimulation site, separated ideally by at least 10 centimetres (cm). This allows an accurate measurement of the motor nerve conduction velocity between these two sites without needing to take the time for transmission of the impulse via the neuromuscular junction into account (see later). The difference in latency between the two stimulation sites therefore represents the conduction time for the fastest conducting nerve fibres between those sites as other factors, such as neuromuscular transmission and muscle activation, are common to both stimulation sites (Cuddon, 2002).

For each stimulation site, the two stimulating electrodes should be placed 2-3cm apart, with the active electrode (cathode) as close to the nerve as possible. The active electrode should also be positioned distally and closest to the recording site (i.e., below the anode and closest to the muscle of interest for a motor nerve conduction study). This is to avoid blockage of impulse conduction at the level of the anode (where the nerve is hyperpolarised) as may occur if the anode were positioned between the cathode and recording site (Cuddon, 2002; Kimura, 2013).

Electrophysiology units allow the clinician to choose either a 'constant voltage' stimulation (in volts [V]) or a 'constant current' (in amperes [A]) (Kimura, 2013). This difference is important as:

- A 'constant voltage' stimulation delivers a chosen (adjustable) voltage across the stimulating electrodes, independent of the stimulus current. The impedance varies with the stimulation site (under the needle electrode and within the extracellular fluids in contact with the needles), and therefore the current delivered will vary with that impedance;
- A 'constant current' stimulation delivers an adjustable current through the stimulating electrodes, independently from the impedance under the needles. In this scenario, the voltage dynamically adjusts to maintain a constant stimulating current.

The 'constant current' provides a more consistent stimulus control and is preferable for studies involving trains of stimuli or averaging. It is therefore, in general, the set-up chosen for companion animals.

Human patients (who undergo nerve stimulation without sedation or anaesthesia) do not tolerate a stimulation longer than 2ms, and a stimulation duration <50μs limits the stimulation effect due to tissue capacitance. Therefore, a stimulation duration between 0.1 and 1-2ms is usually accepted (stimulation rate of 1-2Hz), with an intensity of 10-500V (1-50mA) (**Table 4.1**). This level of stimulation is perfectly safe except when delivered near pacemakers that can be inhibited by such stimulation. In cases with a pacemaker, a ground electrode should be placed between the stimulation site and the pacemaker. In cases with catheters near the heart, such as central venous pressure lines, the current could be directed via the catheter to the heart and make electrical stimulation contra-indicated (in theory this is for catheters that are actually reaching the heart). The bandwidth is similar to EMG, being from 2-10Hz. The sweep speed and amplification can be changed manually during recording.

Stimulation parameters	Value
Duration	0.1-2ms
Rate	1-2Hz
Intensity	10-500V (1-50mA) – supramaximal

Table 4.1. Stimulation parameters for motor nerve conduction studies

The stimulating current is gradually increased from baseline so that more and more nerve action potentials are generated. This in turn means that more muscle fibre action potentials are generated, with the CMAP being the summation of all the individual muscle fibre action potentials. Practically, supramaximal stimulation is achieved when no additional increase in CMAP amplitude is observed with increased stimulation intensity (Michell, 2013). If the intensity is too low, only a proportion of the total number of available/functional nerve fibres will be recruited, creating a small and/or unusually shaped waveform. If the intensity is too high, the current can spread down the axon to depolarise the nerve away from the stimulation point (i.e., closer to the recording site), leading to artefactual shortening of the latency (Kimura, 2013). Therefore ideally, a stimulus intensity that is only slightly higher (supramaximal) than that resulting in the largest CMAP should be used (**Figure 4.1**).

(ii) Recording

In people, surface electrodes are routinely used for recording (Michell, 2013). In dogs and cats, needle electrodes are routinely used but surface electrodes can also be considered (Crespo *et al.*, 2020).

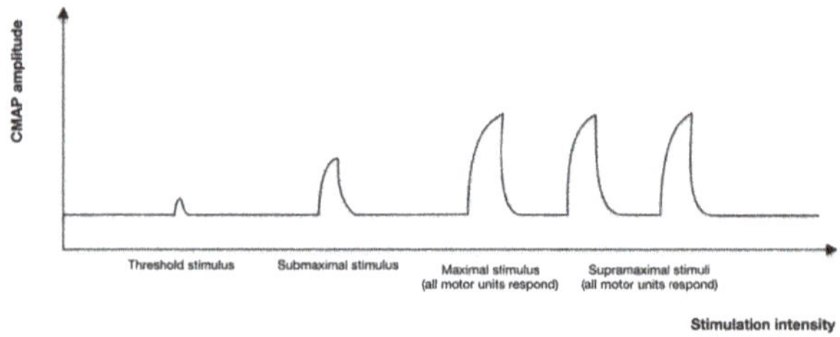

Figure 4.1. Amplitude of the compound muscle action potential with increasing stimulus intensity. The threshold stimulus is the lowest intensity of stimulating current necessary to elicit a compound muscle action potential. With submaximal stimuli, not all the motor units are recruited. Maximal and supramaximal stimulations are reached when an increase in stimulus intensity does not lead to a further increase in CMAP amplitude. *Source: Dr Francesca Samarani.*

The recording electrodes are placed in one of the muscles innervated by the nerve being stimulated, typically as a belly-tendon montage. The active electrode (cathode) is placed within the muscle as close as possible to the muscle belly motor point (see below). The anode electrode is then placed on an electrically inactive site – this can be in the muscle tendon distally, which is electrically silent and close enough to the active electrode to be affected by similar background noise, or subcutaneously 1-2cm from the active electrode (Shapiro and Preston, 2013). It is helpful to remember that the recording and stimulating cathodes end up facing each other, both connected to the black ports of the amplifier and stimulator respectively (**Figure 4.2**).

Figure 4.2. Electrode set up for motor nerve conduction studies. The stimulation site is along the nerve innervating the muscle, with the cathode placed distally and the anode placed proximally. The recording site is in the muscle itself, with the cathode placed in the muscle belly and the anode placed at an electrically inactive site (e.g., in a tendon or subcutaneously).

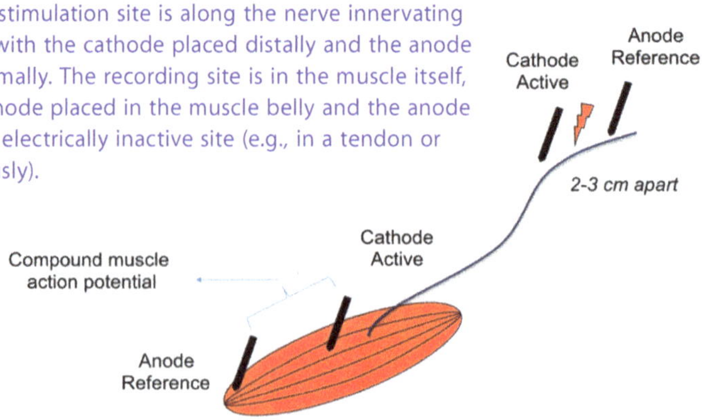

The reference ('ground') electrode is usually placed over a bony prominence between the stimulation and recording sites (e.g., over the stifle or hock for pelvic limb testing, or over the elbow or carpus for the thoracic limb).

Motor responses are in the range of several millivolts and the gain is usually set at 2-5 millivolts per division. The duration of the CMAP is several milliseconds and the sweep speed is usually set to 2-10 milliseconds per division (**Table 4.2**).

Recording parameter	Value
Gain (i.e., amplification, vertical axis)	2-5mV/cm
Sweep speed (horizontal axis)	2-10ms/cm
High frequency filter	10kHz
Low frequency filter	20Hz

Table 4.2. Recording parameters for motor nerve conduction studies.

(iii) Optimisation of recording and stimulation sites

To optimise the recording site, the recording electrode (cathode) is inserted into the body of the muscle and repositioned until the initial deflection of the compound muscle action potential is upward (negative) indicating that the electrode is close to the motor point.

To optimise the stimulation site, one should:

- Place the active electrode as close as possible to where the nerve should run based on anatomical landmarks (see below);
- Gradually increase the intensity of stimulation until a CMAP is obtained;
- Keep a constant stimulation intensity and move the active stimulating electrode until the largest response is observed;
- Then keep the needle in the same place and gradually increase the stimulation intensity to supramaximal (until no further increase in CMAP amplitude);

To optimise the recording site, move the active recording electrode in the muscle belly to achieve the best waveform and largest amplitude (see above).

2. Anatomy for motor nerve conduction studies

(i) Thoracic limb

a. Radial nerve

The motor portion of the radial nerve is derived from the C7, C8 and T1 ventral nerve roots that originate from motor neuron cell bodies in the ventral horn of their respective spinal cord segments. It innervates the *triceps brachii, extensor carpi radialis, ulnaris lateralis, extensor digitorum communis* and *extensor digitorum lateralis* muscles (Evans and de Lahunta, 2012).

The proximal stimulation site is at the level of the brachial plexus, with the stimulating needles being inserted horizontally, medial to the scapula and lateral to the C6 transverse process. The distal stimulation site is located laterally, at the level of the distal third of the humeral diaphysis. The recording site is in the belly of the *extensor carpi radialis* muscle (Walker *et al.*,1979) (**Figure 4.3**).

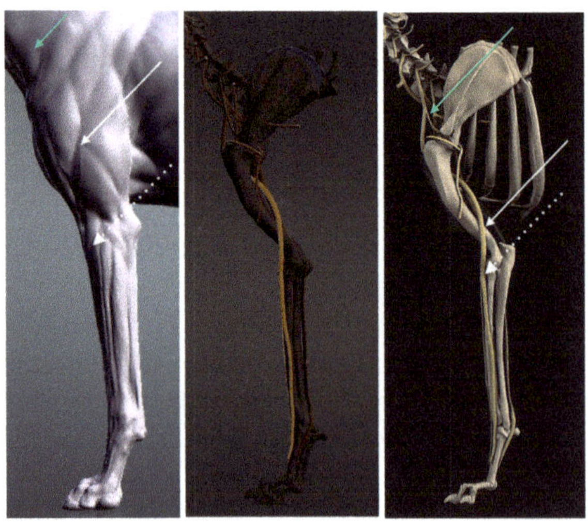

Figure 4.3. Lateral view of the left thoracic limb. Radial nerve stimulation (proximal stimulation site = green plain arrow, distal stimulation site = white plain arrow) and recording in the *extensor carpi radialis* muscle (dotted arrow). *Adapted with permission from Ivalalearn (part of the Veterinary Information Network® family).*

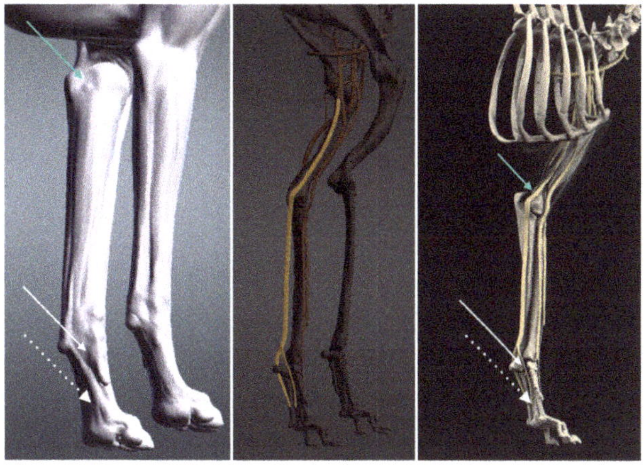

Figure 4.4. Medial view of the left thoracic limb. Ulnar nerve stimulation (proximal stimulation site = green plain arrow, distal stimulation site = white plain arrow) and recording in the *palmar interosseous* muscle (dotted arrow). *Adapted with permission from Ivalalearn (part of the Veterinary Information Network® family).*

b. Ulnar nerve

The motor portion of the ulnar nerve originates from the C8 and T1 spinal cord segments/ventral nerve roots. It innervates the *flexor carpi ulnaris, flexor digitorum profundus* and *palmar interosseous* muscles (Evans and de Lahunta, 2012).

The proximal stimulation site is at the caudomedial aspect of the elbow joint between the medial epicondyle of the humerus and the olecranon. The distal stimulation site can be medial to the carpal joint or just proximal to the accessory carpal bone, deep to the tendon of *flexor carpi ulnaris*. The recording site is in the *palmar interosseous* muscle (Walker *et al.*, 1979; Nafe and Lee, 1983) (**Figure 4.4**).

c. Median nerve

The motor fibres in the median nerve also originate from the C8 and T1 spinal cord segments/ventral nerve roots. It innervates *flexor carpi radialis* and the *flexor digitorum superficialis* muscles (Evans and de Lahunta, 2012).

The proximal stimulation site is medial to the humerus, halfway along the humeral diaphysis. The distal stimulation site is medial to the elbow joint. The recording site is in the *flexor carpi radialis* muscle (Walker *et al.,* 1979) (**Figure 4.5**).

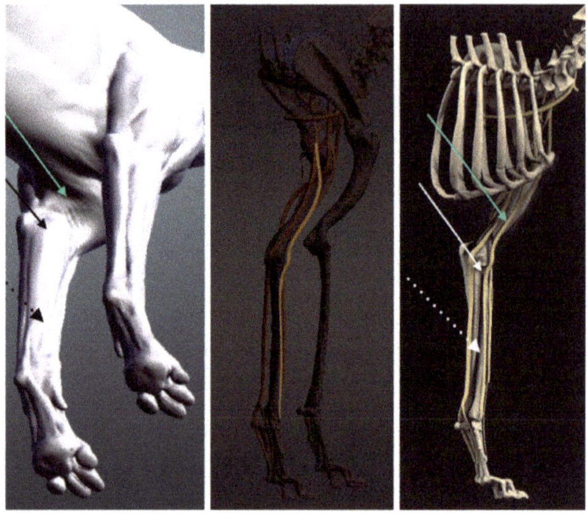

Figure 4.5. Medial view of the left thoracic limb. Median nerve stimulation (proximal stimulation site = green plain arrow, distal stimulation site = black plain arrow [left]/white plain arrow [right]) and recording in the *flexor carpi radialis* muscle (dotted arrows). *Adapted with permission from Ivalalearn (part of the Veterinary Information Network® family).*

(ii) Pelvic limb

a. Sciatic-tibial nerve

The motor portion of the sciatic-tibial nerve originates from the L6 to S1 spinal cord segments/ventral nerve roots. Distally, it innervates the *gastrocnemius, popliteus, flexor digitorum superficialis, flexor digitorum profundus* and *plantar interosseous* muscles (Evans and de Lahunta, 2012).

There are three main stimulation sites for this nerve. The proximal stimulation site is just caudal to the proximal femur between the greater trochanter and the ischiatic tuberosity. The middle stimulation site is midway along the caudal aspect of the femur, although stimulation caudal to the stifle is also possible. The distal stimulation is just above the calcaneal tuberosity of the hock, over the neurovascular bundle between the gastrocnemius tendon and the caudal tibia. Recording is performed in the *plantar interosseous* muscle (Walker *et al.,* 1979; Cuddon, 2002) (**Figure 4.6**).

Direct stimulation of the lumbar spinal nerve roots at L7-S1, with recording in the *gastrocnemius* muscle, has also been described and reference values established (Turan *et al.*, 2014).

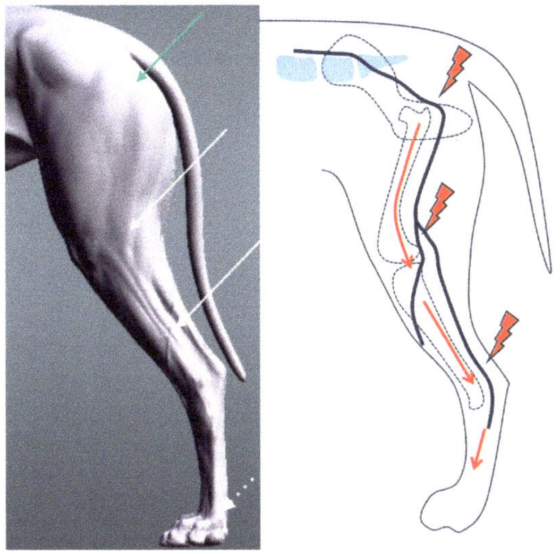

Figure 4.6. Lateral view of the left pelvic limb. Sciatic-tibial nerve stimulation (proximal stimulation site = green plain arrow, middle and distal stimulation sites = white plain arrows), with recording in the *plantar interosseous muscle* (dotted arrow). *Adapted with permission from Ivalalearn (part of the Veterinary Information Network® family).*

b. Sciatic-peroneal nerve

The motor portion of the sciatic-peroneal nerve also originates from the L6 to S1 spinal cord segments/ventral nerve roots. It innervates the *extensor digitorum lateralis, extensor digitorum longus* and *tibialis cranialis* muscles (Evans and de Lahunta, 2012).

The proximal stimulation site is the same as for the sciatic-tibial nerve, as this involves the common trunk of the sciatic nerve before the tibial and peroneal branches divide. The distal stimulation site is lateral to the stifle. Recording is from the *tibialis cranialis* muscle (Walker *et al.*, 1979) (**Figure 4.7**).

c. Femoral nerve

The motor portion of the femoral nerve originates from the L4 to L6 spinal cord segments/ventral nerve roots. It innervates the *iliopsoas, sartorius* and *quadratus femoris* muscles (Evans and de Lahunta, 2012).

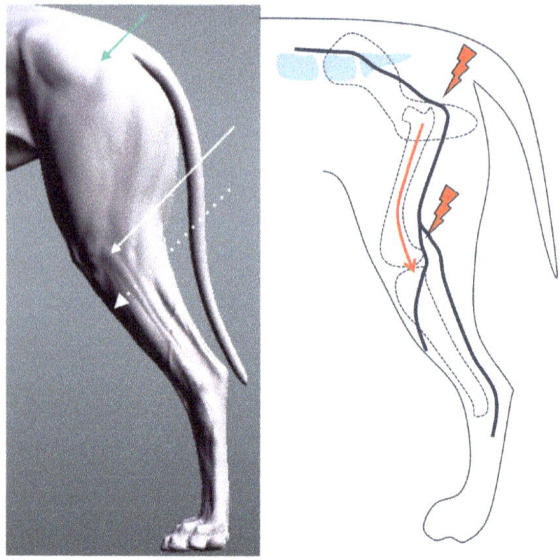

Figure 4.7. Lateral view of the left pelvic limb. Sciatic-peroneal nerve stimulation (proximal stimulation site = green plain arrow, distal stimulation site = white plain arrow), with recording in the *tibialis cranialis* muscle (dotted arrow). *Adapted with permission from Ivalalearn (part of the Veterinary Information Network® family).*

The proximal stimulation site is the 5th lumbar nerve root at the level of the L5-L6 interarcuate space. Distal stimulation can be performed using surface stimulating electrodes placed just proximal to the femoral artery pulsation on the medial aspect of the pelvic limb in the inguinal region. Recording is from the *sartorius* muscle (Ünsal *et al.*, 2017).

d. Obturator nerve

The obturator nerve also originates from the L4 to L6 spinal cord segments. It innervates the *obturatorius externus, pectineus, adductor magnus* and *gracilis* muscles (Evans and de Lahunta, 2012).

Proximal stimulation involves the 6th lumbar nerve root at the level of the L6-L7 interarcuate space. Distal stimulation has been reported using bipolar surface stimulating electrodes with the active electrode 1-2cm caudo-lateral to the side of the ventral pubic tubercle and the reference electrode placed cranially. Recording is made from the *gracilis* muscle (Ünsal *et al.*,2017).

3. Interpretation of motor nerve conduction studies

Determining the differences between two sides of the body, or between two nerves in the same limb, serves as the most sensitive means of examining a patient with a unilateral disorder affecting a single nerve.

(i) Compound muscle action potential

a. Characteristics

The recording trace will initially show a stimulation artefact that reflects the electrical impulse used to stimulate the nerve. However, with modern fast-recovering amplifiers, the extent of the stimulation artefact is minimised. If the stimulation artefact is too large, it might be the result of the active and anode electrodes being too close. If this persists, placing the reference ('ground') electrode between the stimulating and recording electrodes can also be tried.

The compound muscle action potential will follow the stimulation artefact at a variable latency dependent on the nerve conduction velocity and distance between stimulating and recording electrodes. It is a biphasic potential with an initial negativity (upward deflection) from the baseline if the active recording electrode is at the level of the muscle motor point; if not, a small positive deflection is seen first. If the active recording electrode is far away from the motor point, the waveform can have a reduced amplitude as it may pick-up positivity from one part of the muscle and negativity from another part leading to phase cancellation. Alternatively, signal from other muscles can be picked up and modify the typical CMAP morphology for that given muscle.

The morphology and duration of the CMAP is both nerve and muscle dependent. However, the shape of a CMAP for a given nerve largely depends on the composition of the nerve (i.e., the proportion of large and small diameter axons), and can be directly compared to the axon-diameter frequency histogram. Such histograms plot the number of axons against the spectrum of their diameters (**Figure 4.8**). At the level of the whole peripheral nerve, or fascicles within a nerve, those with more axons will generate larger currents but also have smaller total resistance due to their larger size. Therefore, there may be little difference in amplitude between a large fascicle and a small peripheral nerve.

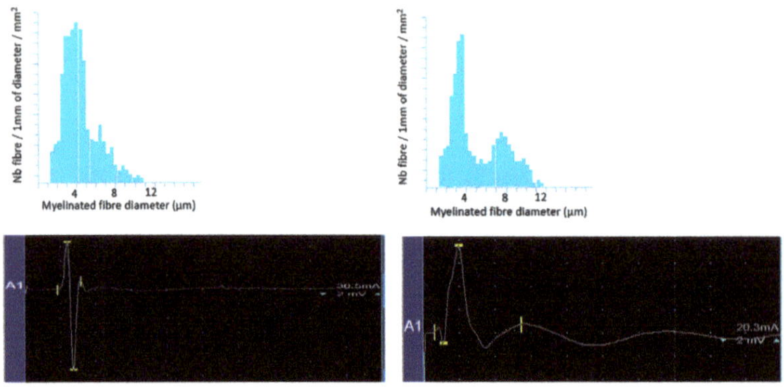

Figure 4.8. Influence of the composition of a motor nerve on the shape of the compound muscle action potential. A. Upper part: morphometry of the sciatic-tibial nerve. Vertical axis: number of fibres/mm of diameter/mm^2, horizontal axis: myelinated fibre diameter (µm). Lower part: shape of the compound muscle action potential obtained following stimulation of the sciatic-tibial nerve. B. Upper part: morphometry of the sciatic-peroneal nerve. Vertical axis: number of fibres/mm of diameter/mm^2, horizontal axis: myelinated fibre diameter (µm). Lower part: shape of the compound muscle action potential obtained following stimulation of the sciatic-peroneal nerve.

The limitations of basic motor nerve conduction studies and what the results mean in terms of which axons they assess should also be considered. Small, myelinated fibres (e.g., Aδ and β fibres) and unmyelinated fibres carry afferent and efferent autonomic information, somatic pain and temperature sensation. Because of their slow conduction velocities, the currents from these fibres are not appreciated with standard nerve conduction studies. Therefore, neuropathies involving only small/unmyelinated fibres may have a normal motor nerve conduction study. Sensory conduction studies (see 'Section 7 – Appendicular sensory nerve conduction studies') record current from nerve fibres innervating the skin and, more specifically, the largest and fastest Aβ fibres. Currents from Ia fibres are not recorded during routine motor or sensory nerve conduction studies. These fibres are afferents from the muscle spindles and mediate the afferent arc of the stretch reflex. They are only recorded during mixed nerve conduction studies because the entire mixed nerve is stimulated. As a consequence, the waveforms recorded via mixed nerve conduction velocities are faster than those recorded during routine motor or sensory nerve conduction studies.

b. Analysis

For each CMAP recording, the latency, amplitude, area, duration, shape and phases can be recorded, calculated and analysed.

• Latency

The latency of a CMAP is the time elapsed between the stimulation artefact and the onset of the waveform (**Figure 4.9**). It represents several consecutive phenomena: the nerve activation (from application of the stimulus to generation of an action potential), the conduction time from the stimulation site to the neuromuscular junction, the neuromuscular transmission at the level of the neuromuscular junction, and the propagation of the CMAP along the muscle membrane (Kimura, 2013; Shapiro and Preston, 2013). The latency represents conduction along the fastest functional motor fibres distal to the level of stimulation, although the shortest fibres might contribute to the initial deflection (Kimura, 2013; Michell, 2013). Compound muscle action potential latencies are within the milliseconds range.

• Amplitude and area

The CMAP amplitude can be measured either from baseline to the largest negative peak, or from 'peak to peak' (**Figure 4.9**). As a compound potential, the amplitude reflects the total number of muscle fibres that depolarise close to the tip of the recording electrode, and is in the millivolt range (Kimura, 2013; Michell, 2013). Published values are ~15 to 20mV for a normal animal, but this depends on the set-up used: for example, many of the normal values published in dogs have used crocodile clips to obtain recordings, which is different to the subcutaneous needles typically used in modern practice. Ideally, each clinic should define their own normal reference values. If not, it is good practice to test a normal limb (ideally the contralateral limb in cases with unilateral signs) to compare to the findings in an affected limb. However, it is also important to note that there can be considerable variation from one patient to another, influenced by factors such as muscle mass between breeds which leads to variation in waveform amplitude/morphology. This is another reason to use a normal limb as an internal control whenever possible, or to have reference values for each breed to use in animals with generalised signs.

The CMAP amplitude is proportional to the number of functional axons and to the number of activated and functional myofibres.

The CMAP area is the area under the curve between the baseline and the negative +/- positive peak(s) and is calculated by the EMG machine. In cases with dispersed waveforms (e.g., longer duration), it is a more consistent estimate of the number of activated myofibres than amplitude alone.

Differential diagnoses for low CMAP amplitudes/areas include axonal neuropathies, demyelinating polyneuropathies with conduction block between the stimulating and recording sites (see below), and certain myopathies and junctionopathies (Michell, 2013; Shapiro and Preston, 2013). Temporal dispersion, when there is a loss of synchrony of action potentials, also leads to decreased amplitudes; in this case, the CMAP duration is prolonged (Michell, 2013). Further discussion regarding the specific electrophysiologic findings for each of these scenarios can be found later in this chapter.

If there is severe focal demyelination or loss of myelin function between the proximal and distal stimulation sites, a conduction block can sometimes be identified when the CMAP amplitudes/areas for the two sites are compared (**Figure 4.10**). Assuming there is no other nerve pathology, if the nerve is stimulated below the level of the block, the CMAP will have a normal amplitude and shape, with a normal conduction velocity. However, when the nerve is stimulated above the level of the block, the CMAP will have a small amplitude (or is even absent), because the induced action potential fails to propagate through and past the level of the block to reach the recording site. The conduction velocity can also be slow, as those that do propagate past the block take longer to do so. To determine the exact location of a conduction block, the proximal site of stimulation can be moved distally; the conduction block will be located just proximal to the stimulating electrode (cathode) at the point at which the CMAP returns to normal. This process may be difficult unless the nerve is superficially located and has a well-defined course.

A 'pseudo-conduction block' can be seen when the nerve conduction study is performed across the lesion in the acute phase of an axonopathy (before Wallerian degeneration occurs). In this scenario, the conduction block will disappear after Wallerian degeneration occurs.

As mentioned above, there is a relatively wide range of normal amplitudes in dogs and cats. Therefore, comparing the CMAP amplitude between the normal side and the affected side is the more precise way to detect abnormalities in dogs without symmetric/generalised signs.

- Duration

The duration of the CMAP is the time elapsed from onset of the waveform to the final return to the baseline (**Figure 4.9**). It reflects the timing of arrival of action potentials down different nerve fibres at the level of the muscle, and therefore the synchronicity of firing of the muscle fibres.

The CMAP duration is frequently affected by disorders that result in slowing of some but not all motor fibres (e.g., demyelination). This leads to desynchronisation of the muscle fibre action potentials as some nerve potentials will arrive at the muscle to activate their myofibres before others, prolonging the response after a single stimulation. An increase in the total number of muscle fibres in a motor unit (e.g., reinnervation) can also increase the CMAP duration (Shapiro and Preston, 2013).

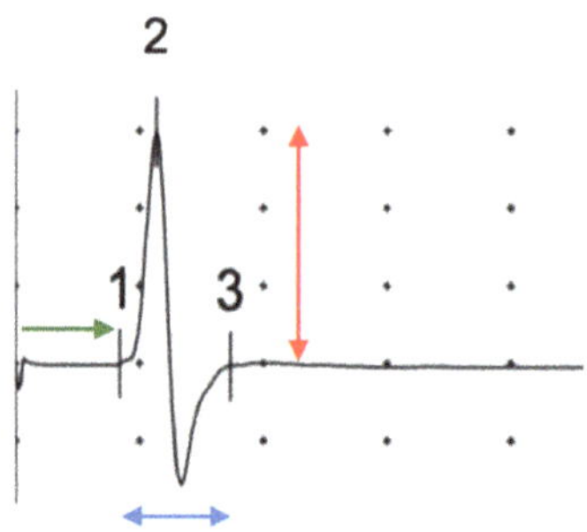

Nerve /	Muscle	Latency ms	Amplitude mV	Amp %	Duration ms
R Tibial - AH					
Ankle	AH	4.22	14.9	100	4.48

Figure 4.9. Compound muscle action potential recorded from the plantar interosseous muscle after distal stimulation of the sciatic-tibial nerve in a normal dog. Horizontal scale = 5ms/division, vertical scale = 5mV/division. Green arrow = CMAP latency. Blue arrow = CMAP duration. Red arrow = CMAP amplitude measured here from baseline to the largest negative peak. These values can be assessed from the graph and are calculated by the electrophysiology software and displayed in a table.

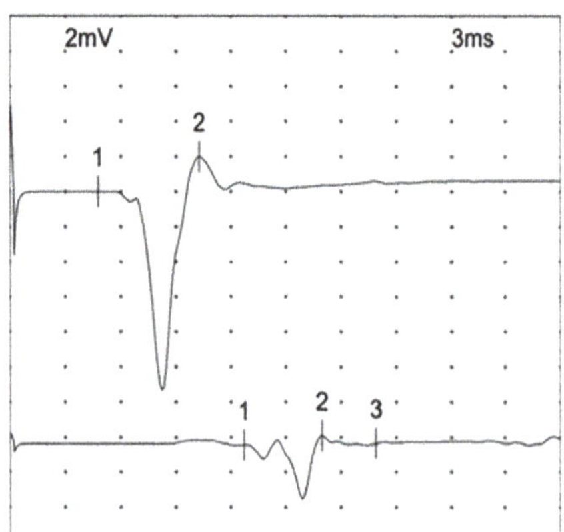

Figure 4.10. Compound muscle action potentials (upper trace: distal stimulation point, lower trace: proximal stimulation point) obtained after stimulation of the ulnar nerve in a dog with a conduction block. The amplitude of the CMAP obtained after proximal stimulation is markedly decreased (less than 50 percent of the CMAP obtained after distal stimulation).

• Shape/phases

The morphology of the CMAP should be the same when comparing the proximal and distal stimulation sites for any given nerve, with only the latency being different (longer for the proximal site). This ensures that the same nerve fibres are tested (same level of myelination) and that comparisons are valid. However, CMAPs generated from proximal stimulation can have a slightly increased duration and lower amplitude. This is because the slower conducting fibres within a nerve will progressively accumulate a lag time as the impulse travels down a longer distance, known as 'physiologic temporal dispersion' (Kimura, 2013).

Polyphasic CMAPs occur when the muscle fibres located close to the tip of the recording needle do not fire in synchrony. As described above for CMAP duration, this means that the stimulated axons are conducting at different speeds (i.e., different degrees of myelination or dysfunction) and impulses arrive to stimulate the muscle at slightly different times (see later in **Figure 4.18**).

(ii) Motor nerve conduction velocity

As described above, the CMAP latency represents the nerve activation time, nerve conduction time between the stimulation site and axonal terminals, the neuromuscular transmission time, and the propagation along the muscle membrane to the recording site. The delay of transmission at the level of the neuromuscular junction and muscle leads to a delay between depolarisation of the distal nerve and recording of the CMAP in the muscle, with the extent of this delay being unknown and imprecise between stimulations (Kimura, 2013).

To overcome this issue and allow recording of an accurate and repeatable conduction velocity, two points of stimulation are used for calculation of the motor nerve conduction velocity (MNCV). The CMAPs produced by proximal and distal stimulation should have similar shapes, but the proximal latency will be longer than the distal latency as there is a longer distance for the action potentials to travel to reach the neuromuscular junction (Shapiro and Preston, 2013). This difference in latency represents the time taken for the action potential to travel from one stimulation site to the other. The influence of the axon terminal conduction time and neuromuscular transmission time are excluded as these are common to both sites (Kimura, 2013). The MNCV along the length of nerve between the stimulation sites can therefore be calculated by dividing the distance between the two stimulation points by the latency difference (**Figures 4.11 and 4.12**). The distance between the stimulation sites is measured using a flexible tape measure and knowledge of the nerve anatomy. Ideally, the two stimulation points should be separated by at least 10 centimetres to increase the accuracy of the conduction velocity measurement.

MNCV (m/s) = distance between stimulation sites (mm)/ (proximal latency [ms] – distal latency [ms]).

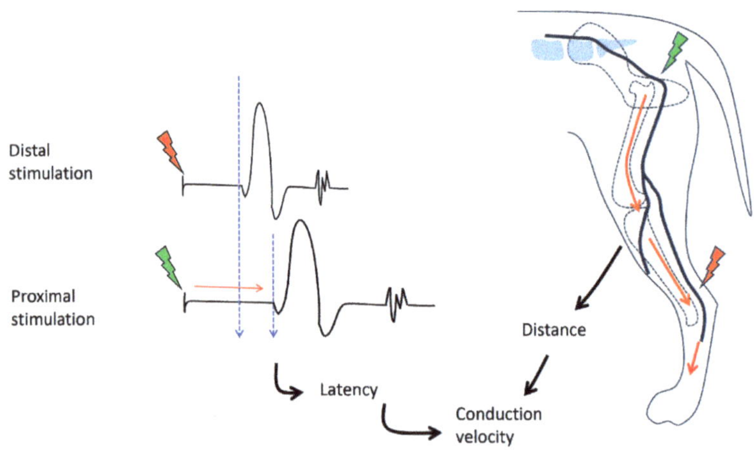

Figure 4.11. Calculation of the motor nerve conduction velocity for the sciatic-tibial nerve. The latencies of the CMAPs following proximal and distal stimulation are recorded by the machine and the difference between latencies is calculated (in milliseconds [ms]). The distance between the proximal and distal active stimulating electrodes (cathodes) is then measured (in millimetres [mm]). The ratio between distance and difference in latencies gives the motor nerve conduction velocity.

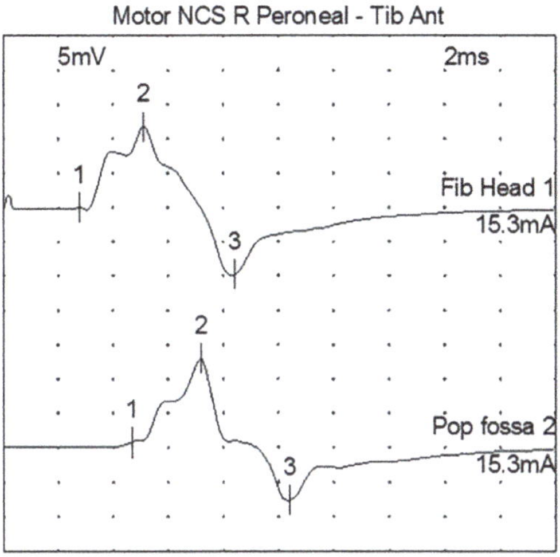

Nerve / Sites	Muscle	Latency ms	Amplitude mV	Amp % %	Duration ms	Segments	Distance cm	Lat Diff ms	Velocity m/s
R Peroneal - Tib Ant									
Fib Head	Tib Ant	2.76	11.8	100	5.68	Fib Head - Tib Ant	15		
Pop fossa	Tib Ant	4.69	12.2	104	5.73	Pop fossa - Fib Head	15	1.93	78

Figure 4.12. Motor nerve conduction velocity for the sciatic-peroneal nerve stimulated at the level of the stifle/fibular head (top) and hip/popliteal fossa (bottom). The latency difference between the proximal and distal stimulation sites (4.69–2.76 = 1.93ms) is calculated by the software. The distance between the proximal and distal stimulation sites (15cm, 150mm) is measured by the operator with a tape measure and entered into the machine, leading to calculation of the motor nerve conduction velocity (78 m/s). Horizontal scale = 2ms/division, vertical scale = 5mV/division.

The MNCV represents the conduction velocity of the fastest conducting motor axons between the proximal and distal stimulation sites (Shapiro and Preston, 2013). Other fibres within the nerve between the stimulation and recording sites will contribute to the CMAP amplitude and area, but are not reflected in the calculated MNCV.

Imprecision in the measurement of conduction velocities can arise from multiple factors:

- Difficulty in determining the onset of the CMAPs – this can be improved by changing the sweep speed of the recording screen during waveform analysis;

- Imprecision of the nerve length measurement, especially when the course of the nerve is not straight;
- Inappropriate stimulus strength (too high) leading to activation of the nerve distal to the measured stimulation point.

Altogether, these errors can lead to variation of +/-10m/s.

Reported motor nerve conduction velocities in dogs and cats are in the region of ~60-70m/s for the sciatic-tibial and ulnar nerves (that are longer with smaller distal axons), and ~70-80m/s for the sciatic-peroneal, radial and median nerves. Normal values for the commonly tested motor nerves can be found in the appendix (Lee and Bowen, 1970; Walker *et al.,* 1979; van Nes, 1986; Steiss and Argue, 1987).

Significantly decreased MNCV usually indicates damage to the myelin, or severe axonal loss leading to loss of large, fastest conducting axons.

(iii) Residual latency

The measured latency following distal stimulation alone ('L_1' in this example) includes the time for neuromuscular transmission and muscle activation. Therefore, without knowing the precise length of these neuromuscular delays, the conduction velocity of the axons along this distal segment cannot be accurately assessed. However, one can estimate the latency within the distal segment of the nerve alone (termed the 'distal latency') by dividing the distance between the distal stimulation site and recording site by the conduction velocity previously obtained for more proximal segments as described above; 'calculated latency', or 'L_2' in this example. This is typically faster than L_1 as it does not take neuromuscular delays into account (**Figure 4.13**). Reference values of the distal latency for the sciatic-tibial nerve in dogs have been published (Schaeppi *et al.*,1982).

Subtracting the calculated latency (L_2) from the measured latency (L_1) provides a measurement called the 'residual latency', which is an estimate of the delays occurring at the level of the nerve terminals and neuromuscular junction (Kimura, 2013). It is also possible to calculate the ratio between the calculated (L_2) and measured (L_1) latencies, which again provides an indication of distal conduction delays.

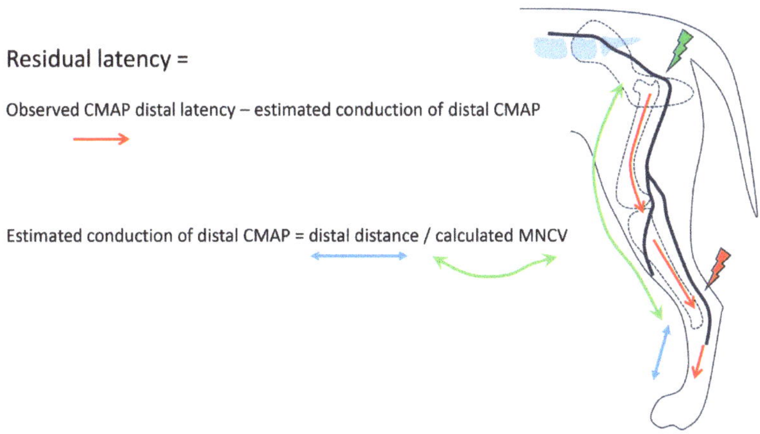

Figure 4.13. Calculation of the residual latency.

(iv) Effect of the age, temperature and size

a. Age

Adult values for MNCV are reached between six months and one year of age. The sharpest increase in MNCV is noted between birth and 2-3 months of age (Swallow and Griffiths, 1977; Sims and Redding, 1980). The MNCV gradually declines from seven years of age in dogs (10 years in cats) and decreases by 10 to 15 percent by 10 years of age. This is also accompanied by a dispersion of the CMAP. Amplitude of the CMAP increases sharply with age, resulting in a final 14- to 18-fold increase by 32 weeks and older (Swallow and Griffiths,1977).

b. Temperature

In dogs, MNCV decreases linearly by 1.7m/s for each degree of temperature drop between 37 and 20 degrees Celsius (Lee and Bowen, 1975). As such, a limb temperature of greater than 36 degrees Celsius should be maintained during testing.

c. Size

Long nerves conduct slightly slower than shorter nerves and the CMAPs will have a decreased amplitude and longer duration due to physiologic temporal dispersion (see above).

4. Patterns of abnormalities

(i) Neuropathies

There are two broad types of pathology that can affect peripheral nerves and lead to the clinical signs and electrophysiologic changes associated with peripheral neuropathies: axonal loss and demyelination. The distinction between the two can be important to guide the diagnosis, prognosis and treatment.

In general, axonal loss results in a decreased amplitude of the CMAP, and demyelination results in a decreased MNCV. However, in nature, the reality can be more complex as:

- Severe axonal loss with loss of the fastest conducting fibres can lead to decreased nerve conduction velocities;
- Demyelination can lead to reduced CMAP amplitudes due to either temporal dispersion and/or conduction block;
- Concurrent axonal loss and demyelination occurs in certain disorders.

a. Axonal neuropathies

In the case of a purely axonal neuropathy, there is a reduction in amplitude and/or area of the CMAP (Cuddon, 2002; Kimura,

2013; Michell, 2013). The conduction velocity of the intact axons remains normal, and the motor nerve conduction velocity often remains within the normal range as long as even a few of the fastest conducting fibres remain functional (**Figure 4.14**). Nerve conduction velocities can be decreased when the largest and fastest axons are lost. In that case, the MNCV will decrease, but typically remains over 70-80 percent of the normal value, which is the MNCV of the slowest conducting axons (Mallik and Weir, 2005). The latencies will be normal or only mildly increased for the same reason.

In practice, a reduction of more than 2/3 of the expected amplitude with normal latency often reflects an axonal neuropathy. However, decreased amplitude of the CMAP can have other causes (e.g., temporal dispersion, conduction block, myopathy, junctionopathy (see later).

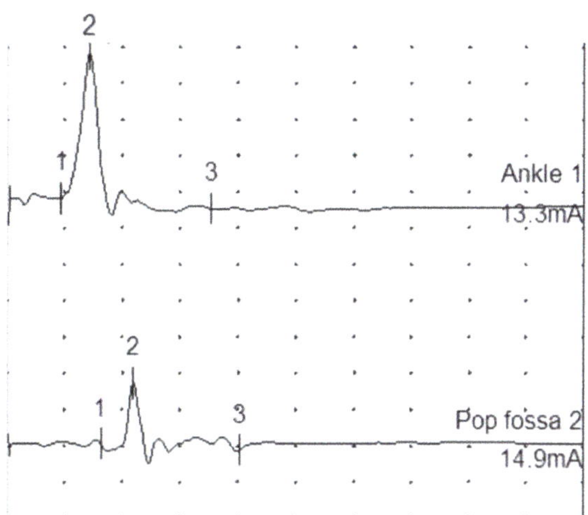

Nerve / Sites	Muscle	Latency ms	Amplitude mV	Amp % %	Duration ms	Segments	Distance cm	Lat Diff ms	Velocity m/s
L Tibial - AH									
Ankle	AH	4.69	2.0	100	12.97	Ankle - AH	16		
Pop fossa	AH	8.13	0.8	42.3	12.03	Pop fossa - Ankle	16	3.44	47

Figure 4.14. Compound muscle action potential recording after distal (top) and proximal (bottom) stimulation of the sciatic-tibial nerve of a cat with an axonal neuropathy. Horizontal scale = 5ms/division, vertical scale = 0.5mV/division. The CMAP amplitudes are markedly decreased (2mV and 0.8mV) following both proximal and distal stimulation, with only mildly reduced motor nerve conduction velocity (47m/s).

Traumatic lesions of the peripheral nerves can be classified using Seddon's scheme dependent on the severity of nerve injury, which has implications for the prognosis and time for recovery (Kamble *et al.*, 2019). Three types of injury are described:

- Neurapraxia, the mildest type of injury, involving no physical disruption of the nerve or perineurium and leading to conduction block but no axonal loss;
- Axonotmesis, where there is a loss of axonal continuity but no disruption of the surrounding connective tissue (endoneurium, perineurium, epineurium);
- Neurotmesis, the most severe type of injury, where the entire nerve and surrounding connective tissues are severed.

Following axonal injury, Wallerian degeneration does not occur immediately. It begins within the 2-3 days following an acute lesion to the nerve and takes 5-10 days to be complete. Therefore, over the first hours and days after injury, the axons distal to the site of injury remain normal before they subsequently undergo gradual degeneration. Consequently, the distal stimulation site for a motor nerve conduction study can be normal if it is performed within the first few days after injury (**Figure 4.15**).

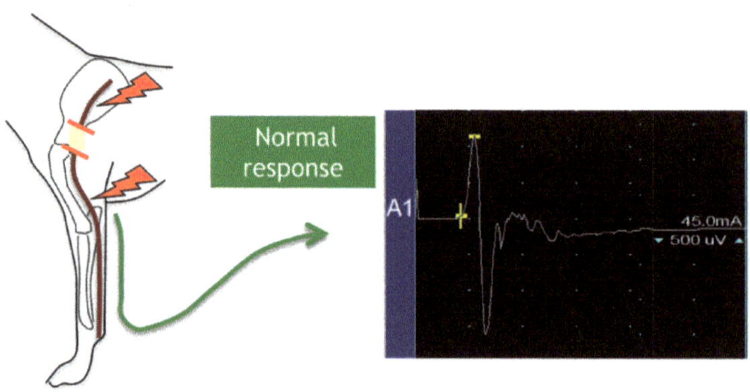

Figure 4.15. Motor nerve conduction study performed immediately following an hyperacute or acute axonal neuropathy (i.e., within 1-2 days). Normal responses are recorded if the nerve is stimulated distal to the site of injury. In contrast, if the nerve was stimulated proximal to the site of injury, the nerve conduction study would immediately be abnormal.

If the nerve is stimulated proximal to the site of injury, the nerve conduction study will be abnormal immediately as the impulse cannot pass through the lesion to reach the muscle where the recording electrodes are placed. The amplitudes of the CMAPs resulting from proximal stimulation will therefore be markedly decreased/absent. A limitation in terms of predicting injury severity and prognosis at that moment in time is that one cannot differentiate a conduction block (where the axon remains intact), from axonal degeneration or axonal transection.

Electrophysiological findings from a few days after the acute injury will then depend on the severity of the injury:

- If the lesion is neurapraxia (conduction block but no axonal loss), distal stimulation will lead to a normal CMAP (no Wallerian degeneration) but stimulation proximal to the site of injury will lead to a CMAP with reduced amplitude because of the conduction block (see previously);
- In case of an axonotmesis, the conduction velocity of any intact axons will remain normal meaning that the MNCV usually remains within the normal range. As mentioned above, MNCV can be decreased if the largest and fastest axons are lost but not more than approximately 35m/s or more than 70 percent of the normal values. In practice, if the latency is normal but there is a reduction of more than 2/3 of the expected amplitude then this often reflects axonal degeneration associated with axonotmesis (partial injury) (**Figure 4.16**). In this case, both the distal and proximal stimulation sites will show similar reduction in CMAP amplitude.
- In the case of a neurotmesis, once Wallerian degeneration has occurred, both proximal and distal stimulation will lead to an absent CMAP as there is no transmission across the site of injury and complete denervation of the muscle, with no intact axons present distal to the injury (Sims *et al.*, 1979) (**Figure 4.17**).

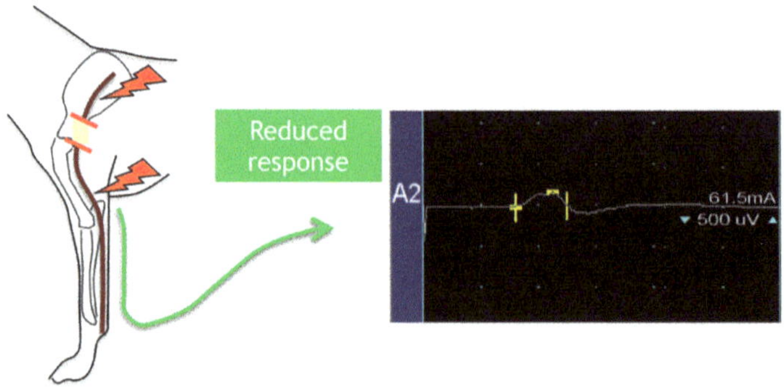

Figure 4.16. Electrophysiological findings in case of an axonotmesis. Reduced CMAP amplitude following proximal and distal stimulation, due to axonal loss and Wallerian degeneration over the first 5-10 days following injury.

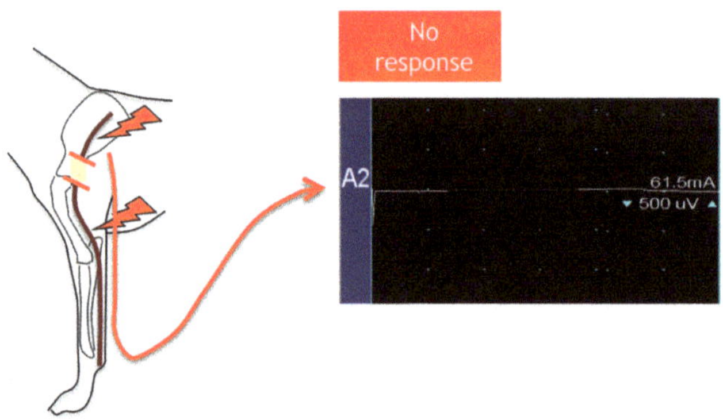

Figure 4.17. Electrophysiological findings in case of a neurotmesis. Proximal and distal stimulation with recording distal to the injury gives no recording.

b. Demyelinating neuropathies

In case of a demyelinating neuropathy, the MNCV is often markedly decreased (to less than 70 percent of the lower reference limit) because the saltatory conduction of the nerve action potential is impaired. A conduction velocity below 70% of the normal value, with a CMAP amplitude of more than 80% of the normal value, is highly suggestive of demyelination in the absence of significant axonal loss (Kimura, 2013).

When demyelination is homogeneous between nerves and between different axons within a nerve, the MNCV is reduced but the nerve potentials in different axons remain synchronised, meaning that there is no temporal dispersion. As a consequence, the morphology of the CMAP remains normal (Shapiro and Preston, 2013).

However, if the demyelinating disease is not homogeneous between axons, there will be heterogeneity of nerve conduction velocities within the nerve following a single stimulation and individual action potentials will reach the recording electrodes at different times. As a consequence, the CMAP will be prolonged and polyphasic (temporal dispersion). There could also be some phase cancellation between individual axons and peaks of opposite polarity, leading to a decreased CMAP amplitude (Shapiro and Preston, 2013) (**Figure 4.18**).

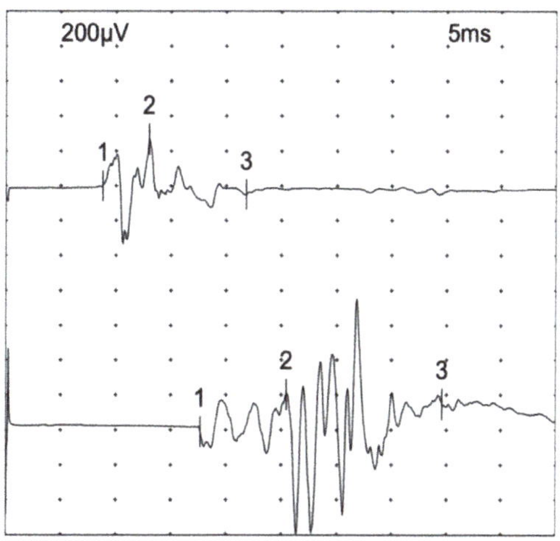

Nerve / Sites	Muscle	Latency ms	Amplitude mV	Amp % %	Duration ms	Segments	Distance cm	Lat Diff ms	Velocity m/s
R Tibial - AH									
Ankle	AH	9.22	6.0	100	35.89	Ankle - AH	8		
Pop fossa	AH	15.10	5.7	94.6	10.36	Pop fossa - Ankle	22	5.89	37

Figure 4.18. Demyelinating polyneuropathy in a 9-year-old Springer Spaniel. Compound muscle action potentials obtained following stimulation of the sciatic-tibial nerve with recording in the plantar interosseous muscle. The motor nerve conduction velocity is reduced (37m/s). The demyelination is not homogeneous in this dog; the CMAPs are polyphasic with a prolonged duration (temporal dispersion), and their amplitudes are reduced.

In case of severe focal demyelination, a conduction block can be identified if the nerve conduction study is performed across the lesion (proximal stimulation point above the lesion and distal stimulation point below the lesion). As described previously, this is accompanied by a marked reduction of either the amplitude or area of the proximal CMAP when compared to the distal CMAP (**Figure 4.10**). When the nerve is stimulated below the block, the CMAP is of normal amplitude and shape, with a normal MNCV. When the nerve is stimulated above the block, the CMAP is of small amplitude (or absent) because some action potentials fail to propagate through the block, and the conduction velocity across the block is also reduced. To determine the exact location of the conduction block, the proximal site of stimulation can be moved distally. The conduction block is located just proximal to the stimulating electrode (cathode) at the point at which the CMAP returns to normal. This can be done more easily if the nerve is superficially located and has a well-defined course.

In cases of chronic demyelinating neuropathy, there can also be some axonal loss due to the importance of myelin for axonal protection. This will result in decreased CMAP amplitudes and abnormal spontaneous electrical activities on EMG (**Figure 4.19**).

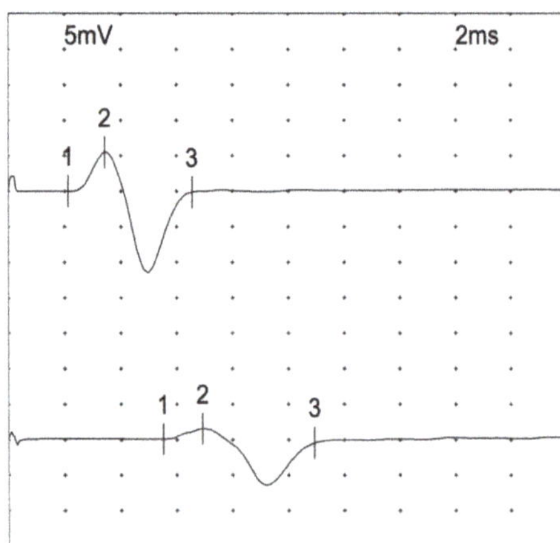

Nerve / Sites	Muscle	Latency	Amplitude	Amp %	Duration	Segments	Distance	Lat Diff	Velocity
		ms	mV	%	ms		cm	ms	m/s
R Ulnar - ADM									
Wrist	ADM	2.14	5.5	100	4.43	Wrist - ADM	7		
B.Elbow	ADM	5.52	1.5	28.9	5.42	B.Elbow - Wrist	15	3.39	44

Figure 4.19. Compound muscle action potentials obtained following stimulation of the ulnar nerve with recording in the palmar interosseous muscle in a 5-year-old dog with a chronic demyelinating polyneuropathy. The motor nerve conduction velocity is reduced (44m/s) and the amplitudes of the CMAPs are also reduced in the absence of significant polyphasia and temporal dispersion (5.5mV and 1.5mV).

(ii) Myopathies

Usually, the diagnosis of myopathy is based on electromyographic abnormalities with a normal motor nerve conduction study, combined with the clinical history, presentation +/- biochemical abnormalities such as increased muscle enzymes. The CMAP amplitudes might be decreased if the muscles where they are recorded (i.e., distal muscles) are involved in the disease and there are fewer functional myofibres to contribute to the compound potential. As the degree of myelination and the axons themselves are normal, the motor nerve conduction velocities are normal, as are sensory nerve studies.

(iii) Junctionopathies

Motor nerve conduction studies (without repetitive stimulation) are generally normal in post-synaptic junctionopathies (e.g., *myasthenia gravis*). However, decreased initial CMAP amplitudes have been recently reported in humans with *myasthenia gravis*, suspected to represented baseline neuromuscular transmission block and stimulation of fewer myofibres to contribute to the potential (Kojima *et al.*, 2022). In case of a pre-synaptic junctionopathy (e.g., botulism), the CMAP amplitude can be decreased as there is reduced release of acetylcholine at the neuromuscular junction which mimics the scenario of axonal loss.

References

Crespo V, Liebel FX, Harcourt-Brown T. Comparison of nerve conduction parameters in canine studies using recording needle and surface electrodes. Vet J. 2020 Oct;264:105534. doi: 10.1016/j.tvjl.2020.105534. Epub 2020 Aug 31. PMID: 33012442.

Cuddon PA. Electrophysiology in neuromuscular disease. Vet Clin North Am Small Anim Pract. 2002 Jan;32(1):31-62. doi: 10.1016/s0195-5616(03)00079-2. PMID: 11785734.

Evans HE and de Lahunta A. Miller's Anatomy of the Dog – 4th Edition. Saunders/Elsevier, St. Louis, Missouri, USA, 2013.

Kamble N, Shukla D, Bhat D. Peripheral Nerve Injuries: Electrophysiology for the Neurosurgeon. Neurol India. 2019 Nov-Dec;67(6):1419-1422. doi: 10.4103/0028-3886.273626. PMID: 31857526.

Kimura J. Electrodiagnosis in Diseases of Nerve and Muscle: Principles and Practice – 4th ed. Oxford University Press, 2013.

Kojima Y, Shibuya K, Uzawa A, Kano H, Nakamura K, Yasuda M, Suzuki Y, Tsuneyama A, Suichi T, Ozawa Y, Misawa S, Noto Y, Mizuno T, Kuwabara S. Decreased initial compound muscle action potential amplitudes in myasthenia gravis. Neurology and Clin Neuroscience. 2022 Sep;10(5):245-251. https://doi.org/10.1111/ncn3.12661

Lee AF, Bowen JM. Evaluation of motor nerve conduction velocity in the dog. Am J Vet Res. 1970 Aug;31(8):1361-6. PMID: 5449896.

Lee AF, Bowen JM. Effect of tissue temperature on ulnar nerve conduction velocity in the dog. Am J Vet Res. 1975 Sep;36(9):1305-7. PMID: 1172401.

Mallik A, Weir AI. Nerve conduction studies: Essentials and pitfalls in practice. J Neurol Neurosurg Psychiatry 2005;76(Suppl II):ii23-ii31. PMID: 15961865.

Michell AW. Understanding EMG. Oxford University Press, 2013.

Nafe LA, Lee AF. Evaluation of evoked-muscle potentials from stimulation of ulnar nerves of the dog. Am J Vet Res. 1983 Apr;44(4):669-73. PMID: 6869963.

Schaeppi U, Teste M, Siegenthaler U. Sensory and motor maximum nerve conduction velocity in the peripheral and central nervous system of the beagle dog. Agents Actions. 1982 Oct;12(4):566-74. doi: 10.1007/BF01965943. PMID: 7180741.

Shapiro BE and Preston DC. Electromyography and Neuromuscular Disorders: Clinical-Electrophysiologic Correlations – 3rd ed. Elsevier Inc, 2013.

Sims MH, Redding RW. Failure of neuromuscular transmission after complete nerve section in the dog. Am J Vet Res. 1979 Jul;40(7):931-5. PMID: 228569.

Sims MH, Redding RW. Maturation of nerve conduction velocity and the evoked muscle potential in the dog. Am J Vet Res. 1980 Aug;41(8):1247-52. PMID: 7447119.

Steiss JE, Argue CK. Normal values for radial, peroneal and tibial motor nerve conduction velocities in adult sheep, with comparison to adult dogs. Vet Res Commun. 1987;11(3):243-52. doi: 10.1007/BF00570922. PMID: 3629945.

Swallow JS, Griffiths IR. Age related changes in the motor nerve conduction velocity in dogs. Res Vet Sci. 1977 Jul;23(1):29-32. PMID: 905650.

Turan E, Unsal C, Oren MU, Dilek OG, Yildirim IG, Sarierler M. Electrical stimulation of lumbar spinal nerve roots in dogs. Vet Res Commun. 2014 Sep;38(3):229-35. doi: 10.1007/s11259-014-9608-z. Epub 2014 Jun 15. PMID: 24930120.

Ünsal C, Turan E, Dilek ÖG, Sabancı SS, Sarıerler M. Evaluation of proximal and distal motor nerve conduction using the electrical root stimulation technique in the femoral and obturator nerves. Vet Comp Orthop Traumatol. 2017 Mar 20;30(2):111-117. doi: 10.3415/VCOT-16-02-0021. Epub 2017 Jan 17. PMID: 28094417.

van Nes JJ. Clinical application of neuromuscular electrophysiology in the dog: a review. Vet Q. 1986 Jul;8(3):240-50. doi: 10.1080/01652176.1986.9694048. PMID: 3018992.

Walker TL, Redding RW, Braund KG. Motor nerve conduction velocity and latency in the dog. Am J Vet Res. 1979 Oct;40(10):1433-9. PMID: 525865.

SECTION 5

The F-wave

Nicolas Granger, Edward Ives, Hélène Vandenberghe

Key points

- The F-wave is a late response that follows the direct motor response (M-wave). It is elicited by supramaximal electrical stimulation of a mixed or a motor nerve and is recorded in a similar way to that used for direct motor responses (M-waves).
- The orthodromic and antidromic volleys of the F-wave travel in motor axons and, therefore, recorded F-waves represent purely motor events.
- Measurement of the F-wave minimal latency allows assessment of the ventral nerve root and the most proximal portion of motor (and mixed) peripheral nerves, and therefore assessment of the motor conduction time along the entire length of the largest and fastest motor fibres.
- F-waves are useful in diagnosis of proximal motor nerve disorders, particularly canine idiopathic polyradiculoneuritis in which the lesions are initially confined to the proximal portions of motor nerves.

1. Definition

When a peripheral nerve is electrically stimulated at any point along its course, there is an orthodromic potential that moves away from the neuronal cell bodies (as also occurs in the natural situation when there is normal firing of a motor neuron). This results in electrical activity in the innervated muscle distal to the point of stimulation in the form of a M-wave (or compound muscle action potential, CMAP), as described previously for motor nerve conduction studies ('Section 4 – Appendicular motor nerve conduction studies'). However, electrical stimulation of the nerve itself also generates an antidromic potential that is not normally present in nature. This potential ascends along the peripheral motor fibres, via the ventral nerve root, to the lower motor neuron cell bodies within the grey matter of the spinal cord. A small proportion (1-5%) of these cell bodies will then backfire, resulting in a subsequent descending potential back down the motor axons. When this potential reaches the muscle, it generates a second, smaller compound muscle action potential (200µV – 1mV) that is recorded with a longer latency compared to the M-wave. This is termed the F-wave, deriving from 'foot wave' in humans (**Figures 5.1 and 5.2**). If the stimulated nerve is a mixed sensorimotor nerve, then the antidromic potential will also travel up the sensory fibres, enter the dorsal sensory root, past the dorsal root ganglion, and into the dorsal horn of the spinal cord. However, this potential will reach the lower motor neuron cell bodies in the ventral horn after the antidromic potential that entered via the ventral root. This means that the earliest F-wave will always originate from the potential that ascends the motor fibres of a mixed peripheral nerve, and that the F-wave is a pure motor event. Unlike the M-wave, which only gives information regarding the portion of the motor nerve distal to the point(s) of stimulation, F-wave studies can provide information on conduction through the ventral roots and proximal part of the motor axons, including the cell bodies of alpha motor neurons (ventral horn cells) (Poncelet and Balligand, 1991).

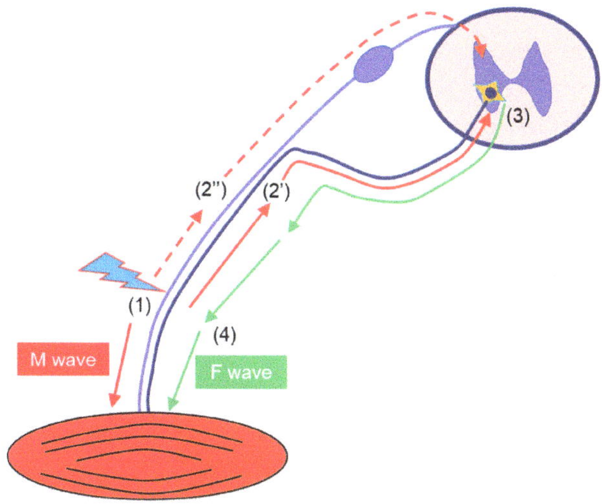

Figure 5.1. F-wave course. Electrical stimulation along a mixed sensorimotor nerve (1) evokes a descending potential creating the M-wave (a muscle contraction) but also an ascending potential along the motor (2′) and sensory (2″) axons; the ascending potential along the motor axons reaches the lower motor neuron cell bodies (3) faster than the ascending potential along the sensory axons. When the potential ascending along the motor axons reaches the lower motor neuron cell bodies, it leads to 'back firing' of the lower motor neurons and a descending, late potential (4; green arrows) recorded after the M-wave, termed the F-wave.

Figure 5.2. M-wave and F-wave recordings following supramaximal stimulation of the ulnar nerve of a normal dog. The M-wave has a shorter latency and larger amplitude (vertical scale = 20mV/division). The F-wave has a longer latency and smaller amplitude (vertical scale = 5mV/division).

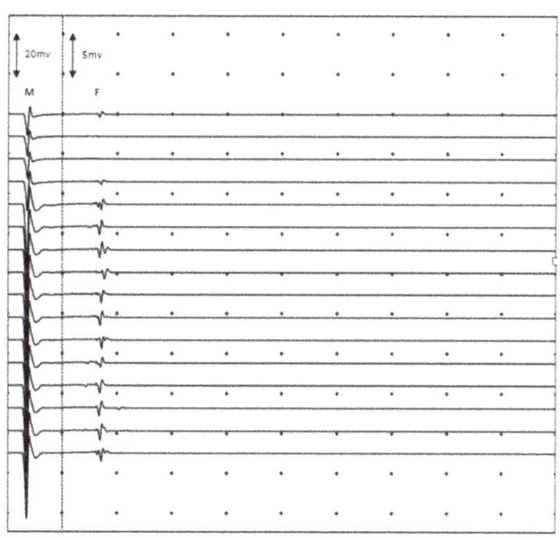

As described above, the electrical activity that initiates the F-wave first travels away from the stimulation site and towards the spinal cord. Therefore, the more proximal the site of nerve stimulation, the earlier the F-wave will be recorded. This is because there will be a shorter distance for the antidromic potential to travel before it reaches the ventral horn motor neurons and stimulates their backfiring. The M-wave, however, will be recorded with a longer latency with proximal stimulation as there is now an increased distance for the orthodromic potential to travel before it reaches the muscle. Therefore, with proximal recordings, the M-wave and the F-wave will become closer together compared to distal recordings (**Figure 5.3**).

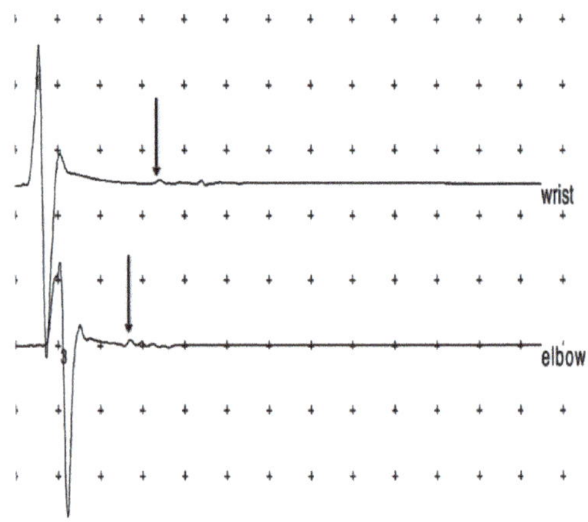

Figure 5.3. F-wave and M-wave recordings following stimulation of the ulnar nerve at the level of the carpus/wrist (distal) and elbow (proximal). The M-wave latency is longer and the F-wave latency (arrow) is shorter following proximal stimulation compared to distal stimulation (horizontal scale = 4ms/division, vertical scale = 4mV/division).

2. Stimulating and recording technique

The stimulating and recording montage for F-waves is the same as for motor nerve conduction studies with supramaximal stimulation, and the same stimulation and recording sites can be used (see 'Section 4 – Appendicular motor nerve conduction studies'). The stimulating cathode electrode remains distal, with the anode being proximal. In theory, this electrode position could block the antidromic impulse (anodal conduction blockade), but in clinical practice anodal hyperpolarisation tends to disappear before the arrival of the antidromic impulse (Knecht *et al.*, 1983).

The F-wave latency will naturally vary between stimulations because different populations of ventral horn cells are activated with each stimulation. Therefore, a series of ~10 to 15 stimulations is used to obtain a good representation of the F-wave latency (Knecht *et al.*, 1983). The authors stimulate at rates less than 0.5Hz (this is usually done manually) to avoid the effects of an earlier stimulus on a subsequent response. This is because the F-wave might fail to cross the axonal hillock if it is still in a depolarised state by the antidromic activation (refractory period of about one second). Concomitant activation of Renshaw cells by the antidromic impulses may also cause transient inhibition of the motor neurons (Knecht *et al.*, 1983). These inhibitory interneurons are the cells that are targeted by the neurotoxin tetanospasmin that is produced following anaerobic infection by the spore-forming bacterium *Clostridium tetani*.

The amplifier display should be set at ~200 µV to 5mV/cm for the amplitude (increase of the gain because the F-wave amplitude is low) and 5 to 10ms/cm for the sweep speed. Most machines can also split the M-wave and F-wave displays so that each part can be set with optimal viewing parameters (displaying the M-wave response and F-wave simultaneously but independently using two optimal gains) (see **Figure 5.2**) (Knecht *et al.*, 1983).

3. Waveform analysis

(i) Latency

The latency of the F-wave is the time elapsed between the stimulus artefact and the onset of the earliest F-wave recorded. It represents the conduction of the impulse via the fastest conducting fibres (as for the M-wave) and is therefore not greatly dependent on the stimulation site (proximal *versus* distal). There is a delay estimated to be ~1ms for central activation of the motor neurons in the spinal cord. The F-wave latency will correlate with the length of the limb/nerve being tested, which can be estimated by the clinician using a tape measure. To account for differences in nerve length between animals of different breeds and sizes, regression equations have been published to calculate the minimum expected F-wave latency.

Steiss (1984) established stimulation techniques needed to produce an F-wave in dogs and reported these linear regression equations to calculate the expected minimum F-wave latencies for the ulnar and sciatic-tibial nerves as follows. These are for formulae that the authors tend to use:

- Sciatic-tibial nerve minimum expected F-wave latency (ms) = 3.45 + (0.33 x pelvic limb length [cm]) where the limb length is measured from the greater trochanter to the tip of the middle toe with the limb in an extended position.
- Ulnar nerve minimum expected F-wave latency (ms) = 6.03 + (0.22 x thoracic limb length [cm]) where the limb length is measured from the cranial angle of the scapula to the tip of the middle toe with the limb in an extended position.

Another regression equation was reported by Okuno *et al.* (2002) for the minimum F-wave latency of the sciatic-tibial nerve in dogs using different distance measurements as follows:

- Sciatic-tibial nerve minimum expected F-wave latency (ms) = 2.799 + (0.029 x length of the tibial nerve [mm]) using a distance measurement from the stimulus point to the cranial border of the spinous process of L5 via the greater trochanter of the femur and the spinous process of L6.

The same group also published a regression equation for the minimum expected F-wave latency of the sciatic-tibial nerve in cats (Okuno *et al.*, 2008):

- F-wave latency (ms) = 2.60 + (0.02 x nerve length [mm]).

Finally, Hirasawa *et al.* (2014) reported a different equation to calculate the expected F-wave latency for the ulnar nerve in dogs:

- Expected F-wave latency (ms) = 2.68 + (0.027 x nerve length [mm]) with the length of the ulnar nerve measured from the cranial angle of the scapula to the acromion of the scapula, then from the acromion of the scapula to the olecranon, and then from the olecranon to the stimulus point.

Further description of how to perform the different measurements of limb length above can be found in the primary sources (see reference list).

(ii) Central latency

The central latency is the conduction time along the proximal portion of the motor nerve between the stimulation site and the spinal cord. It can be calculated by:

- Subtracting the M-wave latency (M) from the F-wave latency (F), and then subtracting an additional 1ms to account for the estimated delay of neuronal backfiring within the spinal cord. This value represents the conduction time in both directions along the proximal segment of the peripheral nerve and ventral nerve roots (**Figure 5.4**).
- This can then be divided by 2 to give the central latency in one direction.

Central latency (ms) = (F – M – 1)/2

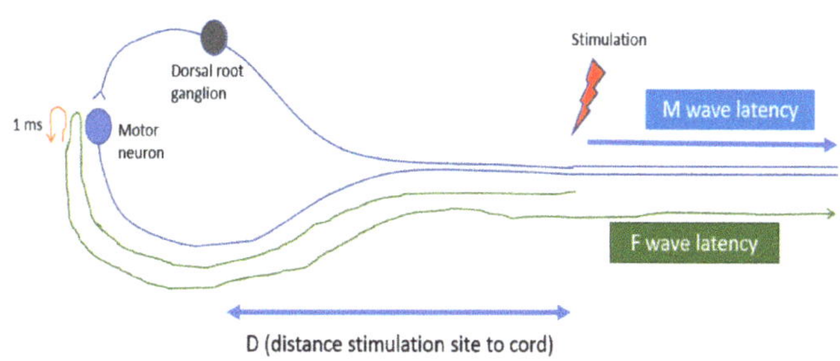

Figure 5.4. Anatomy for calculation of the central latency. This corresponds to the F-wave latency minus the M-wave latency (which represents a common path for both the F-wave and M-wave distal to the stimulation site), minus an additional 1ms to allow for transduction of the signal within the spinal cord and neuronal backfiring. Dividing this value by 2 gives the conduction time in only one direction along segment 'D' (the central latency).

(iii) Conduction velocity

The conduction velocity of the F-wave along the proximal segment (stimulation site to the spinal cord) is calculated by dividing the distance (D) between the stimulation site and the spinal cord (mm) by the central latency (ms).

F-wave conduction velocity (m/s) = D/([F – M – 1]/2)

= 2D/(F – M – 1)

Normal data have been published for the sciatic-tibial and ulnar nerves in dogs:

- Sciatic-tibial nerve mean F-wave conduction velocity = 77.98 +/- 8.62m/s (Okuno *et al.*, 2002).
- Ulnar nerve mean F-wave conduction velocity = 79.4 +/- 5.7m/s (Hirasawa *et al.*, 2014 – using the same measurements for ulnar nerve length as described above for the minimum F-wave latency).

In cats, a value of 97.1 +/- 5.0m/s has been reported for the mean F-wave conduction velocity in the sciatic-tibial nerve (Okuno *et al.*, 2008).

(iv) Chronodispersion

The F-wave chronodispersion is the interval of a few milliseconds between the latencies of the earliest and the latest F-waves. This is a measure of the difference between fast and slow conducting fibres.

(v) Persistence

This is the percentage of trials with detectable F-waves calculated by dividing the number of recorded F-waves by the number of stimuli. It assesses the level of motor neuron excitability and number of functional axons. A normal value is 80-100%, with values of 98.7 +/- 2.3% reported for the tibial nerve in clinically normal cats (Okuno *et al.*, 2008) and 92.5 +/- 9.8% for the ulnar nerve in clinically normal Beagles (Hirasawa *et al.*, 2014).

(vi) F-ratio

The F-ratio compares the conduction time along the proximal segment (from the stimulation site to the spinal cord) to that for the distal nerve segment (between the stimulation site and the muscle). As this is a ratio, it should be independent of limb length if the assumption is true that the relative proportion of the proximal and distal segments is stable for different leg lengths at any given stimulation point. The value can be used to estimate the relative distribution of pathology along the nerve (i.e., whether the proximal or distal parts are more affected, or whether the disease process is evenly distributed along the entire length).

By studying **Figure 5.4** and understanding the anatomic basis of the F-wave, it should be possible to work out that the F-ratio is obtained by dividing the [F-latency *minus* M-latency *minus* 1ms] by [2 times the M-latency]:

$$\textbf{F-ratio} = (F - M - 1)/2M$$

Reference values for the F-ratio have been published for the sciatic-tibial nerve in dogs (Poncelet and Balligand, 1991):

- F-ratio = 1.954 +/- 0.086 when stimulating at the hock;
- F-ratio = 0.883 +/- 0.052 when stimulating at the popliteal fossa.

(vii) Interpretation of F-waves

- Latencies and conduction velocities

As for the M-wave interpretation, if the clinical signs are asymmetric then the normal side can be used as an internal control and compared to the abnormal side whenever possible.

F-waves and M-waves share a common pathway distal to the stimulation site and can therefore be affected concurrently by the same disease. However, F-waves allow the study of a longer segment of nerve than M-waves and provide complementary information. Because abnormalities accumulate in proportion to the nerve length for diffuse/multifocal disease processes, and measurement errors decrease with the length of the segment studied, F-wave latencies are more accurate than M-wave latencies; they have a narrower normal range and can reveal borderline conduction velocity abnormalities in dogs with normal M-waves. For example, if the motor nerve conduction velocity is normally 60m/s, then a 20% reduction in velocity over a 10cm length of nerve would be a difference of only 0.4ms in the onset latency. In comparison, a 20% reduction over a 100cm length of nerve would equate to a delay of 4ms. However, the *minimum* F-wave latency can be normal if just a few of the fastest conducting axons remain unaffected. For this reason, the latency may be normal or only mildly increased in some axonopathies. In contrast, F-wave latencies and conduction velocities may be significantly affected by diseases that cause demyelination (e.g., diabetic neuropathy).

As may be expected, F-waves are also suggested to be more sensitive at assessing disorders involving the proximal segment and ventral motor nerve roots that normal motor nerve conduction studies recording only an M-wave cannot. This is again because they can exaggerate borderline abnormalities that may be observed in the M-wave latencies (e.g., plexopathies, radiculopathies).

• F-ratio

If the motor nerve conduction studies are abnormal (i.e., increased F-wave/M-wave latency), we can draw these assumptions:

- A decreased F-ratio indicates predominant involvement of the distal nerve segment;
- An increased F-ratio indicates predominant involvement of the proximal nerve segment;
- A normal F-ratio indicates equal distribution of the abnormalities between the proximal and distal nerve segments.

If the EMG, M-wave and F-wave studies are normal, then a normal F-ratio would be expected and consistent with no detectable disease.

4. Patterns of abnormalities

For the F-wave to be abnormal (i.e., delayed minimum latency), many motor fibres must be affected. This may not be the case in some radiculopathies or plexopathies and the F-wave study may therefore be normal. However, expected patterns of abnormality have been reported for several conditions:

(i) Acute canine idiopathic polyradiculoneuritis

In dogs with acute idiopathic polyradiculoneuritis, increased minimum F-wave latencies, increased F-ratios and decreased F-wave amplitudes can be seen in the majority of dogs early in the course of disease (67% [8/12 dogs], 92% [11/12 dogs] and 67% [8/12 dogs], respectively) (**Figure 5.5**) (Cuddon, 1998). These abnormalities are followed by electromyographic changes and decreased CMAP amplitudes once denervation has occurred.

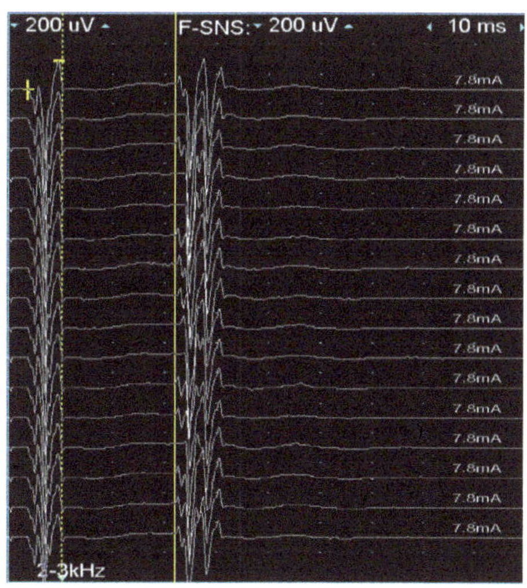

Figure 5.5. F-waves recorded after stimulation of the tibial nerve at the level of the hock in a dog with acute idiopathic polyradiculoneuritis (limb length of 712mm). The M-wave latency was 3.6 ms and the F-wave latency was 32.1 ms. The minimum expected F-wave latency for the tibial nerve should be 3.45 + (0.33 x 71.2) = 26.9ms, therefore the F-wave latency is increased. The F-ratio should be (32.1 – 3.6 – 1)/(2 x 3.6) = 3.8, which is also increased compared to the reference value (1.954). This would be consistent with a predominant involvement of the proximal nerve segment/ventral nerve roots as reported for this condition.

(ii) *Brachial plexus trauma*

In case of severe injury (most likely avulsion) of the motor nerve root(s) following trauma to the brachial plexus, if the electrophysiological examination is performed before distal degeneration of motor axons takes place, the EMG and motor nerve conduction study will be normal. However, the F-waves can be absent as the antidromic potential cannot reach the spinal cord *via* the damaged nerve roots, resulting in a markedly reduced persistence.

(iii) *Degenerative lumbosacral foraminal stenosis*

In dogs with degenerative lumbosacral foraminal stenosis and associated pain, even without neurological deficits, the F-wave latency and the F-ratio were found to be increased compared to dogs without the disease in one study, although there was some overlap of the values between groups (Harcourt-Brown *et al.*, 2019).

(iv) *Myelopathies*

In people, early after a severe spinal cord injury, spinal shock can suppress the ability to generate an F-wave below the level of the lesion despite normal M-wave responses, suggesting an influence of spinal shock on the excitability of motor neurons. The F-waves can remain absent for weeks in these patients. F-waves have been studied in miniature Dachshunds with and without acute thoracolumbar intervertebral disc herniation (Okuno and Orito, 2020). The authors found that the mean F-wave duration was positively correlated to the degree of pelvic limb dysfunction, perhaps reflecting the severity of inhibitory descending motor tract dysfunction.

References

Cuddon, P. A. 1998. Electrophysiologic assessment of acute polyradiculoneuropathy in dogs: comparison with Guillain- Barré syndrome in people. *J. Vet. Intern. Med.* 12: 294–303.
doi: 10.1111/j.1939-1676.1998.tb02125.x. PMID: 9686390.

Harcourt-Brown TR, Granger NP, Fitzpatrick N, Jeffery ND. Electrodiagnostic findings in dogs with apparently painful lumbosacral foraminal stenosis. J Vet Intern Med. 2019 Sep;33(5):2167-2174. doi: 10.1111/jvim.15589. Epub 2019 Aug 5. PMID: 31381186; PMCID: PMC6766485.

Hirasawa S, Shimizu M, Marui Y, Kishimoto M, Okuno S. Establishment of a method to measure length of the ulnar nerve and standardize F-wave values in clinically normal beagles. J Vet Med Sci. 2014 Dec;76(12):1603-7. doi: 10.1292/jvms.14-0089. Epub 2014 Sep 5. PMID: 25649942; PMCID: PMC4300375.

Knecht CD, Redding R, Hyams D. Stimulation techniques and response characteristics of the M and F waves and H reflex in dogs. Vet Res Commun. 1983 Mar;6(2):123-32. doi: 10.1007/BF02214904. PMID: 6868351.

Okuno S, Kobayashi T, Orito K. F-wave latency and F-wave conduction velocity for the tibial nerve in clinically normal dogs. Am J Vet Res. 2002 Sep;63(9):1262-4. doi: 10.2460/ajvr.2002.63.1262. PMID: 12224857.

Okuno S, Kobayashi T, Orito K. F-wave conduction velocity, persistence, and amplitude for the tibial nerve in clinically normal cats. Am J Vet Res. 2008 Feb;69(2):261-4. doi: 10.2460/ajvr.69.2.261. PMID: 18241024.

Okuno S, Orito K. F-wave parameters for the tibial nerve in Miniature Dachshunds with and without naturally acquired thoracolumbar intervertebral disk herniation. Am J Vet Res. 2020 May;81(5):422-427. doi: 10.2460/ajvr.81.5.422. PMID: 32343176.

Poncelet L, Balligand M. Nature of the late potentials and F-ratio values in dogs. Res Vet Sci. 1991;51:1-5. doi: 10.1016/0034-5288(91)90021-f. PMID: 1896622.

Steiss JE. Linear regression to determine the relationship between F-wave latency and limb length in control dogs. Am J Vet Res. 1984 Dec;45(12):2649-50. PMID: 6524757.

SECTION 6

Repetitive nerve stimulation

An Vanhaesebrouck, Hélène Vandenberghe,
Edward Ives, Nicolas Granger

Key points

- Repetitive nerve stimulation involves repeated supramaximal stimulation of motor fibres in a peripheral nerve, with recording of a train of compound muscle action potentials in a muscle innervated by that nerve.
- A belly-tendon montage the same as for motor nerve conduction studies is used, with the active electrode in the muscle placed as close as possible to the muscle belly motor point.
- Typically, low frequencies of 1-5Hz are used, which is an effective way to cause acetylcholine depletion at the neuromuscular junction and reveal abnormalities of neuromuscular transmission, if present.
- A decremental response of more than 10 percent between the first potential and the fifth is suggestive of acquired *myasthenia gravis*. This may resolve with acetylcholinesterase inhibitor administration.
- Single fibre EMG allows selective recording of action potentials from single muscle fibres and measurement of the jitter, which is the mean absolute value to the consecutive

differences in latency of 40-100 single muscle fibre action potentials.

Repetitive nerve stimulation is designed to test the neuromuscular junction and to help diagnose diseases affecting neuromuscular transmission.

1. Physiology of the neuromuscular junction and response to nerve stimulation

The neuromuscular junction transforms electrical signals from the pre-synaptic motor nerve terminal into a chemical signal, which then travels across the neuromuscular junction and binds to the post-synaptic region of the muscle fibre to stimulate muscle contraction (Wood and Slater, 2001). The chemical neurotransmitter at the neuromuscular junction is acetylcholine (Ach).

The nerve terminal contains many synaptic vesicles, with each vesicle containing thousands of molecules of acetylcholine (Kuffler and Yoshikami, 1975). At rest, spontaneous leakage of individual vesicles into the synaptic cleft occurs at a rate of several per minute. Binding of 'leaked' acetylcholine to post-synaptic acetylcholine receptors (AChRs) gives rise to a small post-synaptic depolarisation, called a miniature end-plate potential (mEPP) (Fatt and Katz, 1952; Del Castillo and Katz, 1954; Boyd and Martin, 1956). This depolarisation is so small that no muscle action potential is elicited, and the physiological role of this leaked acetylcholine is unclear (see 'Section 3: Electromyography' for further information regarding the recording of mEPPs).

Upon nerve stimulation, a nerve action potential is generated that reaches the nerve terminal, where it activates voltage-gated calcium channels. This allows the entry of calcium into the pre-synaptic nerve terminal, which in turn leads to the release of several vesicles of acetylcholine into the synaptic cleft (Dodge and Rahamimoff, 1967) (**Figure 6.1**). The released acetylcholine then binds to nicotinic acetylcholine receptors (nAChRs) on the

Figure 6.1. Neurotransmission at the neuromuscular junction, with the red spheres representing acetylcholine. AChE, acetylcholinesterase; AChR, acetylcholine receptor; VGCC, voltage-gated calcium channels; VGNC, voltage-gated sodium channels.

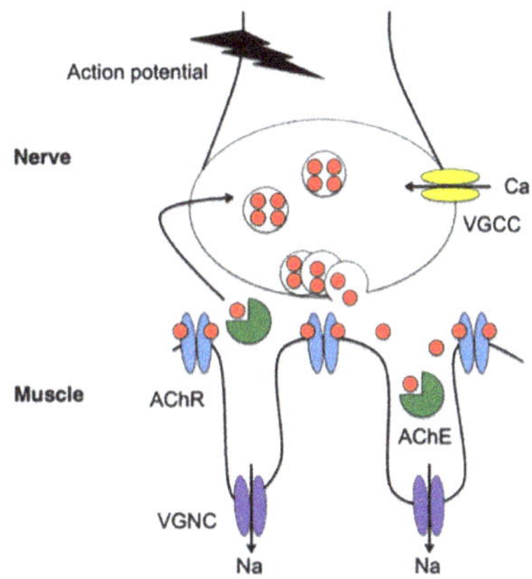

post-synaptic muscle membrane, resulting in a focal depolarisation called the end-plate potential (EPP) (Jones *et al.*, 2016).

If the amplitude of the end-plate potential reaches a certain threshold, voltage-gated sodium channels open, resulting in a muscle action potential (**Figure 6.2**). The muscle action potential is considered an 'all-or-none' event, meaning that once the threshold is reached, the action potential will always be maximal. The action potential is propagated along the muscle membrane resulting in subsequent muscle contraction.

Figure 6.2. End-plate potential and muscle action potential. Stimulation of the nerve produces end-plate potentials and once a threshold is reached, this triggers a muscle action potential.

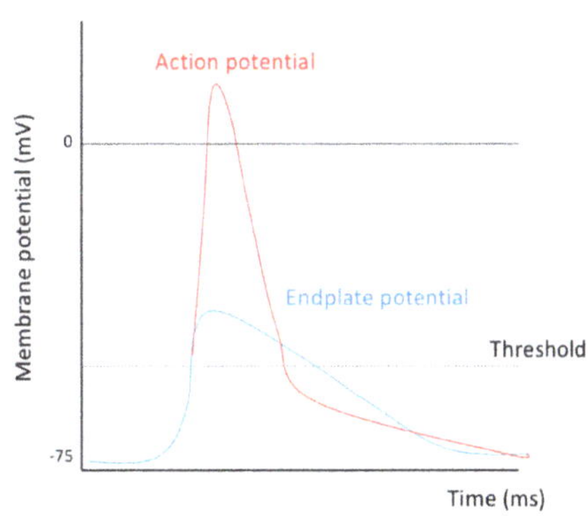

The enzyme acetylcholinesterase terminates signal transmission by rapid hydrolysis of acetylcholine within the synaptic cleft (**Figure 6.1**). Choline is then taken back into the nerve terminal, making it available for re-synthesis of acetylcholine by choline acetyltransferase.

In the nerve terminal, the acetylcholine pool is divided into three compartments: (i) a small portion of acetylcholine – the 'readily releasable pool' – which is immediately available for release; (ii) another compartment called the 'recycling pool', which supplies the immediate pool; and (iii) a large compartment called the 'reserve pool', which is thought to only supply the readily releasable pool on high nerve stimulation frequencies. During continuous nerve stimulation, the readily releasable pool depletes faster than it is replenished (Moyer and van Lunteren, 1999; Moyer and van Lunteren 2001; Rizzoli and Betz, 2005; Denker and Rizzoli, 2010). Consequently, the release of acetylcholine decreases with repeated nerve stimulation. However, under normal circumstances, this reduced amount of neurotransmitter released (e.g., during a train of 10 stimulations over a short period of time) is still well above what is required to reach the threshold for activation of voltage-gated sodium channels, and thus to elicit an action potential and normal muscle contraction. This is called the safety factor of the neuromuscular junction (Wood and Slater, 2001).

Of note, only muscle action potentials can be recorded on repetitive nerve stimulation in a clinical setting. End-plate potentials can be recorded, but only when the action potential is blocked using a toxin. This is clinically not feasible and thus recordings of EPPs are usually only performed *ex vivo* on freshly taken biopsies in specialised research centres. In contrast, mEPPs can occasionally be detected during EMG when the concentric recording needle is in close proximity to the end-plate (see 'Section 3 – Electromyography').

Neuromuscular transmission in dogs is mature by the age of two months (Gödde *et al.*, 1993).

2. Stimulating and recording technique for repetitive nerve stimulation

Repetitive nerve stimulation (RNS), also called the decrement test, is used to measure signal transmission at the neuromuscular junction. In animals, this is performed under general anaesthesia. As this transmission is temperature sensitive, a normal temperature needs to be maintained during the procedure.

To perform repetitive nerve stimulation, a belly-tendon montage the same as for a motor nerve conduction study is used to record a train of compound muscle action potentials (CMAPs) that is elicited by repetitive stimulation (**Figure 6.3**). Two monopolar stimulating needles, a cathode and anode, are inserted close to the motor (or mixed) peripheral nerve to be stimulated. To record the evoked CMAPs, one monopolar needle (the active electrode/cathode) is inserted into the belly of a muscle innervated by this nerve, and the other monopolar needle (anode) is placed in the tendon of the muscle. Alternatively, the anodal electrode can be placed subcutaneously close to the cathode (1-3cm away). Ideally, the active electrode is placed as close as possible to the muscle belly motor point, which is the area of the muscle in which an electrical pulse evokes a muscle twitch with the least current. Mapping of motor points in dogs has been published (Thomson *et al.*, 1971). A reference ('earth/ground' electrode) is

Figure 6.3. Belly tendon montage used for repetitive nerve stimulation studies.

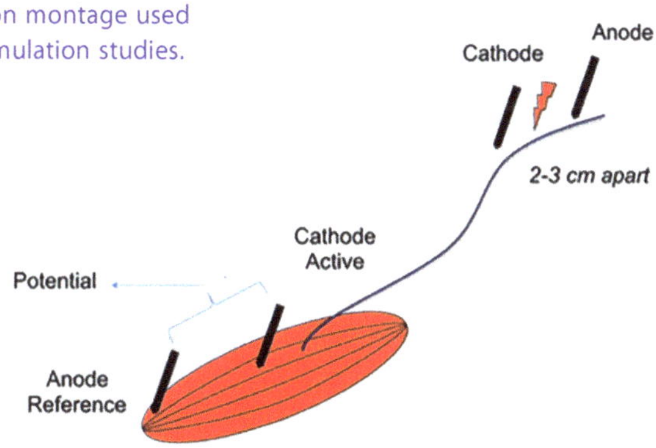

placed subcutaneously between the stimulating and recording electrodes at an electrically silent region (e.g., over the stifle or point of the elbow when testing the limb muscles).

The choice of nerve and muscle combination should be based on the clinical presentation and the distribution of the muscle weakness. The most common nerves and muscles used for repetitive nerve stimulation in dogs and cats are: (i) the ulnar nerve and *palmar interosseous* muscle; (ii) the sciatic-tibial nerve and *plantar interosseous*, or sciatic-peroneal nerve and *tibialis cranialis* muscle (Malik and Church *et al.*, 1989; Sims *et al.*, 1990: Gödde *et al.*, 1993). In humans, eye muscles are particularly affected clinically, for which the underlying reason is not well understood. Similarly, the facial nerve and *orbicularis oculi* muscle could be used for repetitive nerve stimulation in veterinary patients (Añor *et al.*, 2000), however, no reference values for this set-up are currently available for dogs or cats. Ideally, a distal muscle is chosen first as it is likely to give the least movement artefact. However, if no decrement is present, then a more proximal muscle can be examined.

Before starting the first train of 10 stimulations, most electrophysiology units will use a 'single stimulus' set-up mode where the montage can be set up and tested to make sure that the examiner can record an adequate compound muscle action potential (CMAP) from the stimulated nerve/recorded muscle. Stimulation intensity needs to be increased beyond the level that achieves a maximal CMAP amplitude (supramaximal stimulus). Once the maximum CMAP is obtained, the examiner can switch to the 'train of stimulations' mode, which is usually a train of 10 stimulations. Different stimulation rates/frequencies can be used (measured in Hz), and these can be tested in turn if needed. A typical stimulation rate of 2-3Hz is used, which is fast enough to deplete the immediate pool of acetylcholine (Waxenberger *et al.*, 1992). A decrement of the response can be observed for a *normal* neuromuscular junction at stimulation rates greater than 10Hz in dogs (Malik and Church, 1989). The limb should be immobilised using a tie to avoid excessive limb movement, as this can result in the needles falling out during the procedure.

As described in 'Section 4 – Appendicular motor nerve conduction studies', the CMAP reflects the summation of action potentials from several muscle fibres in the area recorded. The term 'decrement' is defined as the % decrease in CMAP amplitude between the 1st and $4^{th}/5^{th}$ or 10th waveforms (see below).

Once a train of 10 CMAPs has been obtained, the repetitive nerve stimulation should be repeated. This is to ensure that the first CMAP amplitude of the second train is of a similar value to that of the first train. If these amplitudes are vastly different, it usually indicates that the needles moved out of position during stimulation and that any decrement recorded during the first train of stimulations may have resulted from needle movement rather than representing a true decrement. To reduce needle movement, the examiner can choose a lower (but still supra-maximal) stimulation intensity that generates less limb movement (Kimura, 2013).

At least 30 seconds between each train of stimulations should be given to allow for recovery of neuromuscular transmission. Also, the muscle length tends to shorten after several contractions, which can affect curve morphology; therefore, these 30 seconds should also be given for muscle relaxation between trains.

3. Waveform analysis

As described above, repetitive nerve stimulation allows the recording of a train of CMAPs (usually 10). Following the recording, it is then possible to analyse either the amplitude or the area of the CMAPs. Measuring the amplitude is usually sufficient, provided that CMAPs observed throughout a train of stimulations are of similar morphology. The amplitude can be measured peak-to-peak or baseline-to-peak, and the electrodiagnostic machine can measure this automatically. The amplitudes (or areas) of CMAPs between the first (baseline) potential and subsequent waves are compared, and the amplitudes of later potentials are expressed as a decrement or increment of the first CMAP.

In humans, the standard approach is to compare the 1st CMAP to 4th and 5th (Kimura, 2013). This is because a process called pseudo-facilitation often occurs at the end of the train (see later), which can mask any decrement. In veterinary medicine, the 1st CMAP is usually compared to the 3rd, 4th, 5th or 10th CMAP (Cuddon, 2002). Some machines will automatically display the difference between the 1st potential and 5th potential, but they can generally be programmed to display either amplitude or area and decrement/increment between any potential.

The % decrement or increment is calculated as follows:

Percentage of decrement = ([amplitude of baseline CMAP – amplitude of lowest CMAP]/amplitude of the baseline CMAP) x 100

Percentage of increment = ([amplitude of highest CMAP – amplitude of baseline CMAP]/amplitude of the baseline CMAP) x 100

In normal animals, the amplitudes and areas of the CMAP do not change significantly after repetitive nerve stimulation over 10 stimuli; i.e., there should not be a decrement of more than 10 percent at stimulation frequencies less than 10Hz (e.g., 2-3Hz) (Sims *et al.*, 1990; Waxenberger *et al.*,1992) (**Figure 6.4**).

Usually, the lowest CMAP amplitude is the 3rd, 4th or 5th CMAP, at which point there is maximum depletion of the stores of readily available acetylcholine. Thereafter, the decrement stays stable (<10% in a normal animal) because other pools of acetylcholine are mobilised to resupply the neuromuscular junction. However, the amplitude of the CMAP will sometimes increase again after the 5th potential due to pseudofacilitation. During pseudofacilitation, the CMAP amplitude increases whilst the area stays the

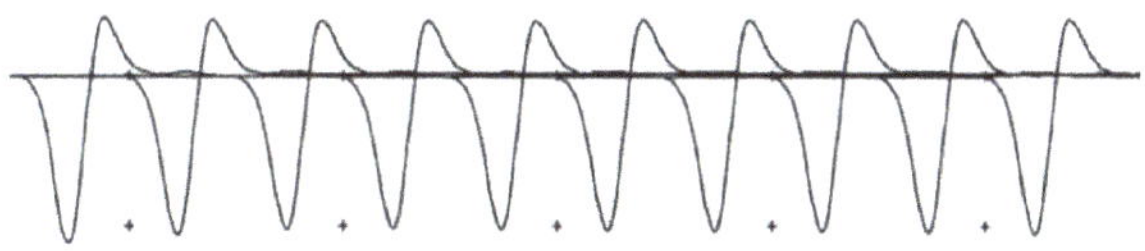

Figure 6.4.
Repetitive nerve stimulation in a normal dog. Note the constant size and shape of the individual CMAPs over the train of 10 stimuli.

same, as the CMAP duration decreases. This is due to synchronisation and summation of individual fibre potentials contributing to the CMAP (Kimura, 2013).

During slow repetitive nerve stimulation (typical 1-3Hz), acetylcholine-loaded vesicles that are docked at the pre-synaptic membrane are released and gradually depleted from the readily available pools. This readily releasable pool is refilled by the reserve pool, however, this is at a slower rate than the actual release. As a consequence, the amplitude of the EPP decreases, although in normal circumstances it remains above the threshold for muscle fibre activation due to the safety factor of the neuromuscular junction described above. Owing to the 'all-or-none' feature of the CMAP, a maximal CMAP will still be obtained after every stimulus in spite of the lower EPP. A significant decrement (>10%) suggests that there is a disorder affecting synaptic transmission that is reducing the safety factor (e.g., *myasthenia gravis*). This results from the EPP no longer being able to reach the threshold required to elicit an action potential at the post-synaptic membrane, meaning that fewer muscle fibres are activated to contribute to the CMAP (reducing the amplitude and/or area over repeated stimulations).

During rapid repetitive nerve stimulation (e.g., 50Hz), calcium accumulates in the pre-synaptic terminal resulting in an increase in the probability of acetylcholine vesicle release into the synaptic clefts. An increment of CMAP amplitudes and area at high stimulation frequencies (called facilitation) can suggest the presence of a pre-synaptic disorder (e.g., botulism, see below).

4. Single-fibre electromyography

Single-fibre EMG is a selective recording technique that allows identification of action potentials from single muscle fibres using a very small recording surface. This is different to RNS, in which a compound potential from multiple myofibres is recorded.

To perform single-fibre EMG, the nerve is stimulated at the motor point, which is where its motor branches enter the muscle belly. The motor point can be located by moving the stimulating electrodes until the place is found where the stimulating current induces a muscle twitch with a minimal stimulation intensity. The recording electrode contains an exposed port on its side and is placed within the muscle belly.

During single-fibre EMG, the latency between nerve stimulation and the onset of muscle fibre action potentials naturally varies. This is due to fluctuations in the time for the end-plate potentials at the neuromuscular junction to reach the action potential threshold and produce a muscle action potential. This variation is called the 'neuromuscular jitter'. Neuromuscular jitter is defined as the mean absolute value of the consecutive differences in latency of 50-100 single muscle fibre action potentials after stimulation of intramuscular nerve bundles at the level of the motor point in at least 20 muscle fibres per muscle. This is a sensitive measure of the safety factor of neuromuscular transmission, and it increases when the ratio between depolarisation threshold and end-plate potential increases (i.e., when the safety factor decreases). Disorders affecting the neuromuscular junction lower the safety factor either because there is less acetylcholine released into the synaptic cleft (i.e., pre-synaptic disease), or because the end-plate is less responsive to acetylcholine (e.g., blockade of nAchRs in myasthenia gravis). This results in increased jitter, or even impulse blocking, when the end-plate potentials cannot elicit a muscle fibre action potential (Añor *et al.*, 2003).

In dogs, values have been reported for the *peroneus longus* (an easily located muscle belly and motor point), the *extensor carpi radialis* and the *orbicularis oculi* muscles (Añor *et al.*, 2003).

In people, another parameter called 'fibre density' can be assessed with single-fibre electromyography. It allows assessment of the local concentration of muscle fibres within a motor unit. Increased fibre density is consistent with reinnervation, (i.e., muscle fibre type grouping following collateral sprouting of motor nerves). This has not yet been assessed in dogs (Juel *et al.*, 2019).

5. Patterns of abnormalities – repetitive nerve stimulation in disease

(i) *Myasthenia gravis*

In *myasthenia gravis* cases, at low stimulation frequencies (typical 1-3Hz) the amplitude of the first CMAP is typically normal. However, the amplitude of subsequent CMAPs will then drop, resulting in an abnormal decrement on waveform analysis. This is because there is a reduced number of available nAchRs on the post-synaptic membrane following antibody-mediated blockade and receptor internalisation. Therefore, as the volume of Ach released into the synaptic cleft reduces with repeated stimulation, the EPP elicited by the nerve impulses becomes reduced in amplitude until it eventually fails to bring the membrane potential above the threshold for action potential generation in some muscle fibres. This results in fewer muscle fibres contributing to the size of the CMAP, causing a reduction in amplitude. The amplitude will drop considerably between the 1st potential and the 2nd, with further decremental responses (but to a lesser extent) to approximately the 5th potential. After this, either a steady state plateau is obtained or pseudofacilitation occurs, with increasing amplitudes to sometimes higher values than the 1st potential.

A decrement of more than 10% between the 1st potential and the 5th (in theory the smallest of the 4th to 6th potentials) is highly suggestive of *myasthenia gravis* (**Figure 6.5**) (Zacks *et al.*, 1966; Johnson *et al.*, 1975; Shelton *et al.*, 2002). However, a negative finding in a distal muscle should lead the examiner to study a proximal (or facial) muscle, particularly if there is a high suspicion of acquired *myasthenia gravis* from the clinical history and examination.

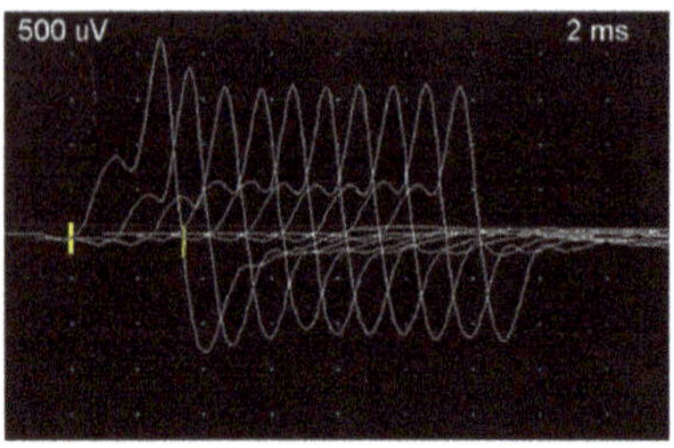

Trace No	Peak Amp (mV)	Amp Decr %	Area mVms	Area Decr %
1	2.23	0	3.01	0
2	1.96	12	2.13	29
3	1.74	22	1.87	38
4	1.66	26	2.10	30
5	1.72	23	2.12	30
6	1.72	23	2.07	31
7	1.73	22	2.04	32
8	1.73	22	2.07	31
9	1.74	22	2.10	30
10	1.72	23	2.07	31

Figure 6.5. Repetitive nerve stimulation (stimulation rate of 3Hz) in a dog with acquired *myasthenia gravis*. Observe the >10% decrement of both the amplitude and area between the 1st and following stimulations.

Once an affected muscle is found, IV injection of either edrophonium (Tensilon® 0.1-0.2mg/kg in dogs or 0.25-0.5mg total dose in cats [no longer available in the UK]) or neostigmine (Prostigmin® 20ug/kg intravenously) can be used to demonstrate a return to a normal recording (**Figure 6.6**). If this test is performed, it is good practice to closely monitor the live ECG from the anaesthetic machine and have some atropine (0.02-0.04 mg/kg) or glycopyrrolate ready when injecting edrophonium (Zacks *et al.*, 1966; Johnson *et al.*, 1975; Shelton *et al.*, 2002). In humans, this test is no longer routinely used, as short-acting acetylcholinesterase inhibitors may result in cardiorespiratory arrest and antibody testing is more extensively developed in humans compared to veterinary patients, making this test no longer required. Cholinergic crisis after neostigmine administration has been described in dogs (Foy *et al.*, 2011).

Figure 6.6. Repetitive nerve stimulation in a dog with acquired *myasthenia gravis* after treatment with edrophonium. Note the normal (<10% decrement) in area and amplitude on repeated tests post-edrophonium separated by >30 seconds.

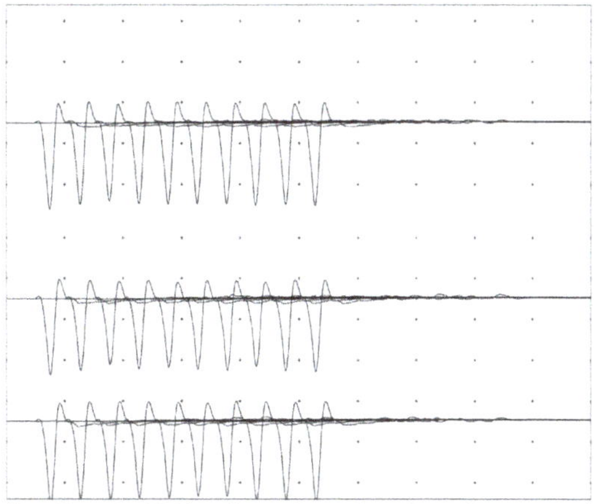

R Peroneal - EDB								
Post edrophonium	2	2.3	9.7	100	8.3	-1	100	0:00:00
Post edrophonium	2	2.2	-3.6	95.2	7.5	-6	90.8	0:00:51
Post edrophonium	2	2.1	10.5	90.8	8.1	-4.9	97.7	0:01:35

In humans, there are rare cases of *myasthenia gravis* (e.g., due to MUSK antibodies) in which specifically proximal muscles are clinically affected. Therefore, in those cases it is preferable to directly test weak proximal muscles rather than distal muscles. As a reminder, EMG in cases with post-synaptic disorders, such as *myasthenia gravis,* is typically normal, as well as sensory and motor nerve conduction velocities and CMAP amplitude after a single stimulation.

(ii) *Congenital myasthenic syndromes*

Mutations in more than 30 genes have been described in humans with congenital myasthenic syndromes (Vanhaesebrouck and Beeson, 2019). Only a few have so far been described in dogs or cats (Mignan *et al.*, 2020), but it is likely that more will be found in the future.

a. Pre-synaptic

Pre-synaptic myasthenic syndromes are the result of defects in proteins involved in acetylcholine synthesis, packaging of acetylcholine into synaptic vesicles, docking of these vesicles and release of acetylcholine at the neuromuscular junction. The most common pre-synaptic congenital myasthenic disorder in humans is due to a mutation in choline acetyltransferase (CHAT), impairing the synthesis of acetylcholine. In dogs, CHAT-associated congenital myasthenia has been reported in Old Danish pointers (Flagstad *et al.*, 1989). In these dogs, a decremental response was observed on low-frequency RNS (3Hz), but only, as in humans, after fatigue had been induced by a long stimulation train (called preconditioning, 5 min at 10Hz) (Proschowski *et al.*, 2007). Many pre-synaptic disorders, but not those due to CHAT mutations, show an *increment* on repetitive nerve stimulation at high frequency stimulation (50Hz). In pre-synaptic disorders in humans, often there is variable response to injection with edrophonium. In dogs with CHAT mutations, no response to edrophonium or pyridostigmine was observed (Proschowski *et al.*, 2007).

b. Synaptic

The best-known example of synaptic congenital myasthenic syndrome is acetylcholinesterase deficiency due to a mutation of the gene coding for the collagen-like tail subunit of the asymmetric acetylcholinesterase gene (ColQ). This is important to anchor acetylcholinesterase to the basal membrane of the synaptic cleft so that it can hydrolyse acetylcholine. This mutation has been reported in Labrador Retrievers, Golden Retrievers, Sphinx cats and Devon Rex cats (Rinz *et al.*, 2014; Abitbol *et al.*, 2015; Gandolfi *et al.*, 2015; Tsai *et al.*, 2019). In animals with this condition, there can be a decremental response on repetitive nerve stimulation in dogs, although repetitive nerve stimulation studies can be normal in cats. In cats, abnormal spontaneous myofibre activity (positive sharp waves and complex repetitive discharges) can sometimes be seen on electromyography. As the disease is caused by insufficient breakdown of acetylcholine, and therefore too high levels of acetylcholine within the synapse, the decrement will worsen after injection of edrophonium (Mignan *et al.*, 2020).

Acetylcholinesterase inhibitors should not be used in this disease, as they will worsen the clinical signs due to further increasing the amount of acetylcholine in the synaptic cleft; the presence of too much acetylcholine for too long within the synaptic cleft will result in breakdown of the structure of the neuromuscular junction (Vanhaesebrouck and Beeson, 2019).

c. Post-synaptic

Congenital myasthenia in humans is most commonly caused by a mutation of the CHNRE gene coding for the epsilon subunit of the acetylcholine receptor. In veterinary medicine, it has been reported in Jack Russell terriers and in a Heide terrier (Rinz *et al.*, 2015; Herder *et al.*, 2017). In these cases, there is a decremental response on repetitive nerve stimulation that improves after injection of edrophonium (Rinz *et al.*, 2015).

(iii) Botulism

Botulinum toxin binds to the pre-synaptic nerve terminal and, once internalised, it inactivates acetylcholine release. Needle EMG recordings may demonstrate abnormal spontaneous electrical activity (e.g., fibrillation potentials), because there is a functional denervation of the muscle. Typical characteristics for botulism on repetitive nerve stimulation are a decremental response at low stimulation rates (1-3Hz) and an incremental response at high stimulation rates (50Hz) (Aleman *et al.*, 2011). The decremental response seen with low stimulation rates may be masked if the 1st CMAP amplitude is markedly reduced (due to functional denervation). High frequency stimulation leads to incrementation following accumulation of calcium at the pre-synaptic terminal and therefore an increased probability of exocytosis of acetylcholine (facilitation). These electrodiagnostic abnormalities might not be found in all the muscles if the intoxication is mild (Van Nes, 1986).

(iv) Myopathies

A decremental response is observed in some cases of polymyositis as the post-synaptic membrane can be damaged by the inflammatory process. It has also been described in several congenital myopathies in people (Rodríguez *et al.*, 2014).

(v) Neuropathies

A decremental response can sometimes be observed when the denervation is severe and involves the nerve terminal, resulting in deficient exocytosis of acetylcholine (Aleman *et al.*, 2014).

References

Abitbol M, Hitte C, Bossé P, *et al.* A COLQ missense mutation in Sphynx and Devon Rex cats with congenital myasthenic syndrome. PLos One. 2015;10(9):e0137019. doi: 10.1371/journal.pone.0137019. PMID: 26327126. PMCID: PMC4556666.

Aleman M, Williams DC, Jorge NE, Magdesian KG, Brosnan RJ, Feary DJ, Hilton HG, Kozikowski TA, Higgins JK, Madigan JE, Lecouteur RA. Repetitive stimulation of the common peroneal nerve as a diagnostic aid for botulism in foals. J Vet Intern Med. 2011 Mar-Apr;25(2):365-72. doi: 10.1111/j.1939-1676.2011.0682.x. Epub 2011 Feb 11. PMID: 21314725.

Aleman M, Dickinson PJ, Williams DC, Sturges BK, LeCouteur RA, Vernau KM, Shelton GD. Electrophysiologic confirmation of heterogenous motor polyneuropathy in young cats. J Vet Intern Med. 2014 Nov-Dec;28(6):1789-98. doi: 10.1111/jvim.12439. Epub 2014 Sep 17. PMID: 25231268; PMCID: PMC4895637.

Añor S, Espadaler JM, Pastor J, Pumarola M. Electrically induced blink reflex and facial motor nerve stimulation in beagles. J Vet Intern Med. 2000 Jul-Aug;14(4):418-23. doi: 10.1892/0891-6640(2000)014<0418:eibraf>2.3.co;2. PMID: 10935892.

Añor S, Lipsitz D, Williams DC, Tripp L, Willits N, Maselli R, LeCouteur RA. Evaluation of jitter by stimulated single-fiber electromyography in normal dogs. J Vet Intern Med. 2003 Jul-Aug;17(4):545-50. doi: 10.1111/j.1939-1676.2003.tb02476.x. PMID: 12892306.

Boyd IA, Martin AR. The end-plate potential in mammalian muscle. J Physiol. 1956 Apr 27;132(1):74-91. doi: 10.1113/jphysiol.1956.sp005503. PMID: 13320373; PMCID: PMC1363540.

Cuddon PA. Electrophysiology in neuromuscular disease. Vet Clin North Am Small Anim Pract. 2002 Jan;32(1):31-62. doi: 10.1016/s0195-5616(03)00079-2. PMID: 11785734.

Del Castillo J, Katz B. Quantal components of the end-plate potential. J Physiol. 1954 Jun 28;124(3):560-73. doi: 10.1113/jphysiol.1954.sp005129. PMID: 13175199; PMCID: PMC1366292.

Denker A, Rizzoli SO. Synaptic vesicle pools: an update. Front Synaptic Neurosci. 2010 Oct 5;2:135. doi: 10.3389/fnsyn.2010.00135. PMID: 21423521; PMCID: PMC3059705.

Dodge FA Jr, Rahamimoff R. Co-operative action a calcium ions in transmitter release at the neuromuscular junction. J Physiol. 1967 Nov;193(2):419-32. doi: 10.1113/jphysiol.1967.sp008367. PMID: 6065887; PMCID: PMC1365607.

Fatt P, Katz B. Spontaneous subthreshold activity at motor nerve endings. J Physiol. 1952 May;117(1):109-28. PMID: 14946732; PMCID: PMC1392564.

Flagstad A, Trojaborg W, Gammeltoft S. Congenital myasthenic syndrome in the dog breed Gammel Dansk Hønsehund: clinical, electrophysiological, pharmacological and immunological comparison with acquired myasthenia gravis. Acta Vet Scand. 1989;30(1):89-102. doi: 10.1186/BF03548072. PMID: 2782236; PMCID: PMC8142211.

Foy DS, Trepanier LA, Shelton GD. Cholinergic crisis after neostigmine administration in a dog with acquired focal myasthenia gravis. J Vet Emerg Crit Care (San Antonio). 2011 Oct;21(5):547-51. doi: 10.1111/j.1476-4431.2011.00672.x. Epub 2011 Aug 24. PMID: 22316202.

Gandolfi B, Grahn RA, Creighton EK, *et al.* A COLQ variant associated with Devon Rex and Sphynx feline hereditary myopathy. Anim Genet. 2015;46:711-715. doi: 10.11111/age.12350. PMID: 26374066. PMCID: PMC4637250.

Gödde T, Jagger A, Vandevelde M, *et al.* Evaluation of repetitive nerve stimulation in young dogs. J Small Anim Pract 30:20-26, 1989

Herder V, Ciurkiewicz M, Baumgärtner M, Jagnnathan V, Leeb T. Frame-shift variant in the CHRNE gene in a juvenile dog with suspected myasthenia gravis-like disease. Anim Genet. 2017;48:625. doi: 10.1111/age.12558. PMID: 28508416.

Johnson RP, Watson AD, Smith J, Cooper BJ. Myasthenia in Springer Spaniel littermates. J Small Anim Pract. 1975 Oct;16(10):641-7. doi: 10.1111/j.1748-5827.1975.tb05790.x. PMID: 1207073.

Jones RA, Reich CD, Dissanayake KN, Kristmundsdottir F, Findlater GS, Ribchester RR, Simmen MW, Gillingwater TH. NMJ-morph reveals principal components of synaptic morphology influencing structure-function relationships at the neuromuscular junction. Open Biol. 2016 Dec;6(12):160240. doi: 10.1098/rsob.160240. Erratum in: Open Biol. 2017 Jan;7(1): PMID: 27927794; PMCID: PMC5204123.

Juel VC. Single fiber electromyography. Handb Clin Neurol. 2019;160:303-310. doi: 10.1016/B978-0-444-64032-1.00019-9. PMID: 31277856.

Kimura J. Electrodiagnosis in Diseases of Nerve and Muscle: Principles and Practice – 4th ed. Oxford University Press, 2013.

Kuffler SW, Yoshikami D. The number of transmitter molecules in a quantum: an estimate from iontophoretic application of acetylcholine at the neuromuscular synapse. J Physiol. 1975 Oct;251(2):465-82. doi: 10.1113/jphysiol.1975.sp011103. PMID: 171380; PMCID: PMC1348438.

Malik R, Ho S, Church DB. The normal response to repetitive motor nerve stimulation in dogs. 1989. https://doi.org/10.1111/j.1748-5827.1989.tb01455.x

Mignan T, Targett M, Lowrie M. Classification of myasthenia gravis and congenital myasthenic syndromes in dogs and cats. J Vet Intern Med. 2020 Sep;34(5):1707-1717. doi: 10.1111/jvim.15855. Epub 2020 Jul 15. PMID: 32668077; PMCID: PMC7517852.

Moyer M, van Lunteren E. Effect of phasic activation on endplate potential in rat diaphragm. J Neurophysiol. 1999 Dec;82(6):3030-40. doi: 10.1152/jn.1999.82.6.3030. PMID: 10601438.

Moyer M, van Lunteren E. Effect of temperature on endplate potential rundown and recovery in rat diaphragm. J Neurophysiol. 2001 May;85(5):2070-5. doi: 10.1152/jn.2001.85.5.2070. PMID: 11353023.

Proschowsky HF, Flagstad A, Cirera S, Joergensen CB, Fredholm M. Identification of a mutation in the CHAT gene of Old Danish Pointing Dogs affected with congenital myasthenic syndrome. J Hered. 2007;98(5):539-43. doi: 10.1093/jhered/esm026. Epub 2007 Jun 22. PMID: 17586598.

Rinz CJ, Levine J, Minor KM, *et al.* A COLQ missense mutation in Labrador retrievers having congenital myasthenic syndrome. PLoS One. 2014;9(8):e106425. doi: 10.1371/journal.pone.0106425. PMID: 2566616. PMCID: PMC4148433.

Rinz CJ, Lennon VA, James F, *et al.* A CHRNE frameshift mutation causes congenital myasthenic syndrome in young Jack Russell terriers. Neuromuscul Disord. 2015;25:921-927. doi: 10.1016/j.nmd.2015.09.005. PMID: 26429099.

Rizzoli SO, Betz WJ. Synaptic vesicle pools. Nat Rev Neurosci. 2005 Jan;6(1):57-69. doi: 10.1038/nrn1583. PMID: 15611727.

Rodríguez Cruz PM, Sewry C, Beeson D, Jayawant S, Squier W, McWilliam R, Palace J. Congenital myopathies with secondary neuromuscular transmission defects; a case report and review of the literature. Neuromuscul Disord. 2014 Dec;24(12):1103-10. doi: 10.1016/j.nmd.2014.07.005. Epub 2014 Jul 30. PMID: 25127990.

Shelton GD. Myasthenia gravis and disorders of neuromuscular transmission. Vet Clin North Am Small Anim Pract. 2002 Jan;32(1):189-206, vii. doi: 10.1016/s0195-5616(03)00085-8. PMID: 11785729.

Sims MH, McLean RH. Use of repetitive nerve stimulation to assess neuromuscular function in dogs. A test protocol for suspected myasthenia gravis. Progress in Veterinary Neurology 1990 1 3 311-319.

Thomson FK, Bowen JM. Electrodiagnostic testing: mapping and clinical use of motor points in the dog. J Am Vet Med Assoc. 1971 Dec 15;159(12):1763-70. PMID: 5128790.

Tsai KL, Vernau KM, Winger K, *et al.* Congenital myasthenic syndrome in Golden retrievers is associated with a novel COLQ mutation. J Vet Intern Med. 2019;34:1-8. doi: 10.1111/jvim.15667. PMID: 31769119. PMCID: PMC6979411.

Vanhaesebrouck AE, Beeson D. The congenital myasthenic syndromes: expanding genetic and phenotypic spectrums and refining treatment strategies. Curr Opin Neurol. 2019 Oct;32(5):696-703. doi: 10.1097/WCO.0000000000000736. PMID: 31361628; PMCID: PMC6735524.

van Nes JJ. Clinical application of neuromuscular electrophysiology in the dog: a review. Vet Q. 1986 Jul;8(3):240-50. doi: 10.1080/01652176.1986.9694048. PMID: 3018992.

Waxenberger MK, Heckmann R, Wiestner T, Hogg HP. Neuromuscular transmission studies in the healthy dog: EMG and muscle force measurement after repetitive nerve stimulation. Zentralbl Veterinarmed A. 1992 Jun;39(5):372-81. doi: 10.1111/j.1439-0442.1992.tb00194.x. PMID: 1323192.

Wood SJ, Slater CR. Safety factor at the neuromuscular junction. Prog Neurobiol. 2001 Jul;64(4):393-429. doi: 10.1016/s0301-0082(00)00055-1. PMID: 11275359.

Zacks SI, Shields DR, Steinberg SA. A myasthenic syndrome in the dog: a case report with electron microscopic observations on motor end-plates and comparisons with the fine structure of end-plates in myasthenia gravis. Ann N Y Acad Sci. 1966 Jan 26;135(1):79-97. doi: 10.1111/j.1749-6632.1966.tb45465.x. PMID: 5221369

SECTION 7

Appendicular sensory nerve conduction studies

Hélène Vandenberghe, Edward Ives, Nicolas Granger

Key points

- Sensory fibres have a lower threshold of activation and faster conduction velocity than motor fibres, therefore activation of a mixed nerve can still allow assessment of sensory nerve conduction.
- Only one stimulation point is necessary for calculation of sensory nerve conduction velocity because, unlike motor nerve conduction velocity calculation, there is no neuromuscular junction or intervening synaptic delay and the sensory latency is derived simply from the nerve conduction time between the stimulus point and the recording point along the same nerve.
- Sensory nerve action potentials are much smaller than compound muscle action potentials and responses are averaged to minimise the effect of background noise on the waveforms.
- Interpretation of sensory nerve conduction studies relies on the same principles as interpretation of motor nerve conduction studies.

- The cell body of sensory nerve fibres (dorsal root ganglion) is located at the level of the intervertebral foramen and sensory nerve fibres only degenerate in case of a lesion located distal to the ganglion. Therefore, normal sensory nerve potentials are obtained in case of a preganglionic lesion (e.g., nerve root avulsion).

1. Recording technique

Sensory nerve conduction studies can be performed from sensory or mixed sensorimotor nerves.

Two types of potential can be recorded dependent on the type of nerve stimulated:

- Sensory nerve action potentials (SNAPs), which are the summation of individual sensory fibre action potentials (i.e., compound potentials) recorded after stimulation of a pure sensory nerve.
- Mixed nerve action potentials (MiNAPs), which are recorded after stimulation of a mixed sensorimotor nerve. Stimulation of a mixed nerve evokes: (i) descending motor potentials distal to the stimulation point; and (ii) ascending motor *and* sensory potentials proximal to the stimulation point (Kimura, 2013). Therefore, MiNAPs recorded proximal to the stimulation point represent a summation of action potentials travelling up both motor and sensory fibres in a mixed nerve. Unlike pure motor or sensory nerve conduction studies, mixed sensorimotor nerve studies also allow assessment of the large diameter, myelinated Ia sensory fibres supplying the muscle spindles (Preston and Shapiro, 2013). Large diameter Ia fibres have a lower threshold of activation and conduct at a faster velocity than motor fibres (by 5-10%); these differences allow separation of the motor and sensory impulses, meaning that activation of a mixed nerve can still provide assessment of sensory nerve conduction (Kimura, 2013).

The same principles apply to sensory nerve conduction studies as for motor nerve conduction studies (see 'Section 4 – Appendicular motor nerve conduction studies').

(i) Stimulation

The most common technique used in animals involves stimulation of the skin (or sub-cutaneous tissue), with recording from near the peripheral nerve innervating that portion of the skin. This is termed an orthodromic nerve conduction study because the recording electrodes measure an action potential that is traveling in the physiologic direction (i.e., proximally for a sensory nerve) (Cuddon, 2002; Kimura *et al.*, 2013; Preston and Shapiro, 2013). The nerve can also be directly stimulated distal to the recording site (Whalen *et al.*, 1986).

In contrast to motor nerve conduction studies, in which a delay for neuromuscular transmission needs to be considered, the sensory latency represents conduction along the nerve alone, from the sensory receptors directly to the recording site. This means that only one stimulation site is needed to calculate the sensory nerve conduction velocity.

The stimulation also requires less current than for motor nerve conduction studies because sensory fibres have a lower threshold of activation compared to motor fibres. Surface electrodes can be used but, as for motor studies, subcutaneous needles are preferred to improve signal-to-noise ratio (Holliday *et al.*, 1977). The current is gradually increased until a compound sensory nerve action potential is recorded. Supra-maximal stimulation of the skin will produce a small twitch of the skin visible around the stimulation site and leads to activation of all large diameter fibres. Increasing the stimulus intensity results in a higher amplitude of the SNAP or MiNAP (van Nes, 1985). However, if the current is too high, co-stimulation of nearby nerves and movement resulting from muscle potentials may interfere with the shape of the recorded wave (Preston and Shapiro, 2013). Neuromuscular blockade under general anaesthesia, using substances such as atracurium, can be used to eliminate muscle artefact and improve the quality of recording. However, ventilation and careful anaesthetic monitoring is essential in these cases, with use typically reserved for specialist centres with veterinary anaesthetists.

(ii) Recording

The pair of recording electrodes is placed over the nerve being studied based on anatomical landmarks. Alternatively, for a mixed nerve, the sensory nerve conduction study can be performed immediately after the motor nerve conduction study by simply using the previous stimulating electrodes left in place as recording electrodes. The active recording electrode (cathode) should be placed distally so that it is closest to the active stimulating electrode (**Figure 7.1**). The two recording electrodes are separated by approximately 2-3cm. Placing the reference ('ground') electrode between the stimulation and recording sites helps to reduce stimulus artefact.

Figure 7.1. Electrode set up for a sensory nerve conduction study (tibial nerve in a dog).

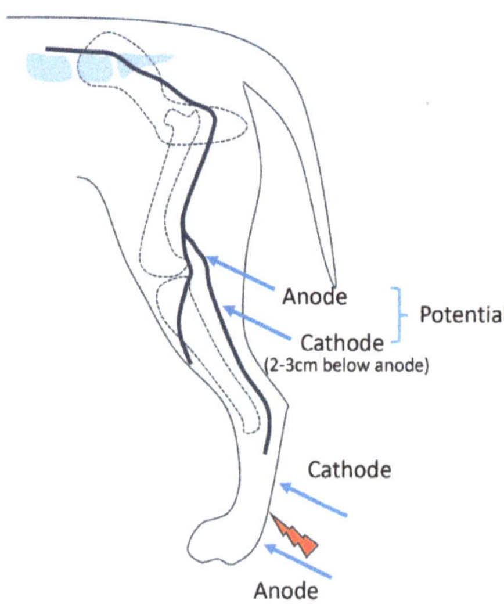

The amplitudes of sensory potentials are typically very small (in the μV range); therefore, electrical noise and technical factors are more likely to interfere with recording and acquisition of good quality SNAPs/MiNAPs compared to motor potentials that are larger. This is why signal averaging is used to extract the compound sensory action potentials from background noise (Holliday et al, 1977). To do this, a train of ~250-500 stimulations is used and stimuli are delivered at a relatively high rate (up to 20Hz) (Holliday *et al.*, 1977). Signal averaging works on the principle that electrical signals detected at the recording site will be maintained and amplified if they are time-locked to the stimulus, whereas background noise will be cancelled out over time as it is randomly detected at the recording electrodes independent of stimulation timing.

A summary of stimulation and recording parameters for sensory nerve conduction studies is shown in **Table 7.1**.

Stimulation parameters	**Value**
Stimulus duration	0.2msec
Stimulation rate	10Hz
Number of stimulations	Signal averaging of 250-500 impulses
Stimulation intensity	Supramaximal
Recording parameters	**Value**
Gain	1-5μV/cm
Sweep speed	1ms/cm
High frequency filter	5kHz
Low frequency filter	2Hz

Table 7.1. Stimulation and recording parameters for sensory nerve conduction studies.

2. Anatomy for sensory nerve conduction studies – stimulation and recording sites

The stimulation and recording sites for different sensory and mixed sensorimotor nerves are as follows:

(i) Lateral superficial radial nerve (sensory nerve)

The area of skin stimulated is the dorsal aspect of the thoracic paw and recording is from the lateral superficial radial nerve at the distal third of the humeral diaphysis, just proximal and cranial to the elbow (**Figure 7.2**) (Redding *et al.*, 1982).

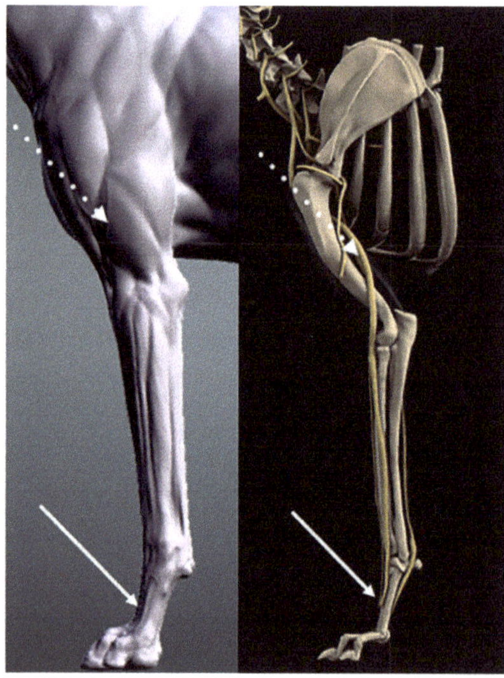

Figure 7.2. Anatomy for lateral superficial radial nerve sensory nerve conduction study. A. Surface anatomy. B. Peripheral nerve anatomy with the skin and muscles removed. Stimulation site = plain arrow; recording site = dotted arrow. *Adapted with permission from Ivalalearn (part of the Veterinary Information Network® family).*

(ii) Ulnar nerve (mixed nerve)

The area of skin stimulated is the lateral aspect of digit V (lateral aspect of the paw, slightly lateral and proximal to the accessory carpal bone) and recording is made from the ulnar nerve, medial to the elbow, between the olecranon and medial epicondyle of the humerus (**Figure 7.3**) (Redding et *al.*, 1982).

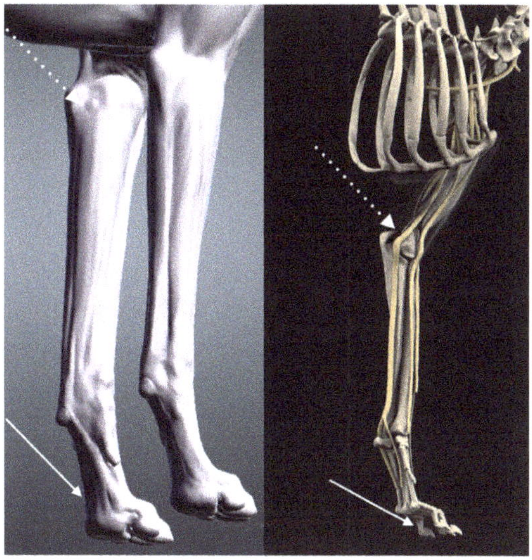

Figure 7.3. Anatomy for ulnar nerve sensory nerve conduction study. A. Surface anatomy. B. Peripheral nerve anatomy with the skin and muscles removed. Stimulation site = plain arrow; recording site = dotted arrow. *Adapted with permission from Ivalalearn (part of the Veterinary Information Network® family).*

(iii) Peroneal nerve (sensory nerve)

The area of skin stimulated is the dorsal aspect of the pelvic limb paw and recording is made from the peroneal nerve caudolateral to the stifle (**Figure 7.4**) (Redding *et al.*, 1982).

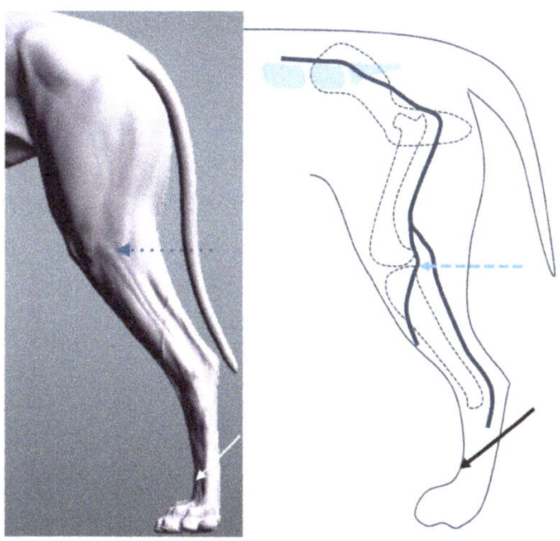

Figure 7.4. Anatomy for peroneal nerve sensory nerve conduction study. A: Surface anatomy. B. Peripheral nerve anatomy with the skin and muscles removed. Stimulation site = plain arrow; recording site = dotted arrow. *Adapted with permission from Ivalalearn (part of the Veterinary Information Network® family).*

(iv) Tibial nerve (mixed nerve)

The area of skin stimulated is the plantar aspect of the pelvic limb paw and recording is made from the tibial nerve proximal to the calcaneus of the hock (in the neurovascular bundle between the gastrocnemius tendon and the tibia), or at the level of the stifle (**Figure 7.5**) (Redding *et al.*, 1982).

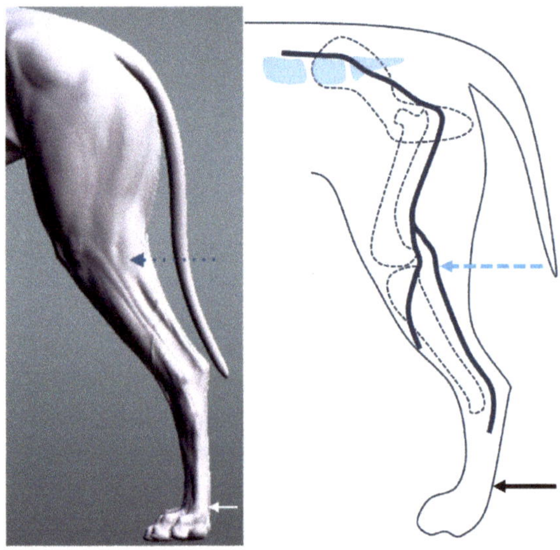

Figure 7.5. Anatomy for tibial nerve sensory nerve conduction study. A. Surface anatomy. B. Peripheral nerve anatomy with the skin and muscles removed. Stimulation site = plain arrow; recording site = dotted arrow. *Adapted with permission from Ivalalearn (part of the Veterinary Information Network® family).*

(v) Saphenous nerve (sensory nerve)

The nerve is directly stimulated on the medial aspect of the pelvic limb, proximal to the stifle, where the saphenous nerve runs in association with the saphenous artery and vein. Recording can be made either distally (antidromically conducted compound action potential) distal to the stifle where the saphenous nerve accompanies the cranial branch of the saphenous artery, or proximally (orthodromic compound action potential) (**Figure 7.6**) (Whalen *et al.*, 1986).

Figure 7.6. Anatomy for saphenous nerve sensory nerve conduction study. Medial aspect of the right pelvic limb. Stimulation site = plain arrow; recording sites = dotted arrows. A. Distal recording site. B. Proximal recording site.

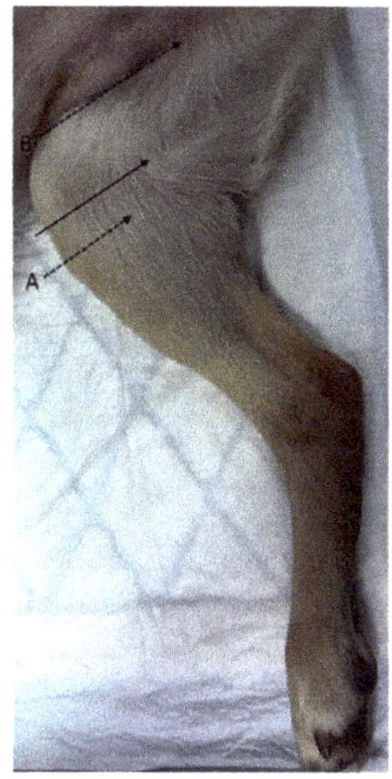

3. Waveform analysis

The interpretation of the amplitude of SNAPs and MiNAPs can be challenging due to their small size in the μV range compared to CMAPs that are in the mV range. There is also a great variation in amplitude between one subject and another in humans, which is an even greater problem in companion animals of varying sizes and body mass.

Sensory nerve action potentials are biphasic or triphasic, with a small positive deflection followed by a large negative deflection (Redding *et al.*, 1982). However, their shape will differ dependent on the stimulation parameters and nerve being tested (Whalen *et al.*, 1986).

The latency, peak latency, duration and amplitude of the SNAPs can all be assessed. The latency is measured from the onset of the stimulus artefact to the initial positive deflection. The amplitude is 'peak-peak' measured from the base of the positive deflection to the top of the negative peak (**Figures 7.7 and 7.8**) (Redding *et al.*, 1982). However, as the amplitude is largely variable between subjects and between sides of the same animal, it is of limited diagnostic value alone and the latency and conduction velocity are primarily used in clinical practice (Kimura, 2013).

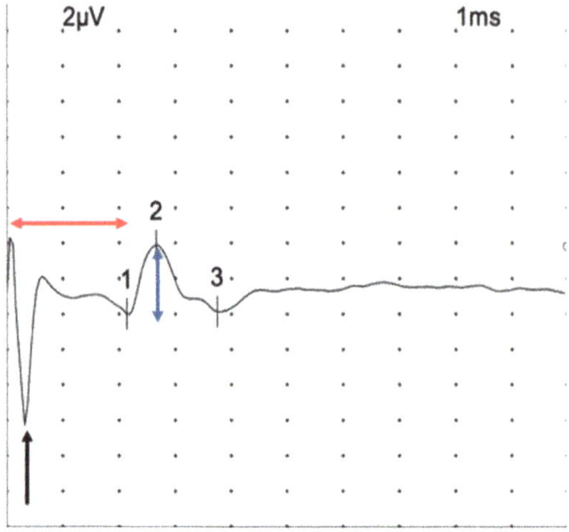

Figure 7.7. Sensory nerve action potential recorded in the peroneal nerve. Horizontal scale = 1ms, vertical scale = 2μV. Black arrow = stimulation artefact. Red double-headed arrow = latency. Blue double-headed arrow = amplitude. Three phases are observed with an initial small positive deflection followed by a larger negative peak.

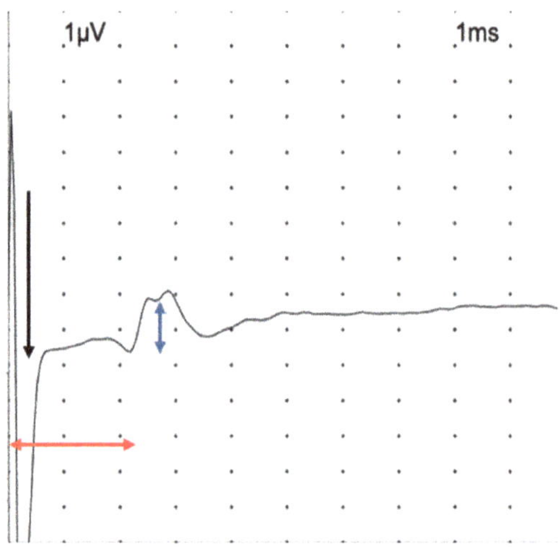

Figure 7.8. Sensory nerve action potential recorded in the ulnar nerve. Horizontal scale = 1ms, vertical scale = 1μV. Black arrow = stimulation artefact. Red double-headed arrow = latency. Blue double-headed arrow = amplitude.

Calculation of the sensory nerve conduction velocity (m/s) is simply performed by dividing the distance between the stimulation point and the recording site (mm) by the latency obtained on the trace (ms). The conduction velocity along sensory nerve fibres reflects the fastest functional fibres in the segment of nerve being tested. There is a minimal 0.15ms delay in activation of the sensory fibres, but this is typically disregarded when calculating the sensory nerve conduction velocity.

Reference values reported in dogs are 60-70m/s for the radial nerve, 55-75m/s for the ulnar nerve, 64m/s for the tibial and peroneal nerves, 62.3 +/- 2m/s for the saphenous nerve with distal recording, and 66.3 +/- 2.2m/s for the saphenous nerve with proximal recording (Lee and Bowen, 1975; Holliday *et al.*, 1977; Redding *et al.*, 1982; Schaeppi *et al.*, 1982; Whalen *et al.*,1986).

Reference values reported in cats are 80-90m/s for the radial nerve, 90-100m/s for the ulnar nerve, 80-90m/s for the peroneal nerve and 75-85m/s for the tibial nerve (Redding and Ingram, 1984).

4. Effect of age, temperature and limb length

The sensory nerve conduction velocity reaches adult values by around 6 months of age. It has also been reported to reduce as the animal gets older (especially after 9-10 years of age in the dog and >14 years in the cat), with slowing by around 10 m/s (Pillai *et al.*, 1991).

Sensory nerve conduction velocity has also been reported to decrease linearly by 1.7m/s for each one degree drop in tissue temperature between 37 and 20 degrees Celsius (Lee and Bowen, 1975). Other authors have published tissue temperature-dependent ranges of sensory nerve conduction velocities in the cutaneous afferents of the ulnar and peroneal nerves (Miyamoto *et al.*, 1990). Distal sensory nerve conduction velocities in cats were reported to be slower than in the proximal segment of the same nerve (Aoki, 1977), likely to be due to a combination of a decrease in temperature of the limb distally and a decrease in fibre diameter in the distal part of the nerve. As discussed for motor nerve conduction studies, it is therefore always good practice to keep a close eye on the animals' temperature while performing electrophysiological studies.

5. Patterns of abnormalities

Sensory nerve conduction studies are less commonly performed in companion animals compared to motor nerve studies. This likely reflects the predominance of motor signs in animals presenting with neuromuscular disorders, the comparative rarity of pure sensory neuropathies, and a clinician's lack of confidence and familiarity compared to EMG and motor nerve studies. However, the same rules described for motor nerve conduction and compound muscle action potentials apply to sensory nerve action potentials.

A significant reduction in conduction velocity typically reflects demyelination, whilst a reduced amplitude reflects axonal loss. However, as described above, it is difficult to interpret a low amplitude for sensory nerve conduction studies compared to CMAPs, and a reduction in conduction velocity can also reflect loss of the largest diameter, fastest-conducting axons rather than demyelination alone.

An important concept to remember is that the SNAP and SNCV will remain normal if a proximal lesion at the level of the nerve root lies between the dorsal root ganglion and spinal cord, as long as the ganglion itself is spared. This is because of the anatomy of peripheral sensory neurons and how they differ from the anatomy of motor neurons (**Figure 7.9A and 7.9B**). Sensory neurons are bipolar neurons with a cell body that is located within a dorsal root ganglion at the level of the intervertebral foramen, rather than within the spinal cord grey matter. Central processes travel proximally from the cell body along the sensory nerve root and enter the dorsal horn of the spinal cord, whilst peripheral processes project distally as the peripheral sensory axons. If a lesion is located proximal to the dorsal root ganglion (i.e., sensory nerve root, sparing the cell bodies), then the peripheral processes will not undergo Wallerian degeneration and the SNAPs recorded at the sites described above (i.e., distally) will remain normal (NB: the cord dorsum potential will be absent in these cases – see

'Section 9 – Somatosensory evoked potentials'). If the lesion lies distal to the dorsal root ganglion, then the SNAP, SNCV and cord dorsum potential can all be affected.

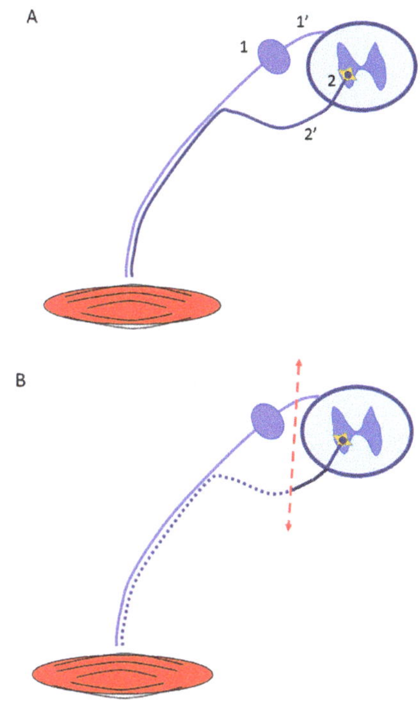

Figure 7.9A. Peripheral bipolar sensory neuron (purple) with its dorsal root ganglion (1) and dorsal sensory nerve root (1') located at the level of the intervertebral foramen. Central processes travel proximally from the cell body along the sensory nerve root and enter the dorsal horn of the spinal cord, whilst peripheral processes project distally as the peripheral sensory axons. Peripheral motor neuron (dark blue) with its cell body in the ventral horn of the spinal cord grey matter (2) and ventral motor nerve root (2'). **B.** Following a proximal lesion at the level of the nerve roots, proximal to the dorsal root ganglion (red dashed arrow), the peripheral processes of the sensory neurons are still connected to the cell body, don't undergo Wallerian degeneration and the SNAP and SNCV remain normal. The peripheral processes of the peripheral motor neurons undergo Wallerian degeneration and motor nerve conduction studies become abnormal. The latter would occur to a peripheral sensory nerve following a lesion distal to the dorsal root ganglion.

Another important consideration is that sensory nerve conduction studies only assess the large diameter, fast conducting sensory fibres (representing around 20 percent of all the sensory fibres within a nerve). Therefore, conventional sensory nerve conduction studies can be normal for disorders affecting the other 80 percent of fibres. These 'small fibre neuropathies' are widely recognised in humans and typically present as pain and/or autonomic dysfunction.

References

Aoki M. Distal slowing of conduction in forelimb and hindlimb myelinated cutaneous afferent fibers in cat. Exp Neurol. 1977 Jul;56(1):200-11. doi: 10.1016/0014-4886(77)90150-9. PMID: 862691.

Cuddon PA. Electrophysiology in neuromuscular disease. Vet Clin North Am Small Anim Pract. 2002 Jan;32(1):31-62. doi: 10.1016/s0195-5616(03)00079-2. PMID: 11785734.

Holliday TA, Ealand BG, Weldon NE. Sensory nerve conduction velocity: technical requirements and normal values for branches of the radial and ulnar nerves of the dog. Am J Vet Res. 1977 Oct;38(10):1543-51. PMID: 931137.

Kimura J. Electrodiagnosis in Diseases of Nerve and Muscle: Principles and Practice – 4th ed. Oxford University Press, 2013.

Lee AF, Bowen JM. Effect of tissue temperature on ulnar nerve conduction velocity in the dog. Am J Vet Res. 1975 Sep;36(9):1305-7. PMID: 1172401.

Miyamoto A, Sumi A, Ishido Y, Nakano T, Yahagi M, Inada S. Sensory nerve conduction velocities in the cutaneous afferents of the ulnar and peroneal nerves of the dog: tissue temperature-dependent reference ranges. Vet Res Commun. 1990;14(2):147-56. doi: 10.1007/BF00346555. PMID: 2345954.

Pillai SR, Steiss JE, Wright JC. Age-related changes in peripheral nerve conduction velocities of cats. Progress Vet Neurol 2:95-104, 1991.

Redding RW, Ingram JT, Colter SB. Sensory nerve conduction velocity of cutaneous afferents of the radial, ulnar, peroneal, and tibial nerves of the dog: reference values. Am J Vet Res. 1982 Mar;43(3):517-21. PMID: 7073069.

Redding RW, Ingram JT. Sensory nerve conduction velocity of cutaneous afferents of the radial, ulnar, peroneal, and tibial nerves of the cat: reference values. Am J Vet Res. 1984 May;45(5):1042-5. PMID: 6732011.

Schaeppi U, Teste M, Siegenthaler U. Sensory and motor maximum nerve conduction velocity in the peripheral and central nervous system of the beagle dog. Agents Actions. 1982 Oct;12(4):566-74. doi: 10.1007/BF01965943. PMID: 7180741.

Shapiro BE and Preston DC. Electromyography and Neuromuscular Disorders: Clinical-Electrophysiologic Correlations – 3rd ed. Elsevier Inc, 2013.

van Nes JJ. Sensory action potentials in the ulnar and radial nerves of dogs: effect of stimulation site and voltage. Am J Vet Res. 1985 May;46(5):1155-61. PMID: 4003890.

Whalen LR, Spurgeon TL, Carsten RE, Gould DH. Conduction velocities and reflexes of the proximal and distal parts of the saphenous nerve of the dog. Am J Vet Res. 1986 May;47(5):1063-70. PMID: 3717727.

SECTION 8

The H-reflex

Nicolas Granger, Edward Ives, Hélène Vandenberghe

Key points

- The H-reflex is the electrical equivalent of the monosynaptic stretch reflex.
- It is elicited by a submaximal stimulus and does not trigger an M- or F-wave.
- The impulse travels up the Ia sensory fibres of a mixed sensorimotor nerve to the spinal cord and synapses with the alpha motor neurons, with subsequent activation of the muscle fibres.
- It is particularly useful for the assessment of neuropathies involving both the afferent and efferent pathways and to quantify motor neuron excitability following spinal cord injury.

1. Definition

The H-reflex is an electrically-elicited monosynaptic reflex which is similar to a stretch reflex induced by tapping a tendon (*e.g.*, the patellar reflex). However, the primary difference is that a tendon reflex involves the stimulation of muscle spindles, whereas the H-reflex is initiated following direct electrical stimulation of peripheral sensory or mixed sensorimotor fibres. The H-reflex was

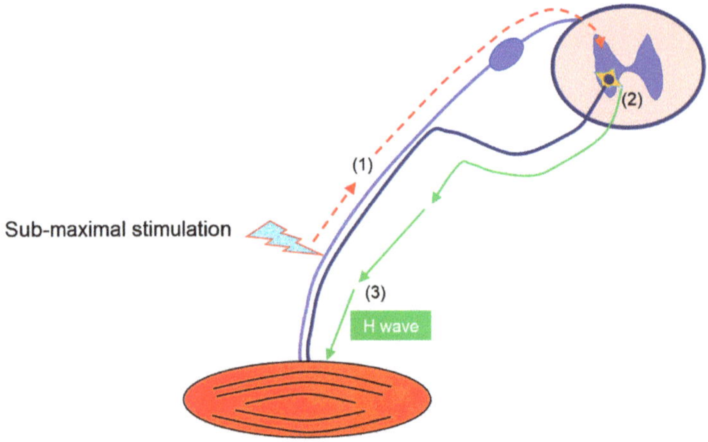

Figure 8.1. H-wave course. Sub-maximal electrical stimulation along a mixed sensorimotor nerve. In contrast to the supra-maximal stimulation used to elicit an F-wave, sub-maximal stimulation does not generate a descending or ascending potential along the motor axons, meaning that there should be no early M-wave or late F-wave in the recording. Sub-maximal stimulation instead evokes only an ascending potential along the sensory axons (1; dashed red arrows); this ascending potential reaches the dorsal root ganglion and enters the spinal cord grey matter to synapse with the lower motor neuron cell bodies in the ventral horn (2). This results in a descending motor potential and the H-wave (3; green arrows), recorded with a delay in comparison to the usual M-wave. The H-reflex is equivalent to a monosynaptic 'stretch' reflex induced by tapping a tendon, except that tapping a tendon involves the initial stimulation of muscle spindles.

first described by Hoffman in 1918 and was thus named after him as the 'Hoffman reflex' (Knecht *et al.*, 1983; Kimura 2013). It is a true reflex involving Ia sensory fibres, a single synapse in the spinal cord grey matter, and α motor neurons as the efferent arm. The ascending impulse enters the spinal cord *via* the dorsal root and synapses with the motor neuron cell bodies in the ventral horn of the grey matter, leading to a delayed motor response called the H-wave. As the initial stimulation used to generate the H-reflex is sub-maximal, the impulse only travels up the sensory fibres and does not stimulate the motor fibres in a mixed nerve, meaning there should be no initial M-wave (or F-wave) in the recording (**Figure 8.1**).

As mentioned above, the H-wave is obtained following sub-maximal stimulation of a mixed sensorimotor nerve (Poncelet and Balligand, 1991). If the intensity of stimulation is progressively increased from sub-maximal to supra-maximal, the Ia sensory fibres will be stimulated along with more and more motor fibres, generating: (i) an initial M-wave and (ii) an antidromic motor volley leading to an F-wave (see 'Section 5 – The F-wave'). The amplitude of the H-wave will decrease as the M-wave amplitude increases (Knecht and Redding, 1981; Sims and Selcer, 1981; Knecht *et al.*, 1983) (**Figure 8.2**). This is because the antidromic ascending motor potentials, that lead to backfiring of the spinal cord motor neurons and generation of the F-wave, collide with the descending potentials that would generate the H-wave. This results in disappearance of the H-reflex and appearance of the

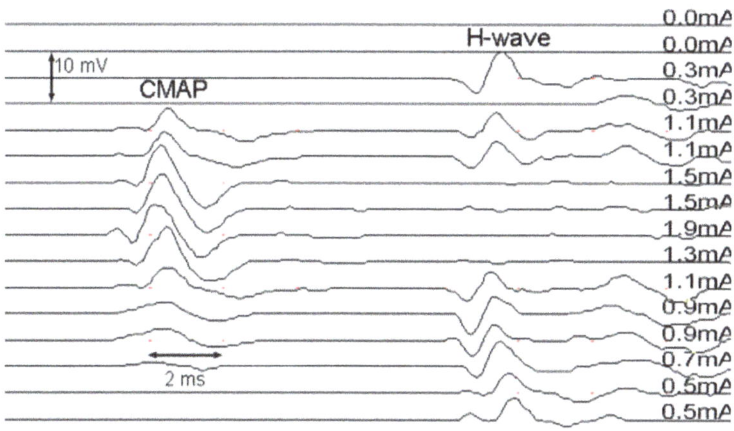

Figure 8.2. H-waves and compound muscle action potentials (M-waves) during repetitive distal sciatic-tibial nerve stimulation at increasing and then decreasing stimulation intensities in a dog under general anaesthesia (see intensity on the right side of the image). For low stimulation intensities (sub-maximal stimulation up to 0.5mA), only the H-wave is generated. For slightly higher stimulation intensities which are still sub-maximal (0.7-1.1mA), the M-wave is also generated, with a shorter latency given the shorter pathway between the stimulation and recording sites for the M-wave *versus* H-wave. The amplitude of the H-wave then decreases and is finally abolished as the stimulation intensity increases, resulting from collision of ascending motor potentials and the descending potentials that would usually result in the H-wave (maximal and supra-maximal stimulations, 1.3 to 1.9mA in this instance).

F-wave that typically has a slightly longer latency. The amplitude of the H-wave is lower than the expected amplitude of the M-wave at supra-maximal stimulation intensities (Sims and Selcer, 1981).

2. Stimulating and recording technique

The H-reflex is obtained by placing stimulating needles near the ulnar nerve or sciatic-tibial nerve, as for motor nerve conduction studies (with the distal stimulation sites preferable). The recording needles are placed in the palmar or plantar interosseous muscles respectively (Knecht *et al.*, 1983).

A sub-maximal stimulation intensity is used initially, which selectively stimulates the Ia sensory fibres and not the motor fibres, with a stimulus rate of one per five seconds (0.2Hz). The optimal duration and voltage of electrical rectangular pulsed stimuli are 0.1-0.2ms and less than 80 volts, respectively (Sims, 1982; Knecht *et al.*, 1983). The same high and low frequency filters are used as for recording of M-waves.

The amplitude of the H-reflex is markedly affected by the type of anaesthesia employed. For instance, the use of halothane and nitrous oxide combination results in a significantly lower amplitude of the H-wave compared to that recorded under pentobarbitone (Malik and Ho, 1991). The length of the H-reflex arc, and therefore latency of the H-wave, also varies with the size of the animal and limb length (Nafe and Lee, 1983).

In humans, the H-reflex is present for most nerves in the first year of life. However, after 2 to 3 years of age it only persists in the plantar and *flexor carpi radialis* muscles, meaning that it is only obtained following stimulation of the tibial and median nerves after that time. This is a good example of the inhibition imposed by the central nervous system on the lower motor neurons as the body matures, and the concept of 'upper motor neurons' inhibiting 'lower motor neurons' (Fisher, 1992; Lewis *et al.*, 2017). The H-reflex can be elicited equally well following stimulation of the sciatic-tibial and ulnar nerves in both neonates and adult dogs (Sims and Selcer, 1981).

3. Waveform analysis

The H-reflex has been studied for the ulnar and sciatic-tibial nerves in dogs and cats, including the latencies, amplitudes, mixed (orthodromic sensory and antidromic motor) conduction velocities and H-reflex latency/limb length ratio.

In dogs, the reported latencies for the proximal and the distal ulnar nerve stimulation sites were 15.4 +/- 2.5ms and 18.3 +/- 2.6ms, respectively (mean +/- SD) (Nafe and Lee, 1983). Mean amplitudes of the H-wave were 1.8 +/- 0.4mV following proximal and 1.6 +/- 0.5mV following distal stimulation of the ulnar nerve (Sims and Selcer, 1981).

The H-reflex recorded from the *plantar interosseous* muscle following stimulation of the sciatic-tibial nerve in the dog had a reported mean latency of 20ms +/- 2ms, with a mean H-wave amplitude of 1.6 +/- 0.9mV (Malik and Ho, 1991). The mixed (orthodromic sensory and antidromic motor) conduction velocity was reported to be 75.2 +/-13.1m/s for the ulnar nerve (Nafe and Lee, 1983).

The thoracic limb length/H-reflex latency ratio has been established for the assessment of proximal neuropathies in the thoracic limb of the dog (Nafe and Lee, 1983) and can be calculated as follows:

Ratio = thoracic limb length (up to C7 vertebra) (mm)/H-latency (proximal or distal stimulation site) (ms).

Reported values were 27.5 +/- 3.9 for the proximal stimulation site (elbow) and 23 +/- 2.7 for the distal stimulation site (accessory carpal bone) for the ulnar nerve (Nafe and Lee, 1983).

In cats, for the ulnar and sciatic-tibial nerves, the conduction velocities of the H-reflex were 49.1 +/- 7.3 and 44.1 +/- 2.7m/s, respectively. The H-wave response of cats was more variable in latency and amplitude than that reported in the dog (Knecht *et al.*, 1985).

4. Patterns of abnormalities

The most interesting clinical application of the H-reflex is that it evaluates both the afferent and efferent pathways (ascending sensory nerve fibres, dorsal root and then motor nerve root function). Therefore, for the sciatic-tibial and ulnar nerves, the H-reflex can provide valuable information that is not available from the M-wave or F-wave recordings. For example, the latency of the H-reflex can be used to document slow conduction velocity found with some peripheral neuropathies.

The amplitude of the H-wave depends on: (i) the intensity of electrical stimulation; and (ii) the α motor neuron excitability. Therefore, if the intensity of the stimulation remains constant, the variation in H-wave amplitude provides a quantitative measure of motor neuron excitability (Sims, 1982). The H-reflex has been used in humans with spinal cord injury (and in dogs in one study) to assess the degree of motor neuron hyperexcitability. The amplitude of the H-wave increases after injury, which constitutes a sign of disinhibition (e.g., loss of upper motor neuron control on the lower motor neuron cell bodies) (*Lewis et al.,* 2017). Subsequent clinical recovery might be associated with a reduction and return to normal of the H-wave amplitude, which could be a topic for further research in dogs.

References

Fisher MA. AAEM Minimonograph #13: H reflexes and F waves: physiology and clinical indications. Muscle Nerve. 1992 Nov;15(11):1223-33. doi: 10.1002/mus.880151102. PMID: 1488060.

Kimura J. Electrodiagnosis in Diseases of Nerve and Muscle: Principles and Practice – 4th ed. Oxford University Press, 2013.

Knecht CD, Redding RW. Monosynaptic reflex (H wave) in clinically normal and abnormal dogs. Am J Vet Res. 1981 Sep;42(9):1586-9. PMID: 7325467.

Knecht CD, Redding R, Hyams D. Stimulation techniques and response characteristics of the M and F waves and H reflex in dogs. Vet Res Commun. 1983 Mar;6(2):123-32. doi: 10.1007/BF02214904. PMID: 6868351.

Knecht CD, Redding RW, Wilson S. Characteristics of F and H waves of ulnar and tibial nerves in cats: Reference values. Am J Vet Res 46:977-979, 1985. PMID: 4014851.

Lewis MJ, Howard JF Jr, Olby NJ. The Relationship between Trans-Lesional Conduction, Motor Neuron Pool Excitability, and Motor Function in Dogs with Incomplete Recovery from Severe Spinal Cord Injury. J Neurotrauma. 2017 Nov 1;34(21):2994-3002. doi: 10.1089/neu.2017.5012. Epub 2017 Jun 16. PMID: 28462632; PMCID: PMC6436022.

Malik R, Ho S. A new method for recording H-reflexes from the plantar muscles of dogs. J Small Anim Pract 32:547 -556, 1991. doi: 10.1111/j.1748-5827.1991.tb00884.x

Nafe LA, Lee AF. Evaluation of evoked-muscle potentials from stimulation of ulnar nerves of the dog. Am J Vet Res. 1983 Apr;44(4):669-73. PMID: 6869963.

Poncelet L, Balligand M. Nature of the late potentials and F-ratio values in dogs. Res Vet Sci. 1991 Jul;51(1):1-5. doi: 10.1016/0034-5288(91)90021-f. PMID: 1896622.

Sims MH. Recovery cycle of the reflex-evoked muscle potential (H reflex): excitability of spinal motor neurons in the healthy dog. Am J Vet Res. 1982 Jan;43(1):89-93. PMID: 7091820.

Sims MH, Selcer RR. Occurrence and evaluation of a reflex-evoked muscle potential (H reflex) in the normal dog. Am J Vet Res. 1981 Jun;42(6):975-83. PMID: 7283248.

SECTION 9

Somatosensory evoked potentials

Nicolas Granger, Edward Ives, Hélène Vandenberghe

Key points:

- Somatosensory evoked potentials are electrical potentials recorded at different levels along the somatosensory pathways following peripheral electrical stimulation of sensory or mixed nerves.
- Somatosensory evoked potentials elicited after stimulation of the tibial nerve are the sciatic root component at L7–S1, the cord dorsum potential at L4-L5, the ascending evoked potential along the entire spinal cord, the medullary component at the level of the cisterna magna, and the scalp somatosensory potential at the level of the contralateral parietal lobe.
- Knowing the correlation between individual potentials and their neuroanatomic origin assists in the localisation of lesions along the somatosensory pathway.

1. Definitions and overview

Evoked potentials are electrical potentials recorded following stimulation of nervous structures. They can be sensory or motor, depending on the anatomical site of stimulation. They also vary dependent on the type of stimulus used. For example, electrical or magnetic stimulation of a mixed peripheral nerve will elicit a compound motor action potential in the muscle(s) innervated by this nerve, in addition to a somatosensory evoked potential (SSEP) at the level of the contralateral sensory cortex following ascending conduction along the spinal cord. In a similar manner, magnetic stimulation of the primary motor cortex will elicit a compound motor action potential in the contralateral appendicular muscles, called a magnetic motor evoked potential (see 'Section 11 – Magnetic motor evoked potentials')

Evoked potentials are useful because they are generally time-locked to the stimulus (i.e., their latencies are predictable) and the anatomical structures responsible for some of these potentials are known along the course of a neural pathway (near-field or far-field potentials – see definitions in 'Section 1 – Anatomy and physiology of the peripheral nervous system and principles of electrophysiology'). There is a nomenclature associated with each nerve in humans that describes the latencies of expected peaks (Kimura, 2013). Field potentials are different to moving action potentials and they represent synchronous, summated electrical activity recorded from the extracellular space adjacent to electrically active cells (e.g., neuronal synaptic activity). They are slightly more challenging to record than moving potentials because the recording needles need to be as close to the neural generator as possible. If the recording electrodes are further away, the amplitude of the recorded waveform will be markedly reduced. However, the latency of field potentials is not dependent on the location of the recording electrodes and therefore constitutes a robust parameter. For moving action potentials, the latency increases as the recording point is moved further away from the stimulation site (Kimura, 2013).

The study of evoked potentials is most widely used to determine whether an area of the brain, spinal cord or the spinal nerve roots can receive/transmit sensory information following electrical stimulation of a peripheral nerve. These somatosensory evoked potentials are small and best separated from background noise by using a series of stimulations and signal averaging (as for other sensory nerve conduction studies, see 'Section 7 – Appendicular sensory nerve conduction studies'). It is also good practice to conduct at least two sets of recordings so that they can be superimposed on the screen of the computer to ensure that the recorded potentials are real. If in doubt, running a recording without any stimulation will allow observation of the background noise alone, to ensure that this has not been misinterpreted as the potential(s) of interest. Motor responses following stimulation of the central nervous system are typically studied following magnetic brain stimulation which is covered in 'Section 11 – Magnetic motor evoked potentials'. The remainder of this chapter will therefore focus on somatosensory evoked potentials.

2. Anatomic and physiologic basis of somatosensory evoked potentials

Somatosensory evoked potentials (SSEPs) are electrical potentials originating from the somatosensory pathways following stimulation of a sensory or mixed sensorimotor peripheral nerve (Holliday, 1992; Cuddon, 2002). Some of these potentials are moving and some are static field potentials. The most common type of stimulation used in the clinic is electrical, but mechanical stimulation (such as a pinprick, vibration or painful stimulus) can also elicit SSEPs (Holliday, 1992; Kimura 2013). The somatosensory pathway (also known as the 'dorsal-column medial lemniscal pathway') is composed of: (1) touch, proprioception and pain receptors from skin, joints or muscles, giving rise to Ia afferents; (2) the sensory axons of the peripheral nerve; (3) the dorsal root ganglion from which the radicular axons emerge, enter the spinal cord and synapse ipsilaterally with the dorsal column nuclei (spinal cord entry zone); (4) the dorsal ascending spinal cord tracts (located ipsilaterally and contralaterally in the dorsolateral funiculus) up to the dorsal column nuclei in the medulla, where the fibres decussate; and (5) the fibres projecting to the thalamus and, finally, the somatosensory cortex (cruciate sulcus and parietal lobe) (Holliday *et al.*, 1979; Cuddon, 2002; Passmore *et al.*, 2014).

Therefore, if one stimulates the tibial nerve for example, this will give rise to five different potentials that can be recorded in dogs or cats (**Figure 9.1**): (i) an ascending (moving) potential, at the level of the L7-S1 intervertebral space, where the sciatic root component enters the spinal canal and forms the *cauda equina*; (ii) a field potential at the level of the L4-L5 intervertebral space, where the dorsal root axons synapse with the interneurons of the lumbar intumescence – this is termed the 'cord dorsum potential', but is also sometimes referred to as the 'root entry zone potential'; (iii) ascending 'moving' potentials that can be followed and recorded along the entire spinal cord, termed 'ascending evoked potentials'; (iv) a field potential from synaptic activity of the nuclei in the medulla at the level of the *cisterna magna;* and (v) a field potential from the sensory cortical grey matter of the parietal lobe, termed the 'scalp somatosensory potential' (Holliday *et al.*, 1979; Besalti *et al.*, 1990). It therefore now becomes clear that recording of these various somatosensory evoked potentials allows the study of the entire ascending (sensory) pathways and gives the possibility to break it down into segments.

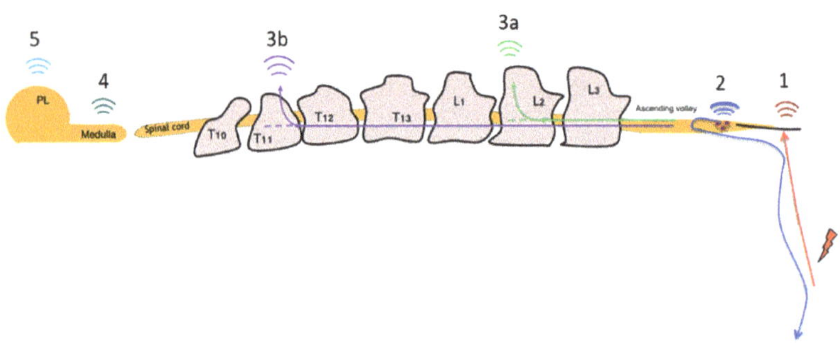

Figure 9.1. Somatosensory evoked potentials and their recording sites following stimulation of the sciatic-tibial nerve. 1. Ascending potential at the level of the L7-S1 intervertebral space (nerve roots entering the spinal canal to form the *cauda equina*); 2. Cord dorsum potential at the level of the L4-L5 intervertebral space; 3a and 3b. Ascending potentials recorded along the spinal cord; 4. Field potential recorded at the level of the cisterna magna; and 5. Field potential recorded from the sensory cortex in the parietal lobe (PL).

3. Cord dorsum potential (CDP) in the lumbar and thoracic regions: recording protocol and utility

Recording of cord dorsum potentials is technically accessible to clinicians wishing to use evoked potentials in the clinic and one that has been studied in a clinical context. In the next section, we focus on the lumbar cord dorsum potential which allows study of the integrity of the sciatic nerve root entry zone, an anatomical region that is commonly affected by stenosis (Cuddon *et al.*, 1999).

(i) Stimulation

The stimulation set-up for cord dorsum potentials is the same as described earlier for motor nerve conduction studies, with a bipolar arrangement using two stimulating electrodes (a cathode and an anode). The needles can be either Teflon coated with a bare-tip (these are longer) or platinum subdermal needles (these are shorter). The choice of needle generally depends on the depth of the nerve to be stimulated and preference of the examiner. However, one advantage of coated needles is that the insulation provided by the Teflon minimises direct stimulation of other tissues, such as muscles, near to the nerve (Holliday, 1992; Cuddon, 2002).

To record a cord dorsum potential in the lumbar region, the tibial nerve (mixed sensorimotor nerve) is typically stimulated (Cuddon *et al.*, 1999). The stimulation site is just above the tarsus between the gastrocnemius tendon and the tibia, with the cathode placed distal to the anode (**Figure 9.2**). It is important to use a distal stimulation site so that the slower ascending impulse travelling through the ventral motor nerve root (i.e., antidromic volley) arrives after the faster sensory impulse and does not interfere with the cord dorsum potential recording by reaching the root first (Cuddon *et al.*, 1999).

The stimulus waveform is a monophasic rectangular impulse of 0.1 – 0.2 millisecond duration (the authors routinely use 0.2

millisecond), at a repetition frequency varying between 3 and 5Hz (the authors routinely use 3Hz). The amplitude of the evoked potential is in the microvolt range, compared to the millivolt range for a compound muscle action potential. Therefore, as for other sensory studies, repetitive stimulation is used and the recordings are averaged to suppress background noise. In addition, possible sources of interference (such as nearby muscles or ECG artefact) must be rejected using a suitable amplification and signal processing system. In the authors' experience, a series of ~1000 repetitions is sufficient, with averaging of at least 256 responses generally recommended (Holliday, 1992).

The stimulation intensity should be such that it just produces a small twitch of the interosseous muscles. It should then be adjusted to 50% greater than that which gave a visible foot twitch, at which point the large myelinated afferent sensory fibres are recruited (Passmore *et al.*, 2014). Using higher intensity stimulation does not change the recorded waveform to a great extent because the large fibres are already recruited and are those that conduct more current with the least resistance.

(ii) Recording

The recording electrodes should be needle electrodes with insulated shafts to minimise their exposure to electrical activity arising from surrounding muscles, and be long enough to reach the vertebral lamina (Holliday, 1992). The best filtering window can be found empirically for each practice, with suggested values being a high pass of 3-20Hz, and low pass of over 2kHz (Poncelet *et al.*, 1999; Passmore *et al.*, 2014) – the authors have successfully used a high pass of 30Hz and low pass of over 3kHz. For the screen display, the gain can be initially set at 10 µV/division and the sweep speed at 5ms/cm.

The active recording needle is placed as close as possible to the source of the signal (i.e., the lumbosacral intumescence for the recording of cord dorsum potential following pelvic limb stimulation). Therefore, the aim is to place the tip of this needle next to the interarcuate ligament between two lumbar spinous processes of interest (Holliday, 1992). The location of the lumbosacral intumescence within the spinal canal varies dependent on the size, breed and species of the animal. The spinal cord of large breed dogs terminates more cranially within the spinal canal than that of small breed dogs, meaning that the lumbar intumescence is also more cranially located in those breeds. Therefore, the active recording needle is placed between the L5 and L6 spinous processes in small breed dogs and between the L4 and L5 processes in large breed dogs (**Figure 9.2**). In support of this, a study by Campbell *et al.* (2013) reported that the largest cord dorsum potentials were recorded from the L4-5 and L5-6 intervertebral spaces in dogs, which is the same as that reported for cats (Nordwall *et al.*, 1979; Cuddon, 2002).

Practically, the active recording needle is inserted in the midline between the two chosen spinous processes and advanced until the bone of the vertebral lamina is felt. The anode is then placed ~2cm away from the active electrode on the opposite side of the stimulated pelvic limb (Holliday, 1992).

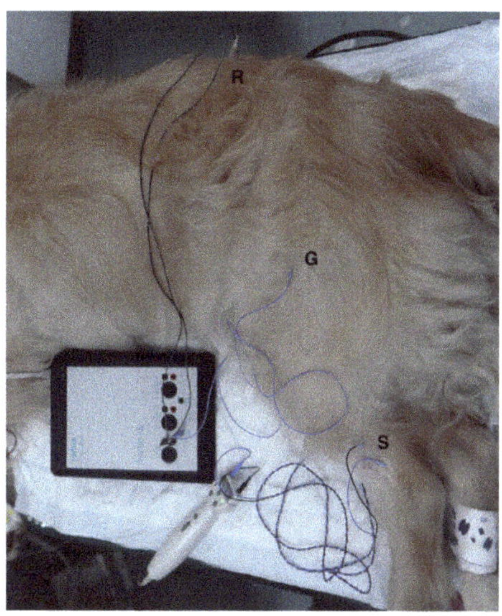

Figure 9.2. Electrode set up for the stimulation and recording of cord dorsum potentials in the pelvic limb. **S**: stimulation site just above the tarsus between the gastrocnemius tendon and the tibia, with the cathode (-) placed distal to the anode (+). **R**: recording site with the active recording needle (-) inserted in the midline between the spinous processes of L4 and L5 in this case, and the anode (+) placed ~2cm away on the opposite side of the stimulated pelvic limb. **G**: reference ('ground') electrode placed subcutaneously between the stimulating and recording electrodes.

Cord dorsum potentials can also be recorded from the cervicothoracic intumescence following stimulation of the radial or ulnar nerve in the thoracic limb – distal ulnar nerve stimulation at the level of the carpus is usually chosen by the authors. However, recording of cord dorsum potentials from the cervicothoracic region is less widely performed than for the lumbar region, perhaps because of the greater prevalence of lumbosacral disorders in dogs, and is not discussed in detail here. Briefly, the active recording needle is placed cranial to the spinous process of T1 with the aim to have the tip of the needle above the C7-T1 interarcuate ligament; the reader is referred to the references and further reading for more detail (Cuddon *et al.*, 1999).

(iii) Cord dorsum potential morphology

A cord dorsum potential is composed of an initial small triphasic wave, followed by a larger negative wave and, finally, a longer but smaller positive wave returning to baseline (**Figure 9.3**) (Holliday, 1992; Cuddon, 2002).

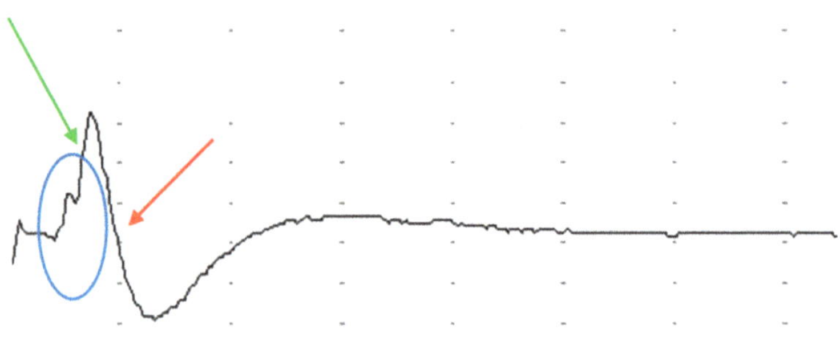

Figure 9.3. Morphology of a normal cord dorsum potential. Triphasic wave (blue circle), followed by a large negative deflection (green arrow) and then a slower positive deflection (red arrow). Horizontal scale = 6ms/division, vertical scale = 2μV/division.

The first triphasic wave is a compound nerve action potential originating from electrical events in the peripheral axons as the sensory wave progresses towards the spinal cord interneurons (dorsal roots and branches towards the spinal cord). It acts as a useful marker to confirm that the recording corresponds to a cord dorsum potential and is composed of the following:

- A small initial downward deflection reflecting a capacitive current flowing outside the axons created by the initial entry of sodium ions at distant nodes of Ranvier and positive charges flowing near/towards the active electrode (meaning that the potential difference between the anode and active recording electrode is negative).
- Then, following the entry of sodium ions at the node of Ranvier closest to the active electrode, the extracellular space becomes negative, which creates an upwards deflection of the trace (the difference in potential between the anode and the active recording electrode now being positive).
- Finally, there is efflux of positive potassium (K^+) charges outside the axons (hyperpolarisation) restoring the extracellular positivity and generating a last downward deflection (Holliday, 1992).

Following the triphasic wave, the interneurons *within* the spinal cord generate a large negative field potential composed of one (or less commonly two) subpeaks of a few milliseconds duration. This is the 'true' cord dorsum potential and originates from the depolarisation of interneurons in the dorsal aspect of the spinal cord grey matter – positive sodium (Na^+) charges enter the interneurons at the level of the synapses and exit more ventrally where these cells project their axons near to the ventral horn of the spinal cord. Therefore, the dorsal region of the spinal cord becomes more negatively charged, the ventral region more positive, and the potential difference between the active recording and the anode electrodes more positive. As described in 'Section 1 – Anatomy and physiology of the peripheral nervous system and principles of electrophysiology' this, perhaps counterintuitively, leads to an upwards deflection of the trace reflecting increased *negative* charge (less positivity) in the extracellular space adjacent to the active electrode. This entry of sodium within the cells, depleting the extracellular space, is also called a 'sink-source' phenomenon (Holliday, 1992).

Eventually, there is a slow, low amplitude positive phase seen as a downward deflection of the trace and a return to (or beyond) baseline. This part of the waveform reflects the movement of positive charges to the dorsal aspect of the spinal cord (regaining positivity), with entry of sodium charges in the pre-synaptic axons in the ventral aspect of the cord and their re-entry into the extracellular space dorsally (Holliday, 1992).

(iv) Normal values of the cord dorsum potential at the lumbar and cervicothoracic level in dogs

As one can see from its anatomical basis and the description above, the cord dorsum potential is a purely sensory event and contains no motor information. The latency of the main negative peak of the cord dorsum potential does not vary because it is a field potential reflecting static electrical activity from interneurons at a specific site. However, the amplitude can be greatly influenced by the distance of the active recording needle from the neurons generating the signal. This makes amplitude data difficult to interpret and of little clinical use between patients. Normal data and formulas that take into account limb/body length have been published to determine the cord dorsum potential onset latency in dogs (Cuddon *et al.*, 1999). Regression equations are not used in cats as there is little variation in limb length for this species.

For the tibial nerve, the expected cord dorsum potential onset latency at L4-5 in dogs is defined as:

-1.194 + (0.014 x pelvic limb length [in mm])

The pelvic limb length is the distance between the greater trochanter and the tip of the middle digit.

Mean +/- SD for CDP onset to peak latency difference = 3.1 +/- 0.3 milliseconds.

For the radial nerve, the expected cord dorsum potential onset latency at C7-T1 in dogs is defined as:

-0.9 + (0.014 x thoracic limb length [in mm])

Mean +/- SD for CDP onset to peak latency difference = 3.0 +/- 0.4 milliseconds.

(v) Clinical utility of the cord dorsum potential at the lumbar level in dogs

In comparison to other tests (e.g., EMG and motor nerve conduction studies), the clinical use of cord dorsum potentials in companion animals has been relatively underreported. Of note, Meij *et al.* (2006) reported an increased latency and reduced amplitude of the cord dorsum potential (CDP) in 21 dogs with L7-S1 foraminal stenosis compared to 11 weight-matched control dogs. In this study, the latency of the main negative peak ('true' CDP) was significantly different in dogs with lumbosacral stenosis (8.6 +/- 0.2ms) compared to control dogs (7.4 +/- 0.2ms) and was suggested to reflect the clinical affectation in those dogs (Meij *et al.*, 2006).

Another more recent study from Harcourt-Brown *et al.* (2019) confirmed and extended these findings: in 25 dogs with lumbosacral stenosis diagnosed from MRI and presenting clinical signs consistent with lumbosacral stenosis (e.g., being reluctant to jump, pain on ventrally directed palpation of the lumbosacral spine, a positive lordosis test etc.), compared to 20 normal dogs with normal lumbosacral MRI, the authors found that cord dorsum potential onset latency was increased: the mean cord dorsum potential onset delay was 1.01ms (SD = 1.55ms) in affected dogs versus 0.02ms (SD = 0.58ms) in unaffected dogs. Interestingly, other electrophysiological parameters were also significantly different between groups: (i) 11 of 25 affected dogs had at least one pelvic limb muscle group affected on EMG compared to 3 of 20 normal dogs ; (ii) the mean F-wave latency delay was longer in MRI-affected dogs compared to MRI-unaffected dogs; (iii) the mean F-ratio of MRI-affected dogs was larger than the mean F-ratio of MRI-unaffected dogs. This altogether demonstrates the utility of electrophysiology alongside advanced imaging when investigating such cases (Harcourt-Brown *et al.*, 2019).

4. Other somatosensory evoked potentials

Various other somatosensory evoked potentials can be recorded in small animals such as ascending evoked potentials along the nerve roots and spinal cord, or static field potentials originating from the medulla at the level of the *cisterna magna*, or from the sensory cortical grey matter in the parietal lobe ('scalp somatosensory potentials') (Holliday, 1992).

(i) The root component

Recording the moving potential as it ascends along a nerve root and enters the spinal canal is possible and corresponds to a sensory nerve compound action potential. This is the same as recording a sensory potential along a peripheral nerve following electrical stimulation of the skin (see 'Section 7 – Appendicular sensory nerve conduction studies'). There is, however, little description of these recordings in dogs. Poncelet (1999) described the L6-7 root component in a normal dog, but it appears that this is rarely performed in practice, perhaps because one can also gather information about sensory conduction along nerve roots via the H-wave and cord dorsum potentials. The root component is therefore not described further here.

(ii) Ascending evoked potentials along the spinal cord

a. Anatomical considerations relating to ascending evoked spinal cord potentials

Ascending evoked potentials are recorded from electrodes placed cranial to the lumbar intumescence and caudal to the atlas, following electrical stimulation of skin, muscle or a sensory nerve carrying afferents from these structures. They are compound action potentials of small amplitude transmitted in spinal cord sensory pathways. Ascending impulses travel in all regions of the spinal cord, but mostly in the dorsal quadrant ipsilateral to the stimulated nerve, particularly in the dorsolateral funiculus and dorsal columns – muscle afferents ascend through the dorsolateral funiculus at velocities ranging from 100-120m/s, whereas skin afferents ascend through the dorsal column axons at velocities ranging from 70-90m/s (Snyder and Holliday, 1984). Some ascending potentials are also associated with synaptic transmission to second order neurons, introducing synaptic delays of ~0.5msec.

Stimulation of a mixed sensorimotor nerve is indiscriminate and will therefore give rise to moving potentials along both muscle and skin afferents from the site of stimulation. Therefore, an important factor to consider is where the peripheral nerve is stimulated along its course (e.g., distal *versus* proximal), as this will dictate which of the dorsolateral funiculus or dorsum column pathways contributes most to the recorded spinal cord potential. In short, because of the difference in conduction velocity along both the peripheral and spinal cord pathways for cutaneous and muscle afferents, the closer to the spinal cord the stimulation site, the greater the contribution of the fastest ascending potentials through the dorsolateral funiculus to the ascending spinal cord potential. Three more factors can also be considered: (i) the muscle mass will influence the morphology of the dorsolateral funiculus (fastest) ascending potentials; (ii) the body temperature (a low temperature increases the latency); and (iii) the conduction velocity in the cervical cord is slower than the conduction velocity more caudally, because some ascending spinal cord axons conduct more slowly in their terminal portions (Park and Hyun, 2015).

The consequence of these various factors is that the appearance and velocities of ascending evoked potentials along the spinal cord may vary and show a degree of temporal dispersion. Clinically, there is little published data in dogs, particularly comparing different techniques in different breeds and normal versus affected dogs, therefore, the utility of ascending evoked potentials along the spinal cord remains unclear. Nevertheless, we will provide a brief description of how to acquire these recordings for clinicians wishing to attempt them.

b. Recording and velocity calculation protocols for ascending evoked spinal cord potentials

A pair of stimulating needles (an anode and cathode) are placed adjacent to a peripheral sensory or mixed nerve in the pelvic or thoracic limb. The active recording needle is placed between two spinous processes to reach the vertebral lamina at the chosen level of recording. The anodal recording electrode is placed ~2cm lateral to the midline, contralateral to the stimulated nerve. Placement of the recording electrodes can be challenging in the thoracic region as the interarcuate space is covered by the dorsal spinous process of the vertebra located immediately cranial to that space, in which case the electrode can be placed just lateral to the base of the spinous process. In the cervical region, the depth of the soft tissues down to the vertebral laminae can also make accurate needle placement challenging, in which case placement of the electrodes can be verified using radiography (Holliday, 1992; Poncelet *et al.,* 1993a). Note that recording of ascending potentials in the cervical spinal cord following stimulation of a thoracic limb peripheral nerve can be obscured by the medullary component described later.

To measure the velocity of an ascending spinal cord potential, the first peak of the evoked potential is used, which will represent either a potential from the ipsilateral dorsolateral funiculus or dorsal column dependent on the site of stimulation along the peripheral nerve (see above). Ideally, the conduction velocity should be calculated by comparing spinal cord potentials of a similar morphology recorded from at least two sites along the spinal cord. If not, one can measure the distance between the L7-S1 site and the spinal cord recording site, and then divide this distance by the latency between the onset of the L7-S1 nerve root potential (or CDP) and the onset of the ascending evoked potential. It is important to interpret the results in light of the type of nerve stimulated, the level of stimulation (e.g., distal *versus* proximal) and the position of the recording electrodes, which all determine if the ascending evoked potential is propagated in the dorsal column or in the dorsolateral funiculus, and therefore the expected conduction velocity (Holliday, 1992). Some normal values have been reported for dogs and cats, and the reader is referred to the references for further reading (Redding *et al.*, 1984; Steiss and Wright, 1990; Poncelet, 1999).

c. Clinical use of ascending evoked spinal cord potentials

It is firstly important to mention that ascending evoked spinal cord potentials extinguish more easily after injury compared to somatosensory evoked potentials recorded from the brain, which may in part explain the paucity of data in companion animals (Schramm *et al.*, 1983a; Schramm *et al.*, 1983b). Historically, ascending spinal cord potentials have been investigated in companion dogs with acute thoracolumbar spinal cord injury caused by disc herniation: the general conclusion is that these potentials are not detectable in dogs that lack 'deep pain' perception, although Shores *et al.* (1987) reported that this was possible in some cases (Shores et al, 1987; Poncelet *et al.*, 1993b). Ascending evoked spinal cord potentials are also inconsistently recorded in other grades of acute thoracolumbar spinal cord injury (in dogs with preserved pain perception in the pelvic limbs) in which we know that the recovery rate is high (Poncelet *et al.*, 1993b). Therefore, there is a high rate of false negative findings in the acute phase, meaning that the absence of detectable ascending spinal cord potentials rostral to the lesion site in a dog with thoracolumbar spinal cord injury does not predict absence of recovery, irrespective of the grade of injury. The presence of detectable ascending spinal cord potentials above the lesion in a dog with thoracolumbar injury and no 'deep pain' suggests that some axons remain functional across the lesion but whether this correlates with recovery is currently unknown.

In the chronic phase of severe injury in dogs with clinically complete spinal cord lesions (i.e., paraplegic with no deep pain perception), ascending spinal cord evoked potentials can be detected above the lesion but do not correlate with recovery of spinal walking or return of deep pain (Hu *et al.*, 2018a; Hu *et al.*, 2018b). With chronic focal lesions (e.g., a slowly growing mass), ascending spinal cord evoked potentials can be detected above the lesion, as well as in ambulatory dogs with chronic thoracolumbar disc herniation (Poncelet *et al.*, 1993b).

Interestingly, a specific waveform called an 'injury potential' can be recorded at the site of spinal cord injury and is recognisable as a large amplitude, long duration, two-peak monophasic positive potential, approximately 40ms in duration, with a slight negative after wave, in experimental cats (Schramm *et al.*, 1983a). This type of injury potential appears as the recording site is moved closer and closer to the lesion site, and then disappears as the recording electrodes are moved away (cranially) from the lesion. The potential also changes polarity either side of the lesion. It was initially thought that the point of appearance and disappearance of the injury potential could be used to predict the extent of spinal cord injury, but this did not correlate with the presence/absence of clinical recovery in subsequent studies (Shores *et al.*, 1987; Poncelet *et al.*, 1998).

(iii) The medullary component

At the level of the cisterna magna, a field potential arising from synaptic activity within nuclei in the medulla occurs. This reflects the significant role this region plays in relaying ascending sensory information ('conscious' proprioception from the dorsal columns and 'unconscious' proprioception from the spinocerebellar tracts) via interneurons to higher brain centres, such as the thalamus, cerebellum and somatosensory cortex. Stimulation is typically performed using a thoracic peripheral nerve, such as the median or ulnar nerve, and recording by placing an active needle electrode dorsal to the arch of C1, with the anode placed ~2cm lateral to the midline and contralateral to the stimulated side.

The clinical utility of medullary potentials remains underreported. In Cavalier King Charles Spaniel dogs, it was found that those with syringomyelia had reduced amplitudes of the first negative peak and first positive peak of the medullary potential compared to those without syringomyelia (Harcourt-Brown *et al.*, 2011).

(iv) Somatosensory evoked potentials from the scalp

a. Anatomical considerations related to somatosensory evoked potentials from the scalp

Somatosensory evoked potentials from the scalp are field potentials originating from the cerebral cortex. They result from stimulation of a peripheral nerve (typically the tibial or ulnar nerve), with the ascending sensory potential entering the spinal cord via the sensory nerve root, ascending along the spinal cord ipsilateral to the stimulated side, decussating in the *medulla oblongata* to the contralateral medial lemniscus and thalamus, and finally reaching the contralateral somatosensory cerebral cortex (cruciate sulcus and parietal region).

b. Stimulation and recording of cortical somatosensory evoked potentials

The influence of different recording locations was reported in 5 dogs following stimulation of the tibial or median nerve: (i) recording contralateral to the site of stimulation generally gave the best recordings, although in 2 of 5 dogs ipsilateral potentials were recorded and not contralateral; (ii) recording at the anatomical point called the 'bregma' (the point of crossing of the coronal and sagittal sutures, at the caudal margin of the frontal bone) and just lateral to the midline gave the best waves (Vanderzant *et al.*, 1989).

Cortical somatosensory evoked potentials are widely regarded to be more resilient/easier to record compared to spinal cord evoked potentials, which is also the experience of the authors. Although some drugs (such as halothane or barbiturates) may partially affect these scalp potentials, with current anaesthetic protocols (propofol/alfaxolone induction maintained with isoflurane/sevoflurane), they are maintained during anaesthesia and therefore give access to electrophysiologic testing of sensory conduction through the whole central nervous system (Allison *et al.*, 1981; Kornegay *et al.*, 1981; Purinton *et al.*, 1983).

Recording is performed using two sub-dermal stainless-steel needles. The tip of the active electrode is placed above the primary somatosensory cortex, contralateral to the stimulated site and slightly lateral to the midline. As mentioned above, just lateral to the bregma is the preferred point. A lack of response should lead the operator to try recording on the ipsilateral side as well. The anode electrode is placed further lateral from the median plane, ~2cm away from the active needle. The reference ('ground') electrode is placed over the tip of the external occipital protuberance (i.e., the inion), in the cervical region, or on a thoracic limb. Stimulation is performed using a pair of sub-dermal needles, as for routine peripheral nerve stimulation, placed close to the nerve of interest in its distal portion. The authors typically use the ulnar or tibial nerve.

The stimulation intensity should be 2 to 3 times the stimulation needed to elicit a motor response. Practically, a pair of recording electrodes is placed in a muscle distal to the stimulation site to record a CMAP and confirm correct placement of the stimulating needles near the nerve. Then, the scalp recording needles over the brain are used instead. The stimulation intensity is slowly increased to visualise a twitch of the muscles below the stimulation point and, once that intensity is found, it is then increased two times for forelimb stimulation and three times for pelvic limb stimulation. Repetitive stimulation is needed (typically 512 stimulations) which are averaged by the software. The authors have successfully used repetitive rectangular impulses of 0.2ms duration applied to the nerve at a frequency of 3Hz, with a bandpass ranging from 30-3000Hz. The band pass can be adjusted during the test to allow the best recording possible. With a low bandpass below 30Hz (e.g., 1-10Hz), cortical somatosensory evoked potentials have a larger amplitude than at 30Hz, and they disappear with a low band pass of 100Hz (Vanderzant *et al;* 1989). Little change is observed in the amplitude of cortical somatosensory evoked potentials with a higher band pass set at 10kHz compared to 3000Hz (3kHz).

c. Morphology of the cortical somatosensory evoked potential

The cortical somatosensory evoked potential in dogs and cats is typically comprised of three main peaks (named P1 [first positive], N1 [first negative] and P2 [second positive]). This morphology is very predictable and constant across animals and recordings. Therefore, the clinician will observe a first small-to-medium size downwards deflection (P1), followed by a large upwards deflection (N1) and then small downwards deflection (P2) (**Figure 9.4**).

The amplitude of cortical somatosensory evoked potentials varies depending on the location of the recording electrodes (site and side – there is usually a natural difference between the right and left sides), the body size of the animal, and likely from one clinic to another because of the varied equipment and settings in place.

Figure 9.4. Morphology of a normal cortical somatosensory evoked potential

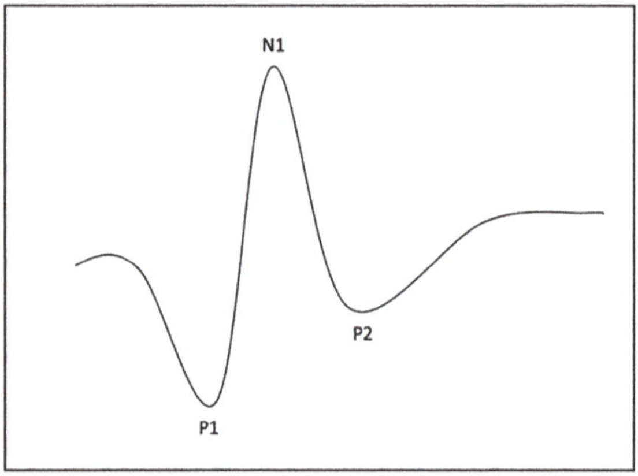

However, the latencies of the peaks are constant and primarily affected by the size of the animal – they therefore constitute a better clinical parameter to assess integrity of the neural pathways, and the mean latencies (and amplitudes) for dogs and cats have been published depending on the stimulated nerve (Poncelet *et al.*, 1993a).

d. Clinical use of cortical somatosensory evoked potentials

Cortical somatosensory evoked potentials have been recorded quite extensively in the experimental setting, such as chronic compression of the feline spinal cord at the L1 lumbar vertebra, demonstrating feasibility in larger mammals (Schramm *et al.*, 1983b). The first clinical report in companion dogs was presented by Bright *et al.* in 1977, which showed a correlation between recovery of ambulation in dogs with natural thoracolumbar spinal cord injury and re-appearance of cortical somatosensory evoked potentials. Later, in a series of 24 companion dogs with acute thoracolumbar injury, Poncelet *et al.* reported that all grade 3 (non-ambulatory paraparetic) dogs had detectable cortical somatosensory evoked potentials, 60% of grade 4 (paraplegic with intact nociception) dogs had detectable cortical somatosensory evoked potentials, and no grade 5 ('deep pain negative') dogs had detectable cortical somatosensory evoked potentials (Poncelet *et al.,* 1993b) (**Figure 9.5**). Lewis *et al.* found no somatosensory evoked potentials in chronically paraplegic deep pain negative dogs, whereas Hu *et al.*, found recordable cortical somatosensory evoked potentials in 12 of 34 chronically paraplegic deep pain negative dogs (Lewis *et al.,* 2017; Hu *et al.,* 2018b). Therefore, and similarly to ascending spinal cord evoked potentials, the detection or absence of cortical somatosensory evoked potentials comes with the possibility of false negative and false positive results and must be interpreted with caution.

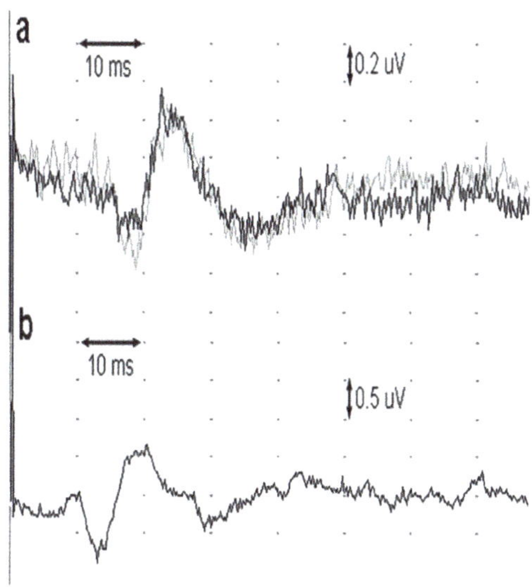

Figure 9.5. Cortical somatosensory evoked potentials recorded following stimulation of the sciatic-tibial nerve (a) and ulnar nerve (b) in a dog with a thoracolumbar spinal cord injury (intervertebral disc extrusion at T13-L1) and non-ambulatory paraparesis (grade 3). The potentials obtained following stimulation of the ulnar nerve are normal. Scalp potentials are detectable following stimulation of the sciatic-tibial nerve, but their amplitude is decreased.

Building on this foundation work, it is interesting to see cortical somatosensory evoked potentials being revisited as a possible method of assessing outcome in dogs with natural thoracolumbar spinal cord injury, in particular through clinical trials testing new therapies, such as those testing 4-aminopyridine, olfactory ensheathing cell transplantation or chondroitinase ABC (Granger *et al.,* 2012; Granger *et al.,* 2014; Hu *et al.,* 2018a; Lewis *et al.,* 2019). For a more detailed review, see Granger *et al.* (2014).

In an attempt to assess spinal cord function during surgery, Okuno *et al.* (2022) recently reported cortical somatosensory evoked potentials (with tibial nerve stimulation) before and during hemilaminectomy decompression surgery in 52 dogs in Japan. This group had previously obtained preliminary feasibility data from dogs with cervical spinal cord diseases and shown an amplitude reduction of the cortical somatosensory evoked potential during surgery using ulnar nerve stimulation (Okuno *et al.*, 2005). In humans, it is proposed that a 60% drop in cortical somatosensory evoked potential amplitude (Fisher *et al.*, 1995) leads to neurological deterioration post-operatively and therefore active functional intraoperative monitoring of the cord is routinely performed. In the 52 dogs studied by Okuno *et al.* (2022), the cortical somatosensory evoked potential amplitude decreased during retraction of the *multifidus* muscles and then increased again after decompression. All cases (ranging from ambulatory paraparesis to paraplegic with intact nociception) recovered following surgery and none had a >50% drop in amplitude (Okuno *et al.*, 2022).

References

Allison T, Hume AL. A comparative analysis of short-latency somatosensory evoked potentials in man, monkey, cat, and rat. Exp Neurol. 1981 Jun;72(3):592-611. doi: 10.1016/0014-4886(81)90008-x. PMID: 6263666.

Besalti O, Ozak A, Senel OO, Eminaga S, Gokce P, Sener O. Scalp and Thoracolumbar Recorded Somatosensory Potentials Evoked by Tibial Nerve Stimulation in Cats. Veterinary Neurology and Neurosurgery. 1990. https://www.vin.com/apputil/content/defaultadv1.aspx?meta=Generic&pId=11157&id=3860423

Bright RM, Breazile JE, Bojrab MJ. Prognostic Application of Cortical Evoked Responses in Dogs with Spinal Cord Injury. Veterinary Surgery 1977. https://doi.org/10.1111/j.1532-950X.1977.tb00562.x

Campbell JO, Olby NJ, Hash JA, Lascelles BD. Assessment of cord dorsum potentials from caudal nerves in anesthetized clinically normal adult dogs without or during neuromuscular blockade. Am J Vet Res. 2013 Apr;74(4):616-20. doi: 10.2460/ajvr.74.4.616. PMID: 23531070.

Cuddon PA. Electrophysiology in neuromuscular disease. Vet Clin North Am Small Anim Pract. 2002 Jan;32(1):31-62. doi: 10.1016/s0195-5616(03)00079-2. PMID: 11785734.

Cuddon PA, Delauche AJ, Hutchison JM. Assessment of dorsal nerve root and spinal cord dorsal horn function in clinically normal dogs by determination of cord dorsum potentials. Am J Vet Res. 1999 Feb;60(2):222-6. PMID: 10048556.

Fisher RS, Raudzens P, Nunemacher M. Efficacy of intraoperative neurophysiological monitoring. J Clin Neurophysiol. 1995 Jan;12(1):97-109. PMID: 7896914.

Granger N, Blamires H, Franklin RJ, Jeffery ND. Autologous olfactory mucosal cell transplants in clinical spinal cord injury: a randomized double-blinded trial in a canine translational model. Brain. 2012 Nov;135(Pt 11):3227-37. doi: 10.1093/brain/aws268. PMID: 23169917; PMCID: PMC3501977.

Granger N, Franklin RJ, Jeffery ND. Cell therapy for spinal cord injuries: what is really going on? Neuroscientist. 2014 Dec;20(6):623-38. doi: 10.1177/1073858413514635. Epub 2014 Jan 10. PMID: 24415275.

Harcourt-Brown TR, Belshaw Z, Parker JE, Jeffery ND, Granger N. Effects of syringomyelia on electrodiagnostic test results in Cavalier King Charles Spaniels. Am J Vet Res. 2011 May;72(5):595-600. doi: 10.2460/ajvr.72.5.595. PMID: 21529209.

Harcourt-Brown TR, Granger NP, Fitzpatrick N, Jeffery ND. Electrodiagnostic findings in dogs with apparently painful lumbosacral foraminal stenosis. J Vet Intern Med. 2019 Sep;33(5):2167-2174. doi: 10.1111/jvim.15589. Epub 2019 Aug 5. PMID: 31381186. PMCID: PMC6766485.

Holliday TA. Electrodiagnostic examination. Somatosensory evoked potentials and electromyography. Vet Clin North Am Small Anim Pract. 1992 Jul;22(4):833-57. doi: 10.1016/s0195-5616(92)50079-1

Holliday TA, Weldon NE, Ealand BG. Percutaneous recording of evoked spinal cord potentials of dogs. Am J Vet Res. 1979 Mar;40(3):326-33. PMID: 475083.

Hu HZ, Granger N, Pai SB, Bellamkonda RV, Jeffery ND. Therapeutic efficacy of microtube-embedded chondroitinase ABC in a canine clinical model of spinal cord injury. Brain. 2018 Apr 1;141(4):1017-1027. doi: 10.1093/brain/awy007. PMID: 29444239.

Hu HZ, Jeffery ND, Granger N. Somatosensory and motor evoked potentials in dogs with chronic severe thoracolumbar spinal cord injury. Vet J. 2018 Jul;237:49-54. doi: 10.1016/j.tvjl.2018.05.007. Epub 2018 May 25. PMID: 30089545.

Kimura J. Electrodiagnosis in Diseases of Nerve and Muscle: Principles and Practice – 4th ed. Oxford University Press, 2013.

Kornegay JN, Marshall AE, Purinton PT, Oliver JE Jr. Somatosensory-evoked potential in clinically normal dogs. Am J Vet Res. 1981 Jan;42(1):70-3. PMID: 7224321.

Lewis MJ, Howard JF Jr, Olby NJ. The Relationship between Trans-Lesional Conduction, Motor Neuron Pool Excitability, and Motor Function in Dogs with Incomplete Recovery from Severe Spinal Cord Injury. J Neurotrauma. 2017 Nov 1;34(21):2994-3002. doi: 10.1089/neu.2017.5012. Epub 2017 Jun 16. PMID: 28462632; PMCID: PMC6436022.

Lewis MJ, Laber E, Olby NJ. Predictors of Response to 4-Aminopyridine in Chronic Canine Spinal Cord Injury. J Neurotrauma. 2019 May 1;36(9):1428-1434. doi: 10.1089/neu.2018.5975. Epub 2018 Dec 12. PMID: 30235970; PMCID: PMC6482892.

Meij BP, Suwankong N, van den Brom WE, Venker-van Haagen AJ, Hazewinkel HA. Tibial nerve somatosensory evoked potentials in dogs with degenerative lumbosacral stenosis. Vet Surg. 2006 Feb;35(2):168-75. doi: 10.1111/j.1532-950X.2006.00128.x. PMID: 16472297.

Nordwall A, Axelgaard J, Harada Y, Valencia P, McNeal DR, Brown JC. Spinal cord monitoring using evoked potentials recorded from feline vertebral bone. Spine (Phila Pa 1976). 1979 Nov-Dec;4(6):486-94. doi: 10.1097/00007632-197911000-00006. PMID: 515839.

Okuno S, Katahira H, Orito K. Somatosensory evoked potentials of the tibial nerve during the surgical decompression of thoracolumbar intervertebral disk herniation in dogs. Front Vet Sci. 2022 Sep 15;9:976972. doi: 10.3389/fvets.2022.976972. PMID: 36187812; PMCID: PMC9519392.

Okuno S, Nakamura A, Kobayashi T, Orito K. Effectiveness of intraoperative somatosensory evoked potential monitoring during cervical spinal operations on animals with spinal cord dysfunction. J Vet Med Sci. 2005 Jul;67(7):719-22. doi: 10.1292/jvms.67.719. PMID: 16082122.

Park JH, Hyun SJ. Intraoperative neurophysiological monitoring in spinal surgery. World J Clin Cases. 2015 Sep 16;3(9):765-73. doi: 10.12998/wjcc.v3.i9.765. PMID: 26380823; PMCID: PMC4568525.

Passmore SR, Murphy B, Lee TD. The origin, and application of somatosensory evoked potentials as a neurophysiological technique to investigate neuroplasticity. J Can Chiropr Assoc. 2014 Jun;58(2):170-83. PMID: 24932021. PMCID: PMC4025087.

Poncelet L. VIN chapter. Electrophysiological Assessment of Spinal Cord Function Through Somatosensory Evoked Potentials in Dogs. (1999)

Poncelet L, Michaux C, Balligand M. Influence of body size on tibial nerve somatosensory evoked potentials in dogs. Am J Vet Res. 1993 Jan;54(1):178-82. PMID: 8427464.

Poncelet L, Michaux C, Balligand M. Somatosensory potentials in dogs with naturally acquired thoracolumbar spinal cord disease. Am J Vet Res. 1993 Nov;54(11):1935-41. PMID: 8291776.

Poncelet L, Michaux C, Balligand M. Motor evoked potentials induced by electrical stimulation of the spine in dogs: which structures are involved? Electroencephalogr Clin Neurophysiol. 1995 Jun;97(3):179-83. doi: 10.1016/0924-980x(94)00330-a. PMID: 7607107.

Poncelet L, Michaux C, Balligand M. Study of spinal cord evoked injury potential by use of computer modeling and in dogs with naturally acquired thoracolumbar spinal cord compression. Am J Vet Res. 1998 Mar;59(3):300-6. PMID: 9522949.

Purinton PT, Oliver JE Jr, Kornegay JN, Bradley WE. Cortical averaged evoked potentials produced by pudendal nerve stimulation in dogs. Am J Vet Res. 1983 Mar;44(3):446-8. PMID: 6838039.

Redding RW, Lee AH, Wilson SG. Spinal-evoked potentials and spinal conduction velocity of the cat: reference values. Am J Vet Res. 1984 Oct;45(10):2175-7. PMID: 6497119.

Schramm J, Krause R, Shigeno T, Brock M. Experimental investigation on the spinal cord evoked injury potential. J Neurosurg. 1983 Sep;59(3):485-92. doi: 10.3171/jns.1983.59.3.0485. PMID: 6886762.

Schramm J, Shigeno T, Brock M. Clinical signs and evoked response alterations associated with chronic experimental cord compression. J Neurosurg. 1983 May;58(5):734-41. doi: 10.3171/jns.1983.58.5.0734. PMID: 6834123.

Shores A, Redding RW, Knecht CD. Spinal-evoked potentials in dogs with acute compressive thoracolumbar spinal cord disease. Am J Vet Res. 1987 Oct;48(10):1525-30. PMID: 3674565.

Snyder BG, Holliday TA. Pathways of ascending evoked spinal cord potentials of dogs. Electroencephalogr Clin Neurophysiol. 1984 Aug;58(2):140-54. doi: 10.1016/0013-4694(84)90027-0. PMID: 6204840.

Steiss JE, Wright JC. Maturation of spinal-evoked potentials to tibial and ulnar nerve stimulation in clinically normal dogs. Am J Vet Res. 1990 Sep;51(9):1427-32. PMID: 2396789.

Vanderzant CW, Schott RJ, Natale JE, Pondo CA, D'Alecy LG. Somatosensory evoked potentials of the dog: recording techniques and normal values. J Neurosci Methods. 1989 Apr;27(3):253-63. doi: 10.1016/0165-0270(89)90087-3. PMID: 2725007.

SECTION 10

Cranial nerve assessment

Hélène Vandenberghe, Edward Ives,
Francesca Samarani, Nicolas Granger

Key points:

- Some cranial nerves and their pathways can be studied with electrophysiology.
- A single test can provide information on more than one cranial nerve, and the results of different tests can be complementary when evaluating cranial nerve function.
- The trigemino-facial reflex, or blink reflex, can be assessed in clinical practice and normal reference values are available.
- Other nerve-specific tests can be conducted for the trigeminal, facial, vagus and recurrent laryngeal nerves, although they have been less studied in companion animals.

Electrophysiologic testing of the cranial nerves is performed using a bipolar montage in a similar way to appendicular nerve conduction studies, with the cathode being the active (stimulating) electrode lying closest to the nerve being stimulated, alongside an anode placed ~2cm away from the active electrode. A pair of recording electrodes is then used to screen the muscle (or nerve) being tested. Assessment of certain cranial nerves has been performed in dogs and cats, with some normal values available

(Steiss and Marshall, 1988; LeDoux *et al.*, 1997; Añor *et al.*, 2000), but little clinical application has been published to date.

Cranial nerve assessment can be broadly divided into the following tests. As for the neurological examination, where different tests are complementary, there are some common components between certain tests and their results can therefore be combined to support a particular lesion localisation:

- Trigemino-facial ('blink') reflex: trigeminal nerve (sensory) – brainstem relay – facial nerve (motor);
- Facial nerve stimulation: facial nerve (motor) and a delayed facio-facial reflex with a brainstem relay;
- Trigemino-trigeminal reflex: trigeminal nerve (sensory) – brainstem relay – trigeminal nerve (motor);
- Vagus and recurrent laryngeal nerve stimulation: vagus nerve (motor);
- Sensory trigeminal nerve conduction study: trigeminal nerve (sensory).

1. Blink reflex

(i) Anatomy

The blink reflex is also called the trigemino-facial reflex and is an electrical analogue of the corneal reflex. The afferent component is composed of the sensory fibres of the ophthalmic branch of the trigeminal nerve (V_1) (**Figure 10.1**). Stimulation of ipsilateral V_1 leads to stimulation of both ipsilateral and contralateral sensory nuclei of the trigeminal nerve in the pons, and also the nuclei of the spinal tract of the trigeminal nerve bilaterally in the medulla oblongata. The nerve impulse then reaches the ipsilateral and contralateral facial motor nuclei in the medulla through a series of interneurons. The efferent component is the motor fibres of the facial nerve which elicits a blink bilaterally in response to unilateral stimulation (**Figure 10.1**) (Añor *et al.*, 2000; Shapiro and Preston, 2013).

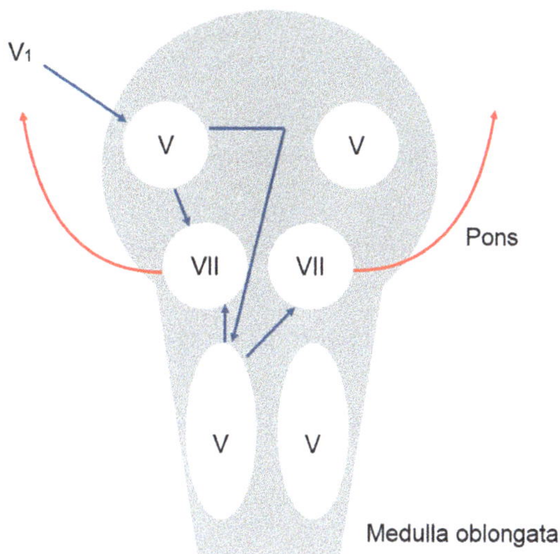

Figure 10.1. Anatomy involved in the blink reflex. V_1 = ophthalmic branch of the trigeminal nerve; V = pontine and medullary sensory nuclei of the trigeminal nerve; VII = motor nuclei of the facial nerve. The afferent pathway (blue arrows) involves the ophthalmic branch of the trigeminal nerve, which synapses with both sensory nuclei of the trigeminal nerve in the pons and the nuclei of the spinal tract of the trigeminal nerve in the medulla oblongata. The efferent pathway (red arrows) involves the motor fibres of the facial nerve bilaterally.

(ii) Procedure

The trigemino-facial (blink) reflex is studied by stimulating the sensory component of the trigeminal nerve at the level of the supraorbital foramen (supraorbital/frontal nerve, branch of the ophthalmic [V_1] nerve) and recording from the *orbicularis oculi* muscles bilaterally, using a two-channel recording apparatus (Añor *et al.,* 2000) (**Figure 10.2**). Surface electrodes can be used for stimulation, with the cathode placed on the supraorbital process of the frontal bone, 1cm dorsal to the medial canthus of the eye. The recording electrodes are placed bilaterally in the *orbicularis oculi* muscles via the ventral eyelids (cathodes) and lateral to the lateral canthus of the eye (anodes). The reference electrode is placed on the dorsal aspect of the muzzle.

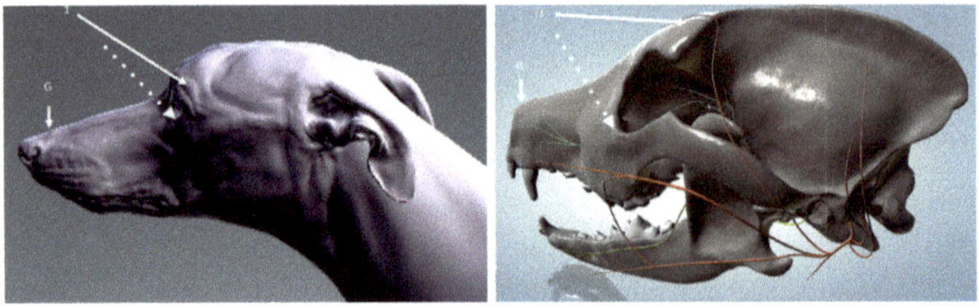

Figure 10.2. Positioning of the stimulating and recording electrodes for the blink reflex. 1 = Stimulation site: frontal nerve; the sensory branches of the trigeminal nerve appear in green on the image on the right. Recording site = *orbicularis oculi muscle*, bilaterally (dotted arrow); the facial nerve course is displayed by the orange lines on the image on the right. G = reference electrode. *Adapted with permission from Ivalalearn (part of the Veterinary Information Network® family).*

(iii) Normal response and recordings

There are three main waveforms that can be recorded when testing the trigemino-facial reflex in sedated dogs: R_1, R_2 and R_c (**Figure 10.3**) (Añor *et al.*, 2000; Shapiro and Preston, 2013).

R_1 is the early response, recorded ipsilateral to the site being stimulated. Its pathway is di-synaptic, involving the ophthalmic branch of the trigeminal nerve, the sensory nucleus of the trigeminal nerve in the pons, the ipsilateral facial motor nucleus in the *medulla oblongata*, the ipsilateral facial nerve, a delay at the neuromuscular junction and conduction along the *orbicularis oculi* muscle fibres. It is a stable and reproducible polyphasic response that could be thought of an electrical analogue of the corneal/palpebral reflex.

The late responses are named R_2 (ipsilateral recording) and R_c (contralateral recording). Their pathways are multi-synaptic, involving the sensory nucleus of the trigeminal nerve in the pons, the nucleus of the spinal tract of the trigeminal nerve in the *medulla oblongata*, the contralateral ventral thalamic nucleus, interneurons connecting to both facial motor nuclei, and both facial nerves. The R_2 and R_c responses are also polyphasic but have a longer duration, smaller amplitudes and more variable latencies compared to R_1; this is a result of multiple synaptic delays and the influence of interneuronal excitability. R_c has a slightly longer latency than R_2 and disappears under general anaesthesia as the polysynaptic reflex pathway to the contralateral facial motor nucleus is suppressed (Whalen, 1985).

Another even later response, called R_3, may appear after high intensity stimulation of the supraorbital nerve. Its pathway likely involves small diameter, high-threshold trigeminal afferent fibres related to nociception and is a long pathway involving the caudal *medulla oblongata* and cranial cervical spinal cord. It is inconsistent and does not appear in all dogs, being recorded in 9 of 15 dogs in one study (Añor *et al.,* 2000).

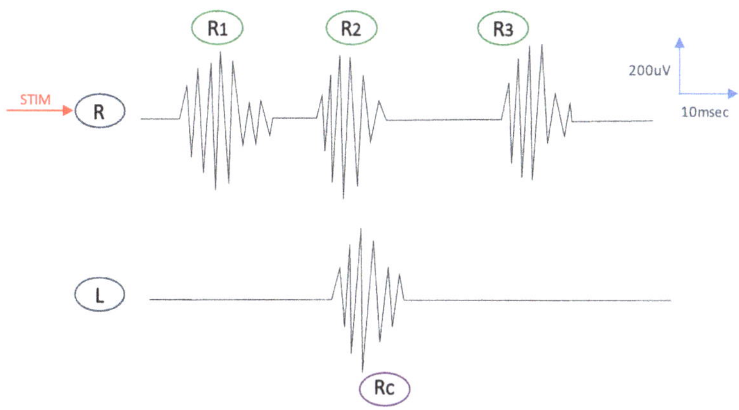

Figure 10.3. Normal blink reflex responses after stimulation of the right supraorbital nerve and recording in both *orbicularis oculi* muscles in a sedated dog. *Source: Francesca Samarani.*

The shortest latencies of each response are assessed, as well as the difference between latencies of the contralateral and ipsilateral responses.

Mean latencies of the blink reflex responses have been published for 8 alert adult male cats (LeDoux *et al.,* 1997) and in a study of 15 sedated adult healthy Beagles (Añor *et al.,* 2000). The reference values for dogs with larger or smaller head sizes may differ, but for unilateral lesions the contralateral (normal) side can be used as an internal control.

(iv) Patterns of blink reflex abnormalities

a. Unilateral trigeminal (sensory) nerve lesion

In this scenario, the signal is interrupted from travelling along the affected trigeminal nerve (ophthalmic branch) towards the nuclei in the brainstem. This means that it cannot stimulate the facial nerve and there will be a delay or absence of all potentials (ipsilateral R_1 and R_2 (+/-R_3), and contralateral R_c) when the affected side is stimulated. All potentials will be normal if the non-affected side is stimulated.

b. Unilateral facial (motor) nerve lesion

Stimulation of the affected side will travel as normal down the sensory fibres of the trigeminal nerve and synapse at the level of the brainstem nuclei. However, as the efferent arm on the affected side is abnormal there will be delayed or absent ipsilateral R_1 and R_2 (+/- R_3) potentials. The contralateral R_c potential will be normal following contraction of the contralateral *orbicularis oculi* muscle via the unaffected facial nerve on the opposite side (**Figure 10.4**).

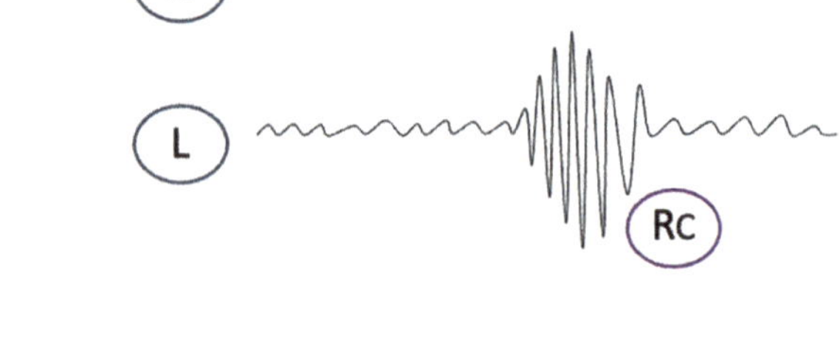

Figure 10.4. Blink reflex responses following stimulation of the right supraorbital nerve in case of a right facial nerve lesion. *Source: Francesca Samarani.*

Stimulation of the normal, unaffected side induces a delayed or absent contralateral R_c potential, but normal ipsilateral R_1 and R_2 (+/- R_3) potentials (**Figure 10.5**).

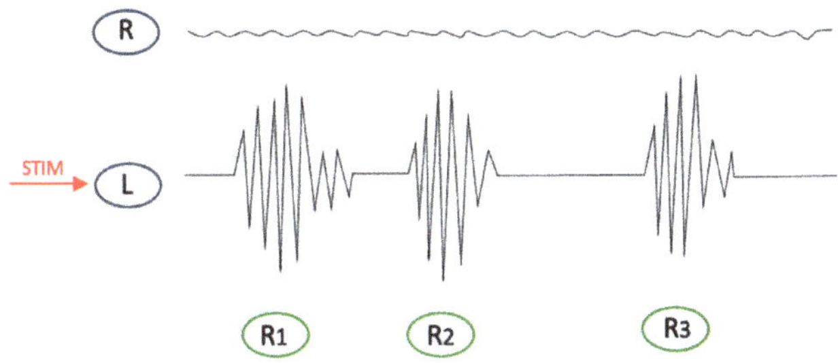

Figure 10.5. Blink reflex responses following stimulation of the left supraorbital nerve in case of a right facial nerve lesion. *Source: Francesca Samarani.*

c. Unilateral pontine lesion

In this situation, the sensory nucleus of the trigeminal nerve and/or the interneurons connecting to the ipsilateral facial motor nucleus may be impaired. This results in a delayed or absent ipsilateral R_1, with normal ipsilateral R_2 and contralateral R_c potentials.

d. Unilateral medullary lesion

In this situation, the nucleus of the spinal tract of the trigeminal nerve and/or the interneurons to the ipsilateral motor nucleus of the facial nerve in the medulla can be impaired. This results in a normal ipsilateral R_1, with a delayed or absent ipsilateral R_2 and contralateral R_C.

2. Facial nerve stimulation

The facial nerve can be stimulated just ventral and caudal to the base of the ear canal, near the tympanic bulla, as it exits the petrous temporal bone via the stylomastoid foramen (internal auricular branches), or at the level of the supraorbital foramen above the eye (palpebral nerve) (Whalen, 1985). The recording electrodes are placed in the ipsilateral *orbicularis oculi* muscle (ventral eyelid), as for the blink reflex, with the reference electrode also placed on top of the muzzle (**Figure 10.6**).

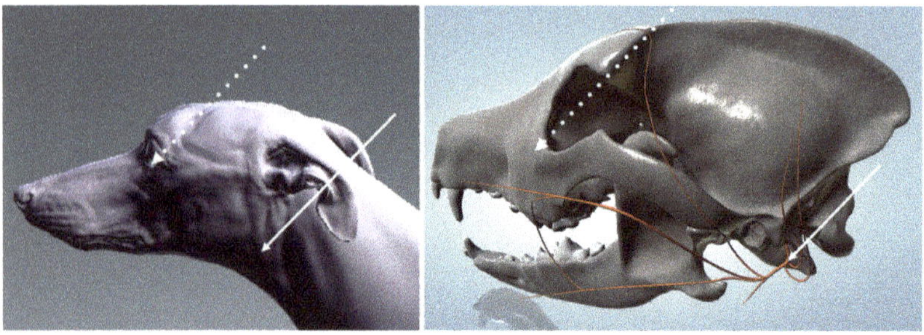

Figure 10.6. Electrode set-up for facial nerve stimulation. Stimulation site: internal auricular branch, plain arrow; recording site = *orbicularis oculi* muscle (dotted arrow); the facial nerve course is displayed by the orange lines on the image on the right. *Adapted with permission from Ivalalearn (part of the Veterinary Information Network® family).*

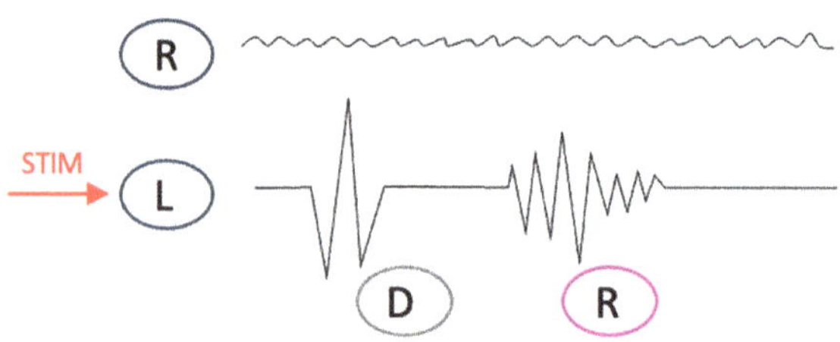

Figure 10.7. Normal facial nerve responses after stimulation of the left facial nerve and recording in both *orbicularis oculi* muscles. D: direct muscle evoked potential. R: facio-facial reflex potential. *Source: Francesca Samarani.*

This set-up allows the study of the direct facial nerve response, being a polyphasic muscle potential in the ipsilateral *orbicularis oculi* muscle following facial nerve stimulation. A reflex response (facio-facial reflex of longer latency) is also noted in the same muscle after the direct response (**Figure 10.7**). Mean latencies for both the direct response and later reflex response in dogs have been published (Añor *et al.*, 2000). For unilateral lesions, the normal side can be used as an internal control to compare amplitudes at the same stimulus intensity.

3. Trigemino-trigeminal reflex

The trigemino-trigeminal reflex can be studied by stimulating sensory fibres of the trigeminal nerve (either at the level of the infraorbital foramen (maxillary branch, V_2), or at the level of the mental foramen (mandibular branch, V_3) and recording in the rostral belly of the ipsilateral *digastricus* muscle (innervated by motor fibres in the mandibular branch) (**Figure 10.8**). This pathway involves interneuronal connections between the trigeminal sensory and motor nuclei in the brainstem.

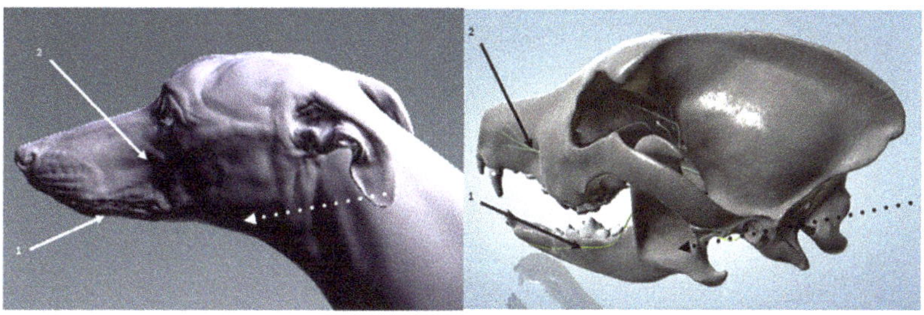

Figure 10.8. Electrode set-up for trigemino-trigeminal reflex testing. Possible stimulations sites: 1: mental foramen; 2: infraorbital foramen; recording site = rostral belly of *digastricus* muscle (dotted arrow). The sensory branches of the trigeminal nerve appear in green on the image on the right. *Adapted with permission from Ivalalearn (part of the Veterinary Information Network® family).*

4. Vagus and recurrent laryngeal nerve stimulation

It is possible to stimulate the *vagus* and recurrent laryngeal nerves along their extra-laryngeal course. For stimulation, the proximal stimulating electrode is placed over the jugular groove to reach the vagal trunk, the distal stimulating electrode (distal segment of the recurrent laryngeal nerve) is placed along the dorsolateral aspect of the trachea. Recording is in the ipsilateral intrinsic laryngeal muscles via percutaneous needle electrodes (**Figure 10.9**).

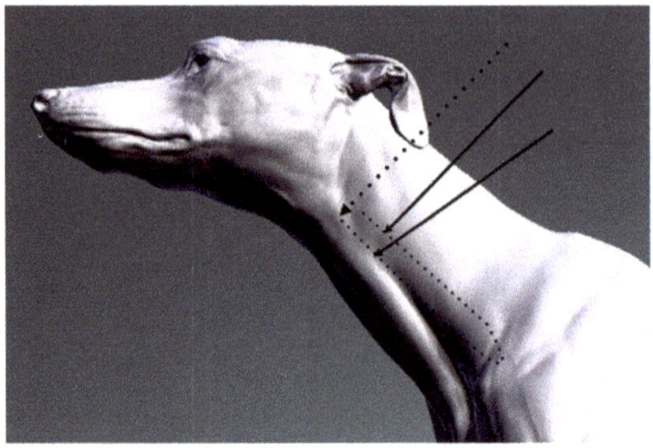

Figure 10.9. Needle electrode placement for stimulation of the left *vagus* nerve, with recording in the ipsilateral intrinsic laryngeal muscles. Proximal stimulation site is the jugular groove; distal stimulation site is dorsolaterally to the trachea (plain arrows); recording site is the ipsilateral intrinsic laryngeal muscles (dotted arrow). *Adapted with permission from Ivalalearn (part of the Veterinary Information Network® family).*

The expected latency calculation for vagus/recurrent laryngeal nerve stimulation has to allow for the nerve length, and therefore needs to be correlated to the neck length. A formula for this correlation and normal latency values (linear regression model) has been published (Steiss and Marshall, 1988).

- **a.** For the left side, latency (ms) = 0.06 x neck length + 1.01
- **b.** For the right side, latency (ms) = 0.04 x neck length + 0.71

Neck length = caudal border of the cricoid cartilage to manubrium, measured on the ventral midline with the neck extended.

The clinical application of this technique has not been investigated (Steiss and Marshall, 1988).

5. Sensory trigeminal nerve conduction study

Stimulation of the mucosa dorsal to the maxillary canine tooth in the mouth can elicit a sensory potential that can be recorded directly from the ipsilateral infraorbital nerve (branch of the maxillary division of the trigeminal nerve, V_2). For recording, the cathode is placed over the infraorbital foramen and the anode slightly distal to this (**Figure 10.10**).

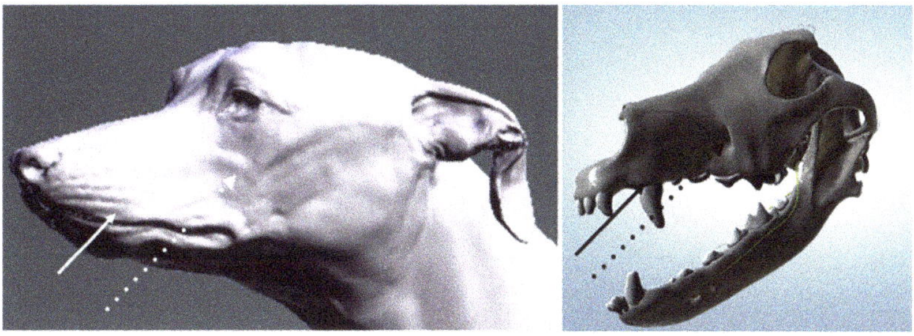

Figure 10.10. Placement of needle electrodes for sensory trigeminal nerve stimulation and recording. Stimulation = next to the maxillary canine in the mouth (plain arrow); recording = infraorbital foramen (dashed arrow); the sensory branches of the trigeminal nerve appear in green on the image on the right. *Adapted with permission from Ivalalearn (part of the Veterinary Information Network® family).*

References

Añor S, Espadaler JM, Pastor J, Pumarola M. Electrically induced blink reflex and facial motor nerve stimulation in beagles. J Vet Intern Med. 2000 Jul-Aug;14(4):418-23. doi: 10.1892/0891-6640(2000)014<0418:eibraf>2.3.co;2. PMID: 10935892.

Kimura J. Electrodiagnosis in Diseases of Nerve and Muscle: Principles and Practice – 4th ed. Oxford University Press, 2013.

LeDoux MS, Lorden JF, Weir AD, Smith JM. Blink reflex to supraorbital nerve stimulation in the cat. Exp Brain Res. 1997 Aug;116(1):104-12. doi: 10.1007/pl00005730. PMID: 9305819.

Shapiro BE and Preston DC. Electromyography and Neuromuscular Disorders: Clinical-Electrophysiologic Correlations – 3rd ed. Elsevier Inc, 2013.

Steiss JE, Marshall AE. Electromyographic evaluation of conduction time and velocity of the recurrent laryngeal nerves of clinically normal dogs. Am J Vet Res. 1988 Sep;49(9):1533-6. PMID: 3223662.

Whalen LR. Electrophysiologic studies of the facial reflexes of the dog. Am J Vet Res. 1985 Jan;46(1):229-34. PMID : 3907430.

SECTION 11

Magnetic motor evoked potentials

Hélène Vandenberghe, Edward Ives, Nicolas Granger

Key points:

- Transcranial magnetic motor evoked potentials are obtained following magnetic stimulation over the motor cortex and recording of the evoked muscle response.
- Transcranial magnetic motor evoked potentials are recorded under sedation in dogs.
- Magnetic motor evoked potentials reflect the functionality of the entire descending motor pathway from the brain to recording site in the muscle.
- Transcranial magnetic motor evoked potentials can be recorded from contralateral appendicular muscles or from head muscles.
- Transcranial magnetic motor evoked potentials have been used in the assessment of dogs with cervical spondylomyelopathy, intervertebral disc herniation, peripheral nerve injuries, and investigated as a treatment option for epilepsy in dogs.

1. Anatomy

Like somatosensory evoked potentials, transcranial magnetic motor evoked potentials assess an entire neurological pathway. A magnetic field is used to stimulate the cerebral cortex (see later), which triggers electric potentials. These descend from: (i) the cerebral cortex and thalamic centers; (ii) the brainstem; (iii) the spinal cord motor pathways (pyramidal and extrapyramidal tracts); (iv) to the motor neuronal cell bodies, ventral nerve roots and axons of the peripheral motor nerves, via the neuromuscular junction, to eventually generate a muscle contraction. This generates a motor unit action potential that can be recorded from the muscle (Van Ham *et al.*, 1994; Nollet *et al.*, 2003; Campos Mello Inglez de Souza 2017).

2. Magnetic stimulation of the brain

Transcranial magnetic stimulation of the motor cortex is performed using a magnetic stimulator and a round coil which can generate a magnetic field of approximately 2 Tesla at its surface. A supramaximal stimulus intensity (usually 70% of the maximum possible magnetic stimulation) is delivered by the magnetic coil that is held tangentially to the scalp. The center of the coil should be placed lateral to the vertex (**Figure 11.1**), pointing towards the parietal motor cortex. Three to five individual pulses can be delivered over the motor cortex on one side to assess repeatability, before repeating the procedure on the opposite side of the head. Clockwise inducing current flow is delivered to stimulate the right motor cortex and counterclockwise flow is delivered to stimulate the left motor cortex (Van Ham *et al.*, 1994; Nollet *et al.*, 2003).

Transcranial magnetic motor stimulation induces some discomfort in the form of a sudden, startling jerking movement of the whole body, and therefore requires the use of chemical restraint in animals. General anaesthesia usually prevents recording of magnetic motor

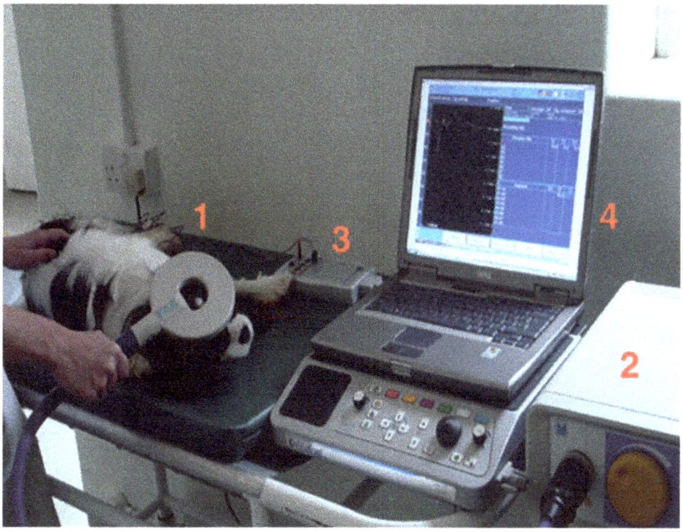

Figure 11.1. Set-up for transcranial magnetic motor stimulation in a Cavalier King Charles spaniel with syringomyelia. The dog was sedated with medetomidine and butorphanol. The left motor cortex is stimulated via a ring coil (1), with its centre placed over the scalp and lateral to the vertex close to the skin (contact with the skin is not needed). This is connected to the magnetic stimulator (2). Recording is obtained via needle electrodes placed in the muscle(s) of interest and connected to the amplifier (3) and electrophysiology unit providing the display (4).

evoked potentials and different sedation protocols have therefore been published, including the use of various combinations of acepromazine, dexmedetomidine, midazolam and opiates (Sylvestre *et al.*, 1993; Van Soens *et al.*, 2009a; Amendt *et al.*, 2016). The authors generally use a sedation with dexmedetomidine and butorphanol (Hu *et al.*, 2018).

3. Recording

(i) Recording parameters

The most commonly used recording parameters are as follows: total recording time of 100ms, gain of 1000μV per division, low and high frequency filters set at 30Hz and 10kHz (da Costa *et al.*, 2006; De Decker *et al.*, 2011; Martin-Vaquero and da Costa, 2014).

(ii) From appendicular muscles

Recording of transcranial magnetic motor evoked potentials is performed using an active recording monopolar needle electrode inserted into the muscle belly of contralateral appendicular muscles: this can be from a single muscle, such as the *extensor carpi radialis* in the thoracic limb, or from multiple muscles at the same time if the amplifier unit has more than one channel (usually 2 to 4). For example, recording from the *extensor carpi radialis* in the right thoracic limb and from the *tibialis cranialis* in the right pelvic limb can be obtained simultaneously from a single stimulation of the left side of the head. The anode electrodes are positioned subcutaneously one centimetre distal to the active recording electrodes. The reference electrode is placed subcutaneously between the stimulation site and the active electrode(s), for example in the dorsal aspect of the cervical region.

(iii) From head muscles

Transcranial magnetic stimulation of the motor cortex can also activate head muscles, therefore allowing evaluation of central conduction pathways: motor cortex, brainstem, cranial nerves exiting the brain, cranial peripheral nerves and the muscles they innervate. Because it is also possible to stimulate some cranial nerves as they exit the skull and obtain a 'peripheral latency', the central delay can also be obtained. This is calculated by subtracting the latency obtained from stimulation of the cranial nerve root/peripheral axon, from the latency of the evoked potentials recorded after cortical stimulation.

For the facial nerve, Estrem *et al.* (1988b) were able to record evoked electromyographic responses from the contralateral *orbicularis oculi* and *orbicularis oris* muscles following magnetic stimulation of the motor cortex. For the peripheral latency, the facial nerve can be stimulated directly just caudal to the external ear canal as it exits the petrous temporal bone via the stylomastoid foramen.

For the laryngeal musculature, Haghighi and Estrem (1991) reported evoked muscle potentials in the contralateral *vocalis* muscle following magnetic stimulation of the motor cortex.

Finally, for the hypoglossal nerve, Estrem *et al.* (1988a) were able to record motor evoked responses from the tongue musculature with magnetic stimulation of the motor cortex.

(iv) Magnetic stimulation of peripheral nerves

Magnetic motor evoked potentials have been recorded after direct stimulation of the radial nerve in a group of dogs with brachial plexus avulsion (Van Soens *et al.,* 2009b). In this study, the magnetic coil was placed in the axillary region, with the flat surface of the coil placed parallel to the skin surface of the limb and the cranial part of the circle of the coil held tangentially to the radial nerve. Recording was made from the *extensor carpi radialis* muscle.

4. Waveform analysis

Transcranial magnetic motor evoked potentials are polyphasic (mainly biphasic or triphasic in shape) (da Costa *et al.,* 2006; De Decker *et al.*, 2011; Martin-Vaquero and da Costa, 2014). Their latencies and amplitudes are measured after placing directed cursors on the oscilloscope. Latencies are measured as the interval from onset of the stimulus to the onset of the response and represent the total motor conduction time from the cerebral cortex to the target muscle. The peak-to-peak amplitude is calculated from the peak of the first negative wave to the nadir of the first positive wave (**Figure 11.2**). The neuronal path length is measured from the site of the transcranial stimulation (vertex) to the active electrode using the estimated course of nerve fibres along the body (Nollet *et al.,* 2003; da Costa *et al.*, 2006; De Decker *et al.,* 2011; Martin-Vaquero and da Costa, 2014).

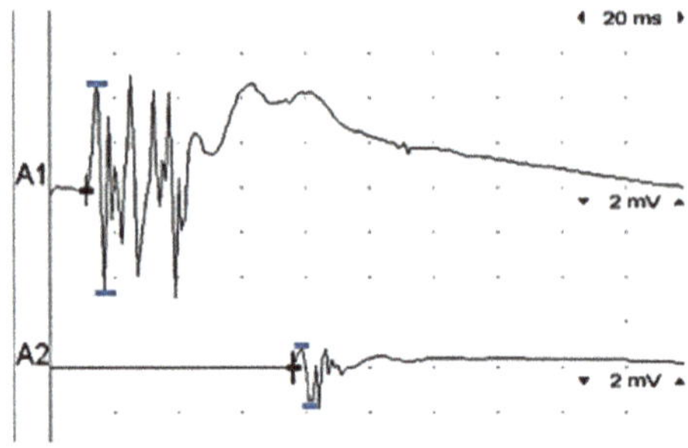

Figure 11.2. Transcranial magnetic motor evoked potentials recorded simultaneously from the left *extensor carpi radialis* (A1) and left *tibialis cranialis* (A2) muscles from a clinically normal Cavalier King Charles spaniel after stimulation of the right motor cortex. The black crosses indicate the onset latency and the horizontal blue bars indicate the peak-to-peak amplitudes, measured from the peak of the first negative wave to the nadir of the first positive wave. Vertical division = 2mV, horizontal division = 20ms.

Reference ranges for transcranial magnetic motor evoked potential latencies and amplitudes have been published in clinically normal large-breed dogs (Poma *et al.*, 2002; Martin-Vaquero and da Costa, 2014). Onset latencies are in the range of 15-20ms with recording in the *extensor carpi radialis* muscle, and 15-30ms with recording in the *tibialis cranialis* muscle. Amplitudes are in the range of 2000-7000µV (2-7mV).

5. Magnetic motor evoked potentials in disease

(i) Cervical spondylomyelopathy

Transcranial magnetic motor evoked potentials can be difficult to record in the acute phase of spinal cord injury in non-ambulatory dogs. However, it has been shown to be a useful screening tool in dogs with chronic cervical spondylomyelopathy and can help to detect slowing of conduction velocity in descending spinal cord motor tracts. Magnetic motor evoked potential latencies and amplitudes have been reported to be abnormal in large breed dogs with cervical spinal cord disease regardless of the severity of their neurological deficits in comparison with normal dogs (Poma *et al.*, 2002). Other studies have found that magnetic motor evoked potential latencies are longer, and tend to correlate with MRI and neurologic findings, in dogs with cervical spondylomyelopathy (da Costa *et al.*, 2006; De Decker *et al.*, 2011; Martin-Vaquero and da Costa, 2014).

(ii) Spinal cord injury secondary to acute intervertebral disc herniation

Magnetic motor evoked potentials have been reported to be abnormal in dogs with type 1 intervertebral disc herniation causing spinal cord injury, even in dogs with spinal pain alone, in which a decreased amplitude may be observed (Sylvestre *et al.*, 1993; Amendt *et al.*, 2017). Significantly prolonged latencies were also associated with the severity of neurologic deficits in these studies. Magnetic motor evoked potentials were recordable in all dogs with mild or no neurologic deficits, but they were recordable in only 50% of ambulatory dogs that were severely ataxic (Sylvestre *et al.*, 1993), and could not be elicited in non-ambulatory dogs (Sylvestre *et al.*, 1993) or paraplegic dogs (Amendt *et al.*, 2017). They could not be used as a predictor of neurologic recovery in one study (Sylvestre *et al.*, 1993) but have been suggested to reflect recovery of function after surgery for type 1 intervertebral disc herniation in others (Amendt *et al.*, 2017; Siedenburg *et al.*, 2018).

(iii) Peripheral nerve injuries

In dogs with traumatic brachial plexus injury, there was a significant difference in magnetic motor evoked potentials following radial nerve stimulation between the normal and affected limb of affected dogs, with a lack of response recorded in the *extensor carpi radialis* being indicative of a poor outcome (Van Soens *et al.*, 2009b).

(iv) Treatment of epilepsy

In people, repetitive transcranial magnetic stimulation of the cortical areas via a series of pulse trains has been proposed as a possible therapeutic tool for genetic epilepsy. The theory being that this procedure has some effect on synaptic plasticity and the type of effect depends on the frequency of stimulation; low frequency stimulation (<1Hz) decreases excitability, whilst high frequency stimulation (>1Hz) increases excitability (Nollet *et al.*, 2003; Nowakowska *et al.*, 2022).

This technique has been studied in dogs and was reported to be well tolerated in 12 dogs with drug-resistant idiopathic epilepsy, with significant reductions in the monthly seizure frequency and monthly seizure day frequency observed in the stimulated patients (Charalambous *et al.*, 2020).

References

Amendt HL, Siedenburg JS, Steffensen N, Söbbeler FJ, Schütter A, Tünsmeyer J, Rohn K, Kästner SB, Tipold A, Stein VM. Transcranial magnetic stimulation with acepromazine or dexmedetomidine in combination with levomethadone/fenpipramide in healthy Beagle dogs. Vet J. 2016 Nov;217:40-42. doi: 10.1016/j.tvjl.2016.06.006. Epub 2016 Jun 17. PMID: 27810209.

Amendt HL, Siedenburg JS, Steffensen N, Kordass U, Rohn K, Tipold A, Stein VM. Correlation between severity of clinical signs and transcranial magnetic motor evoked potentials in dogs with intervertebral disc herniation. Vet J. 2017 Mar;221:48-53. doi: 10.1016/j.tvjl.2017.01.015. Epub 2017 Feb 1. PMID: 28283080.

Campos Mello Inglez de Souza MC, Ferreira RJR, Patricio GCF, Matera JM. Neurophysiological assessment of spinal cord injuries in dogs using somatosensory and motor evoked potentials. Acta Vet Scand. 2017 Jun 12;59(1):37. doi: 10.1186/s13028-017-0305-0. PMID: 28606109; PMCID: PMC5469055.

Charalambous M, Van Ham L, Broeckx BJG, Roggeman T, Carrette S, Vonck K, Kervel RR, Cornelis I, Bhatti SFM. Repetitive transcranial magnetic stimulation in drug-resistant idiopathic epilepsy of dogs: A noninvasive neurostimulation technique. J Vet Intern Med. 2020 Nov;34(6):2555-2561. doi: 10.1111/jvim.15919. Epub 2020 Oct 3. PMID: 33009717; PMCID: PMC7694858.

da Costa RC, Poma R, Parent JM, Partlow G, Monteith G. Correlation of motor evoked potentials with magnetic resonance imaging and neurologic findings in Doberman Pinschers with and without signs of cervical spondylomyelopathy. Am J Vet Res. 2006 Sep;67(9):1613-20. doi: 10.2460/ajvr.67.9.1613. PMID: 16948610.

De Decker S, Van Soens I, Duchateau L, Gielen IM, van Bree HJ, Binst DH, Waelbers T, Van Ham LM. Transcranial magnetic stimulation in Doberman Pinschers with clinically relevant and clinically irrelevant spinal cord compression on magnetic resonance imaging. J Am Vet Med Assoc. 2011 Jan 1;238(1):81-8. doi: 10.2460/javma.238.1.81. PMID: 21194326.

Estrem SA, Haghighi S, Levy WJ, Wertheimer R, Kendall M. Motor-evoked potentials of tongue musculature in dogs. Laryngoscope. 1988 Jun;98(6 Pt 1):628-31. doi: 10.1288/00005537-198806000-00010. PMID: 3374238.

Estrem SA, Haghighi S, Levy WJ, Wertheimer R, Kendall M. Motor-evoked potentials of facial musculature in dogs. Laryngoscope. 1988 Sep;98(9):1012-5. doi: 10.1288/00005537-198809000-00017. PMID: 3412086.

Haghighi SS, Estrem SA. Comparison of evoked electromyography of the larynx to electrical and magnetic stimulation of the motor cortex of the dog. Laryngoscope. 1991 Jan;101(1 Pt 1):68-70. doi: 10.1288/00005537-199101000-00012. PMID: 1984554.

Hu HZ, Granger N, Pai SB, Bellamkonda RV, Jeffery ND. Therapeutic efficacy of microtube-embedded chondroitinase ABC in a canine clinical model of spinal cord injury. Brain. 2018 Apr 1;141(4):1017-1027. doi: 10.1093/brain/awy007. PMID: 29444239.

Martin-Vaquero P, da Costa RC. Transcranial magnetic motor evoked potentials in Great Danes with and without clinical signs of cervical spondylomyelopathy: association with neurological findings and magnetic resonance imaging. Vet J. 2014 Sep;201(3):327-32. doi: 10.1016/j.tvjl.2014.05.035. Epub 2014 May 28. PMID: 24929532; PMCID: PMC4160397.

Nollet H, Van Ham L, Deprez P, Vanderstraeten G. Transcranial magnetic stimulation: review of the technique, basic principles and applications. Vet J. 2003 Jul;166(1):28-42. doi: 10.1016/s1090-0233(03)00025-x. PMID: 12788015.

Nowakowska M, Üçal M, Charalambous M, Bhatti SFM, Denison T, Meller S, Worrell GA, Potschka H, Volk HA. Neurostimulation as a Method of Treatment and a Preventive Measure in Canine Drug-Resistant Epilepsy: Current State and Future Prospects. Front Vet Sci. 2022 Jun 16;9:889561. doi: 10.3389/fvets.2022.889561. PMID: 35782557; PMCID: PMC9244381.

Poma R, Parent JM, Holmberg DL, Partlow GD, Monteith G, Sylvestre AM. Correlation between severity of clinical signs and motor evoked potentials after transcranial magnetic stimulation in large-breed dogs with cervical spinal cord disease. J Am Vet Med Assoc. 2002 Jul 1;221(1):60-4. doi: 10.2460/javma.2002.221.60. PMID: 12420825.

Siedenburg JS, Wang-Leandro A, Amendt HL, Rohn K, Tipold A, Stein VM. Transcranial magnetic motor evoked potentials and magnetic resonance imaging findings in paraplegic dogs with recovery of motor function. J Vet Intern Med. 2018 May;32(3):1116-1125. doi: 10.1111/jvim.15058. Epub 2018 Mar 22. PMID: 29566440; PMCID: PMC5980462.

Sylvestre AM, Cockshutt JR, Parent JM, Brooke JD, Holmberg DL, Partlow GD. Magnetic motor evoked potentials for assessing spinal cord integrity in dogs with intervertebral disc disease. Vet Surg. 1993 Jan-Feb;22(1):5-10. doi: 10.1111/j.1532-950x.1993.tb00360.x. PMID: 8488675.

Van Ham LML, Vanderstraeten GGW, Mattheeuws DRG. Transcranial magnetic motor evoked potentials in sedated dogs. Prog Vet Neurol. 1994;5:147–154.

Van Soens I, Struys MM, Polis IE, Tshamala M, Nollet H, Bhatti SF, Van Ham LM. Effects of sedative and hypnotic drug combinations on transcranial magnetic motor evoked potential, bispectral index and ARX-derived auditory evoked potential index in dogs. Vet J. 2009 Aug;181(2):163-70. doi: 10.1016/j.tvjl.2008.02.014. Epub 2008 Aug 3. PMID: 18682332.

Van Soens I, Struys MM, Polis IE, Bhatti SF, Van Meervenne SA, Martlé VA, Nollet H, Tshamala M, Vanhaesebrouck AE, Van Ham LM. Magnetic stimulation of the radial nerve in dogs and cats with brachial plexus trauma: a report of 53 cases. Vet J. 2009 Oct;182(1):108-13. doi: 10.1016/j.tvjl.2008.05.007. Epub 2008 Jul 7. PMID: 18602850.

SECTION 12

Electroretinography

Maria Vanore

Key points:

- Electroretinography (ERG) is a test that measures the electrical response of the retinal cells (retinal action potentials) following light stimulation.
- Different protocols can be used in order to assess more specifically the different cell types within the retina.
- Rods are very sensitive to light and function at scotopic levels of illumination. To assess the rod response, a dim flash ERG is performed on a dark-adapted eye.
- Cones are less sensitive to light and function at photopic levels of illumination. To assess the cone response, flash ERG is performed on a light adapted eye.
- The a-wave (initial negative deflection) is generated by the photoreceptors.
- The b-wave (initial positive deflection) is mostly generated by the bipolar cells and Müller cells.
- ERG is indicated for investigations of retinal diseases and can also help identify a cause of blindness (e.g., to differentiate sudden onset retinal degeneration and optic neuritis).

Assessment of vision is crucial for localising and diagnosing numerous ocular and neurological disorders, in addition to helping guide the prognosis and treatment. Vision assessment is also an important part of the neurological examination because a large part of the visual pathway belongs to the central nervous system, and the optic disc is the only part of the central nervous system that can be viewed directly by the examiner. An animal with normal vision will have functional visual pathways from the retina to the lateral geniculate body, and then to the striate (visual) cortex (Aguirre, 1973). In animals with subnormal or absent vision, it is important to determine the anatomical origin of visual dysfunction to produce a list of differential diagnoses, which then allows the choice of the most appropriate investigations to reach a definitive diagnosis and give a prognosis for the return of vision. In this context, the flash electroretinogram (ERG) is an essential test to explore the visual state of the animal and to understand if the visual deficit comes from the retina or from the optic nerve.

1. What is flash ERG?

Flash ERG represents an electrical response of the retinal cells following light stimulation and is useful for both clinical and research activities to assess retinal function. To investigate specific retinal diseases, different retinal cell populations can be stimulated depending on the flashlight intensity and the environment light: rod, mixed rod-cone, and cone cells. Flash ERG can also assess visual function in animals with corneal and lens opacities that preclude observation of the ocular *fundus* (Gum, 1980).

Guidelines for clinical ERG protocols for humans have been provided by the International Society for Clinical Electrophysiology of Vision, and for animals by the European College of Veterinary Ophthalmologists (Ekesten *et al.*, 2013). In animals, two different protocols are available: a long and a short protocol. The long protocol (i.e., full-field ERG) is recorded under general anaesthesia and is useful for investigating retinal disorders. The short protocol is generally indicated for pre-operative evaluation of retinal function in conjunction with cataract surgery (Ekesten *et al.*, 2013).

The full-field ERG is an ophthalmologic test that provides non-invasive, objective, quantitative measures of the electrical activity in the retina (Asanad and Karanjia, 2023). It generates a response from the whole retina with the contribution of several retinal layers, summed throughout the retina. This is a useful tool for diagnosing diseases that present with generalised retinal dysfunction, such as rod/cone dystrophies, immune-mediated retinopathy, sudden acquired retinal degeneration (SARD), and toxic retinopathies (e.g., ivermectin). Importantly, the full-field ERG is not indicated for detecting small and localised retinal lesions.

2. The retinal cells contributing to electroretinogram signal generation

The retina includes the neuroretina, which is made of 3 layers of cells encoding light stimulation: the pre-receptor layer, the receptor layer, and the post-receptor layer (**Figure 12.1A**).

The pre-receptor layer includes the retinal pigment epithelium and its relationship to the photoreceptor cells in the subretinal space. The retinal pigment epithelium has a supportive role, including exchanges with the vasculature of the choroid and ion exchanges.

The receptor layer consists of the photoreceptor cells (rods and cones) that are specialised in the photo-transduction process, transforming light energy into electro-ionic energy. The canine retina is dominated by rod receptors. The rods are very light-sensitive and responsible for vision at low light levels, also called scotopic vision. The cones are responsible for vision at higher light levels, called photopic vision.

The post-receptor layer is responsible for transmitting the generated nervous signal to the primary visual cortex, with bipolar cells and ganglion cells that encode visual information in the form of an action potential.

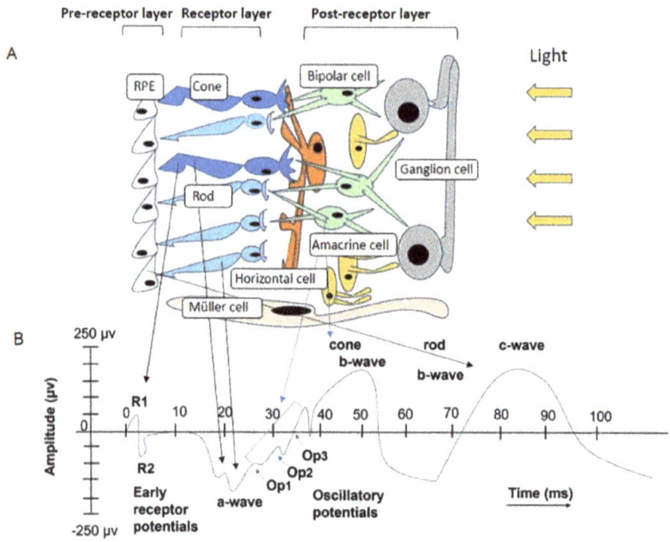

Figure 12.1. Schematic showing the cells of the retina and their electrophysiologic response to a spotlight flash. **A.** The retinal pigment epithelium is the layer of cells located just outside the receptor layer (in the pre-receptor layer, left of the image). The photoreceptors of the receptor layer are the rods and cones in which a negative receptor potential is elicited following stimulation by light. This drives the bipolar cells of the post-receptor layer to become either depolarised or hyperpolarised, and action potentials are transmitted to ganglion cells. The amacrine cells have a negative feedback effect by the release of inhibitory neurotransmitters. The horizontal cells release both excitatory and inhibitory neurotransmitters. **B.** Lower portion of Figure representing the flash ERG: The photopic a-wave is generated by the photoreceptors. The photopic b-wave is generated by the bipolar cells and Müller cells. Op1, Op2 and Op3 represent oscillatory potentials on the ascending part of the photopic b-wave, they are also generated by the bipolar cells. The c-wave derives from changes in the transepithelial potential of the retinal pigment epithelium. The c-wave is mostly recorded in flash ERG research protocols.

The Müller cells (or radial glial cells) span across the thickness of the retina and provide various physiological support to the cells of the neuroretina.

3. Polarisation and depolarisation of the cell membrane following light stimulation: phototransduction

The electrical signal is generated by a repeated alternating polarisation and depolarisation of cell membranes. The polarisation is characterised by a higher concentration of sodium ions (Na^+) in the extracellular space than in the intracellular space, and a higher concentration of potassium ions (K^+) in the intracellular space than in the extracellular space.

When light stimulation of retinal cells occurs, an increase in the permeability of the neuronal membrane is observed in the stimulated area. The sodium ions begin to come into the cell through specific ion channels, which are generally closed in the resting state. At the same time, potassium ions leave the cell via their own specific ion channels. The electrical charges on either side of the cell membrane have therefore an inversion point, which is the point of depolarisation. Photoreceptor cells are polarised in the light and depolarised in the dark. Light stimulation causes a series of repeatable polarisation changes in the retinal pigment epithelium, photoreceptors, and post-receptor layer cells. After light stimulation, hyperpolarisation leads to polarisation and then depolarisation of post-receptor layer cells. With regards to the pre-receptor layer cells, following light stimulation, there is hyperpolarisation of the retinal pigment epithelium, progressing to depolarisation, followed by a state of stable potential after 2 hours.

4. ERG waves

Three major ERG waves can be identified (see **Figure 12.1B**): the a-wave is the initial negative deflection (with a photopic recording) generated by hyperpolarisation of the photoreceptors; the b-wave is the initial positive deflection following the a-wave and is mostly generated by the bipolar cells and Müller cells – the b-wave also contains oscillatory potentials (e.g., Op1, Op2, Op3) along its ascending part; and the c-wave, which is a late positive deflection after the b-wave, reflecting the function of the retinal pigment epithelium. The c-wave is not always obtained and is not assessed in most cases. Each wave has its own amplitude, latency, and an implicit time.

5. Amplitude, latency and implicit time of the a-wave and b-wave

The amplitude, latency, and implicit time of the ERG waves are the main parameters of interest for the interpretation of the ERG. The amplitude (in µv) represents the wave height and is measured from the baseline to the peak of the wave. The latency (in ms) is measured from the onset of the light stimulus to the beginning of the wave. The implicit time (in ms) is the time from the stimulus onset to the peak of the wave (**Figure 12.2**). Amplitudes, latencies, and implicit times of the a-wave and b-wave are recorded in both scotopic (low light level) and photopic (high light level) conditions.

The amplitudes of ERG waves and their latency change during development: the amplitudes of ERG waves increase with age, and latencies decrease until maturation is complete. In a diseased eye, the inverse of this relationship becomes apparent, as the implicit times increase, and waveform amplitudes decrease (Gum, 1980).

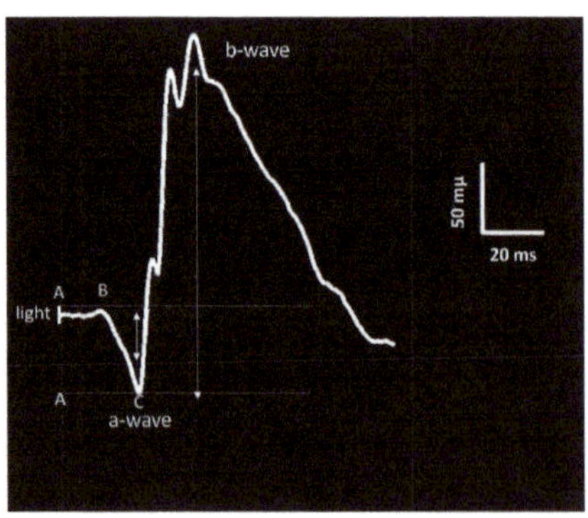

Figure 12.2. Photopic recording of a light-adapted retina showing the a-wave and b-wave. The amplitude of the a-wave (from B to C), the a-wave latency (from A to B) and a-wave implicit time (from A to C) are shown.

6. Methodology of ERG

All ERG units have a contact lens electrode and a built-in light source (LED-electrode). The waveform morphology and amplitude, implicit time, and latency results may differ depending on the ERG unit. It is therefore important that each clinic or laboratory performing diagnostic ERGs for generalised retinal diseases obtains its own normal values using its ERG equipment and establishes normal baseline values for the breeds and for the age groups studied. To monitor the evolution of retinal diseases or to compare different individuals, it is essential to always use the same ERG equipment for each study.

(i) Anaesthesia

Flash ERG should be performed under general anaesthesia in all animals, according to the recommendations of the European College of Veterinary Ophthalmologists guidelines (Ekesten *et al.*, 2013). However, for a short protocol, the flash ERG can be performed under sedation (Ekesten *et al.*, 2013). General anaesthesia prevents muscular movement, reduces stress levels, and reduces the movement of the electrodes which all improve the quality of the recordings (Acland, 1988).

Various sedation and anaesthesia protocols have been documented to affect ERG responses. The amplitude is generally reduced, and the latency increased depending on the protocol (Kommonen, 1988; Kommonen *et al.*, 1988). It is also important to be aware of species variations that may dictate the suitable types and doses of anaesthetics (Yu *et al.*, 2007; Freeman *et al.*, 2013). In the study by Freeman *et al.* (2013), ERG amplitudes were highest in awake dogs and lowest in anesthetised dogs, implicit times were shortest in awake dogs and longest in anesthetised dogs, and differences in b-wave amplitudes and a-wave implicit times were reported to be significant (Freeman *et al.*, 2013). In the study by Violette *et al.* (2022), high doses of trazodone (20mg/kg) and the combination of gabapentin (30mg/kg) and trazodone (5mg/kg) given orally significantly decreased a-wave and/or b-wave amplitudes in clinically normal dogs (Violette *et al.*, 2022).

(ii) Dark adaptation, mydriasis, eye position, electrodes, and standard flash

Both rod and cone functions can be evaluated using flash ERG – dark adapted (scotopic) tests are used to assess rod-driven retinal function, whilst light-adapted (photopic) tests are used to assess the cone-driven responses. Twenty minutes of dark pre-retinal adaptation time are essential before performing an ERG because this will allow all retinal cells to depolarise and therefore full evaluation of rod-driven retinal function. This is because rods are responsible for vision at low light levels, and their visual pigments are quickly used up under photopic conditions. In doing so, this also increases the mean amplitude and implicit time of the waveform ERG recording (Yu *et al.*, 2007).

To perform an ERG, both pupils are first dilated with 1% tropicamide drops. Pupil dilation is essential to obtain the optimal waveform, to avoid recording artefacts produced by reflex pupillary constriction, and to be able to stimulate the whole retina with light (Aguirre, 1973).

Dogs and cats are typically placed in ventral or lateral recumbency to record from either both eyes or one eye at a time, respectively. To achieve full retinal stimulation, the eyeballs should be centred in the orbit. If the eyes show a slight tendency to rotate due to sedation or anaesthesia, the globes can be immobilised with a retention wire.

A topical anaesthetic eyedrop (0.5% proparacaine hydrochloride) is applied to the eye(s) being tested before placing a corneal contact electrode (cathode), with the eyelids kept open using a lid speculum. A methylcellulose gel is applied between the corneal electrode and the cornea to protect the cornea and to ensure proper electrical contact between the electrode and the cornea (Yu *et al.*, 2007).

The electrical activity is recorded between two electrodes in response to retinal light stimulation, which intensity is measured in candelas (cd) (see **Figure 12.3**). The anode electrode is a subcutaneous needle placed under the skin 3-5cm from the lateral canthus, and the active electrode (cathode) is placed on the corneal surface (see above). This corneal contact electrode is a jet electrode comprising a disposable plastic lens with a gold-plated peripheral circumference (Ekesten *et al.*, 2013). Finally, a subcutaneous needle reference electrode is placed near the occipital protuberance.

A standard flash is used as the light stimulator, which is placed a couple of centimetres away from the tested eye (**Figure 12.3**). The strength (time-integrated luminance) of the flash stimulus is calculated by candelas seconds per meter squared (cd·sec/m^2). For a standardised bright white flash (photopic stimulation), the stimulus should have a luminance of 3cd·sec/m^2 to mainly stimulate the cones; and a dim-white flash at a luminance of 0.01 or 0.02cd·sec/m^2 mostly stimulates the rod component. The reason for lowering the intensity is to reduce cone-driven contamination of the dark-adapted rod responses (Ekesten *et al.* 2013). The intensity of the light stimulus can vary (acceptable

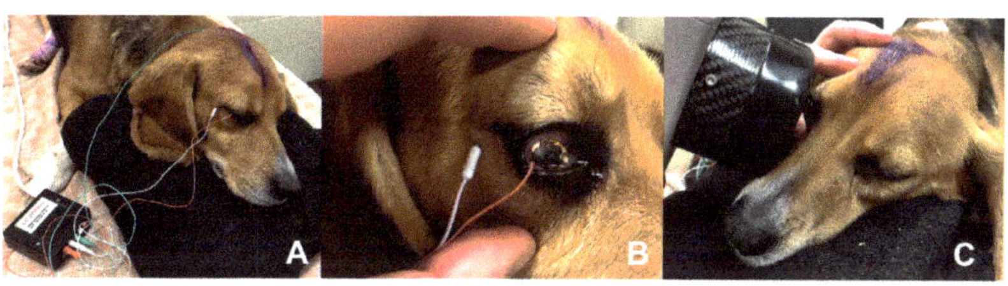

Figure 12.3. Electroretinogram procedure (short protocol under sedation rather than general anaesthesia as used for the standard long protocol). **A.** Under sedation, the dog is positioned in sternal recumbency. A reference subdermal needle electrode (green wire) is placed near the occipital protuberance and the anode electrode (white electrode here) is placed 3-5cm from the lateral canthus of the tested eye. **B.** A contact lens electrode (connected to the red wire in this example), cushioned with 0.3% hydroxypropyl methylcellulose, is applied to the cornea. **C.** The light stimulator is placed a couple of centimetres away from the eye.

range for the standard flash strength) while remaining within the limits indicated by the recommendations of the guidelines. For this reason, it is not possible to compare recorded results between different devices.

(iii) ***Bandpass for ERG recording***

The signal amplification and bandpass filter parameters can affect the quality of the recorded signal. Filtering is used to remove background noise, thus enhancing the signal-to-noise ratio and resulting in a cleaner ERG recording. Electrode impedance should be maintained below 2K-ohms (kΩ) and must be no more than 5kΩ (Ekesten *et al.*, 2013). The preamplifier's bandpass is generally set at 1-300Hz to record standard flash ERG, and in a second channel at 100-300Hz to record and isolate the oscillatory potentials (Ekesten *et al.*, 2013).

7. Morphology of the normal ERG

The shape of the waves generated by retinal stimulation depends on both the strength of the stimulation flash and the state of adaptation of the retina. As described above, scotopic measurements to assess rod pathway function are made from the dark-adapted eye, while photopic measurements that target cone pathway function are made from an eye adapted to light.

- The scotopic a-wave produced by rod stimulation in dim light background, and induced by a low light stimulation is negligible and followed by a slow (upwards) b-wave.
- The photopic a-wave is a downwards deflection induced by a higher light stimulation and it is generated by stimulation of all photoreceptors, in dim light background.
- The photopic b-wave follows the photopic a-wave and is a large amplitude upwards deflection. The origin of the b-wave is in the inner nuclear layer, with bipolar cells and Müller cells suggested to be the source of this

potential. Oscillatory potentials can be observed as small wavelets mainly on the rising phase of the b-wave using high-intensity light stimulus (**Figure 12.4**). If a specific study of the oscillatory potentials is required, it is recommended that a second dark-adapted, mixed rod–cone response is recorded using a high-pass filter setting at 70–100Hz (one flash every 15 seconds) after the dark-adapted, 3.0cd·sec/m^2, mixed rod–cone response (Ekesten *et al.,* 2013). Oscillatory potentials are helpful in the evaluation of disturbances of retinal circulation (Speros and Price, 1981).

- The c-wave is a positive potential of low amplitude with a long latency period; it is generated by the retinal pigment epithelium but is not generally assessed in standard ERG recordings (Gum, 1980).

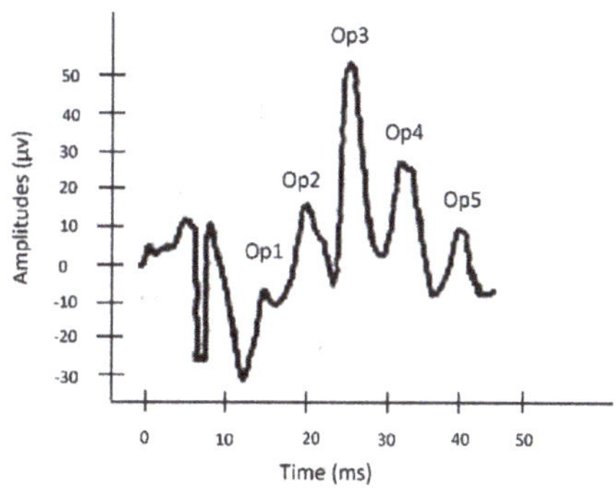

Figure 12.4. Oscillatory potentials of a standard scotopic full field flash electroretinogram.

8. Rod, mixed rod-cone, cone function and flicker

Rod function (**Figure 12.5A**) is recorded after stimulating the dark-adapted retina with low levels of light in a completely dark room, although a dim red room light may be used briefly (Ekesten *et al.,* 2013). The use of white light is recommended for the stimulus, with an intensity of the white flash being 0.01–0.02cd.sec/m^2 (Ekesten *et al.,* 2013). A single flash, repeated at 4-minute intervals, tests rod function and the dynamic process of dark adaptation. Regarding the averaged responses, usually not more than 4 responses are recorded and presented at a rate of 0.2-0.5Hz (Ekesten *et al.*, 2013).

A mixed rod-cone response (**Figure 12.5B**) is recorded after stimulating the retina with a single high-intensity flash of 3cd.sec/m^2. Averaged responses are recorded after 5 flashes; not more than one flash every 15 seconds is recommended in order not to light adapt the rods (Ekesten *et al.*, 2013).

Cone function (**Figure 12.5C**) is tested by light adapting the retina with a fixed multiple of the brightness of the standard flash to desensitise the rod system, and then stimulating the cones with high-intensity light stimuli. It is recommended that the dog be light adapted for 10 minutes using white background light of 30cd/m^2 (Ekesten *et al.,* 2013). The function of the cones is tested using a flash of 3cd.sec/m^2, presented on the white light-adapting background of 30cd/m^2 (Ekesten *et al.,* 2013). Averaging of responses is often required to reduce artefacts and background noise sufficiently, because the amplitudes are normally lower than dark adapted rod and mixed rod–cone responses. If averaging is used, the stimulus frequency should be <5Hz (Ekesten *et al.,* 2013).

Cone flicker responses in the dog (**Figure 12.5D**) should be evaluated at a frequency of 30Hz using a flash of 3cd.sec/m^2 presented on the white, light-adapting background of 30cd/m^2. The best way to obtain reliable and stable responses to the flickering stimulus is to discard the response to the first flash, as this will be a single-flash cone response that interferes with

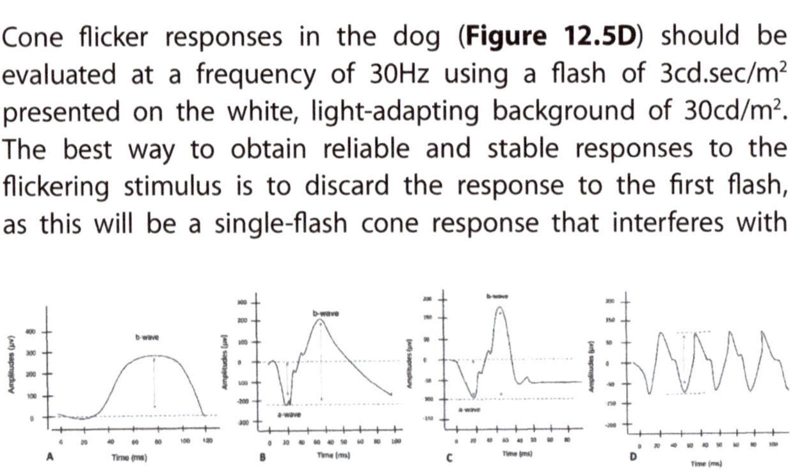

Figure 12.5. Rod, mixed rod-cone, cone responses and flicker in a dog under dark adapted conditions (0.01cd·sec/m^2 stimulus intensity for **A**, 3.0cd·sec/m^2 for **B**) and under light adapted conditions (3.0cd·sec/m^2 stimulus intensity) (**C** and **D**).

the waveform of the subsequent flicker responses. Flicker is used to selectively investigate the cone's function, under photopic conditions (Ekesten *et al.*, 2013).

9. Clinical application, retinal pathologies, and abnormal waves

Electroretinography is valuable for the detection of numerous retinal disorders, including hereditary retinal degeneration (known as progressive retinal atrophy), retinal detachments, hemeralopia (day blindness), and some systemic disorders (Gum, 1980). Some of these diseases can be detected with ERG months, and sometimes years, before any clinical abnormalities are exhibited (Gum, 1980).

Another important use for the ERG is that it can allow differentiation of a retinal disorder from other (neurologic) causes of acute vision loss, such as optic neuritis and intra-cranial neoplasia, in which ocular fundoscopic examination may be normal and ERG is generally not affected (**Figure 12.6**) (Montgomery *et al.*, 2008; Smith *et al.*, 2018).

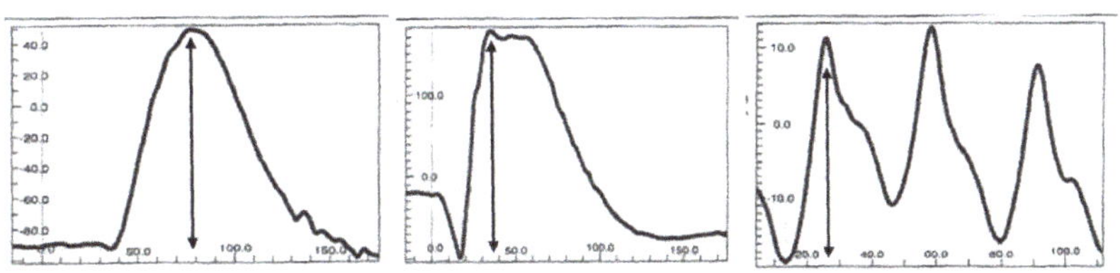

Figure 12.6. Normal ERG in a dog with optic neuritis showing (from the left to the right) the rod response mixed rod-cone response), and flicker.

(i) *Sudden acquired retinal degeneration syndrome*

Dogs affected by sudden acquired retinal degeneration syndrome (SARDS) typically present for assessment of rapid vision loss, that develops over a period of days to weeks, and may also show signs similar to dogs with hyperadrenocorticism (e.g., polyphagia, polyuria/polydipsia, lethargy) (Carter *et al.*, 2009; Auten *et al.*, 2018; Komáromy *et al.*, 2016). In the early stage, affected dogs have a normal retina on fundoscopic examination, with normal to absent pupillary light reflexes. The main differential diagnoses for this condition include optic neuritis, progressive retinal atrophy and immune-mediated retinitis. An absent ('extinguished') flash ERG, when seen in conjunction with a clinically normal appearing fundus, is considered the hallmark of SARDS (Komáromy *et al.*, 2016; Grozdanic *et al.*, 2008). Dogs that have SARDS do not have detectable rod (scotopic ERG) or cone (photopic ERG) electrical activity (Grozdanic *et al.*, 2008) (**Figure 12.7**).

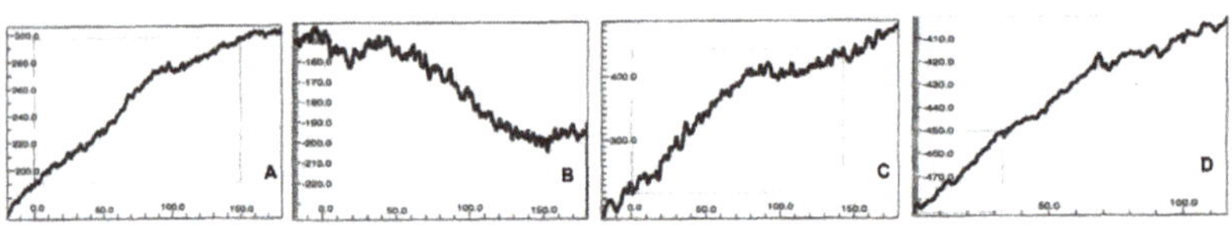

Figure 12.7. ERG in a case with sudden acquired retinal degeneration, showing from the left to the right (A-D) that there are no representative waveforms.

(ii) Immune-mediated retinitis

Immune-mediated retinitis is another retinal disease that must be considered in dogs presenting with a sudden loss or decrease of vision. Clinically, in the early stages, dogs can present with a normal fundoscopic examination, the dazzle reflex can be present, and the pupillary light reflexes normal. Dogs with immune-mediated retinitis can have normal, supranormal, or decreased amplitudes on scotopic and photopic ERG (**Figure 12.8**). It is not unusual to detect completely extinguished ERG amplitudes in one eye and barely detectable or normal amplitudes in the opposite eye (Grozdanic *et al.*, 2008).

The proposed molecular mechanisms underlying the retinal damage seen in SARDS and immune-mediated retinitis are similar, involving activation of T-cells, macrophages and B-cells, with

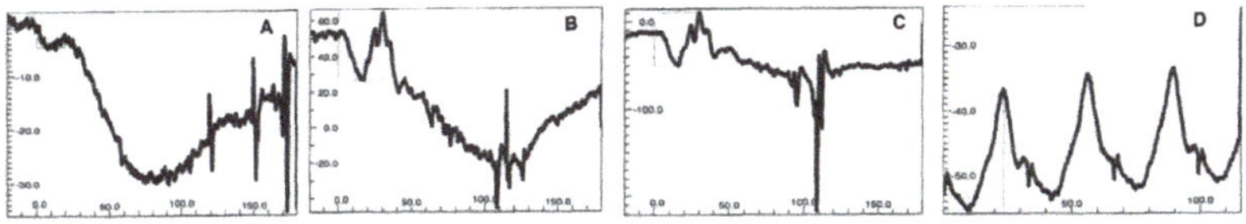

Figure 12.8. ERG in a dog with immune-mediated retinopathy, showing from the left to the right. **A.** Rod-response (dark adapted 0.01cd.sec/m^2) (scotopic b-wave: 1.7µv; 19.9ms). **B.** Mixed rod-cone response (dark adapted 3cd.sec/m^2) (photopic a-wave: 25.4 µv; 17.3ms, b-wave: 37.5 µv; 30.2ms). **C.** Cone response (light adapted 10cd.sec/m^2) (photopic a-wave: 38.1µv; 15.2ms, b-wave: 60.0µv; 29.5ms). **D.** Flicker (light adapted 3cd.sec/m^2) (18.6 µv; 23.5ms). The amplitudes and the implicit times are decreased compared to a normal ERG.

auto-antibodies attacking the retina coming from the systemic circulation or being produced locally (Grozdanic *et al.*, 2008).

(iii) Progressive retinal atrophy

Progressive retinal atrophy is an inherited disease caused by mutation of variants that impact rod functioning first, resulting in loss of rod-mediated ERG responses, prior to significant retinal thinning that can be detected on fundoscopic examination (Millichamp, 1990; Kelawala *et al.*, 2017). In the early stages of the disease, dogs appear to have vision loss in dim light background levels, sluggish pupillary light reflexes and the ERG is affected in rod but not cone responses (Millichamp, 1990; Kelawala *et al.*, 2017). As the retinal atrophy progresses, dogs have dilated pupils and start to also show a decrease in daylight vision. In the advanced stages, cone responses are also affected manifesting as a complete retinal degeneration and the ERG amplitudes continue to decrease until all waveforms are extinguished (Gum, 1980; Millichamp, 1990; Kelawala *et al.*, 2017). The ERG is sensitive enough to diagnose progressive retinal atrophy in dogs even before they begin to show obvious clinical signs of dim light background vision loss (**Figure 12.9**)(Kelawala *et al.*, 2017).

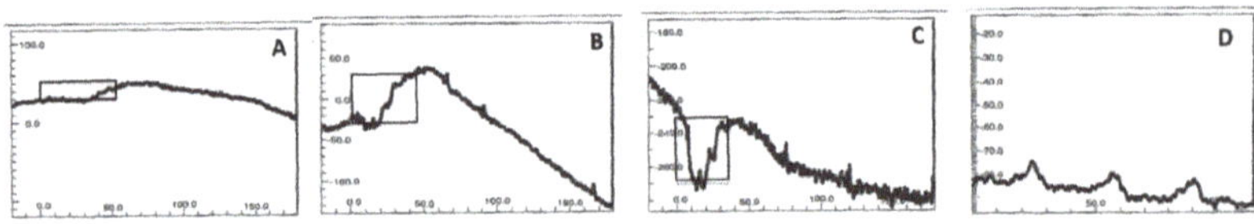

Figure 12.9. Electroretinogram in a dog with progressive retinal atrophy, showing from the left to the right: **A**. Rod-response (dark adapted 0.02cd.sec/m^2) (scotopic b-wave: 21.2μv; 61.3ms); **B**. Rod-cone mixed response (dark adapted 2cd.sec/m^2) (photopic a-wave: 6.6μv; 16.5ms, b-wave: 68.1μv; 44.1ms); **C**. Cone response (light adapted 2cd.sec/m^2) (photopic a-wave: 45.3μv; 17.2ms, b-wave: 37.0μv; 36.5ms) and **D**. Flicker (10.0μv; 24.5ms). The amplitudes and the implicit times are decreased compared to a normal ERG.

(iv) Retinal detachment and cataracts

Electroretinography can be used as a prognostic indicator for postoperative vision in dogs undergoing retinal reattachment surgery, as a recordable pre-operative ERG, even if attenuated, is associated with the return of vision in these dogs (Hoffman *et al.*, 2018).

In a study by Maehara *et al.* (2007), no significant difference was found in ERG amplitude between incipient, immature and hyper mature cataractous eyes. However, in mature cataractous eyes a decreased amplitude was confirmed in all responses compared to control eyes. The effect of lens induced uveitis (LIU) on ERG was only seen as a decreased b-wave amplitude, possibly related to an effect on choroidal and retinal circulation (Maehara *et al.*, 2007).

(v) Optic neuritis

Optic neuritis is a condition caused by uni- or bilateral inflammation of the optic nerves. It is most commonly immune-mediated and attributed to a focal form of meningoencephalitis of unknown origin (e.g., granulomatous meningoencephalitis) (Smith *et al.*, 2018). Dogs will typically present with a sudden, unilateral or bilateral, partial or complete loss of vision, sometimes with concurrent neurologic abnormalities. Pupillary light reflexes are often abnormal, but they may also be normal, particularly in the early stages of the disease. Fundoscopic examination may be abnormal and reveal peripapillary retinal oedema, a swollen optic nerve head, and/or haemorrhage of the retinal vasculature (Smith *et al.,* 2018). As described above, an important differential diagnosis for optic neuritis is SARDS given the similarity in clinical presentation. However, unlike in dogs with SARDS, the ERG is normal in dogs with optic neuritis. Therefore, referral to an ophthalmologist for examination and ERG is always recommended for dogs with acute vision loss, followed by referral to a neurologist for an MRI scan of the brain and cerebrospinal fluid analysis if the ERG is normal (Smith *et al.,* 2018). In humans, standard ERG cannot distinguish the normal eye from one affected by unilateral optic neuritis. However, differences between eyes may be highlighted by the N95 amplitude wave of pattern electroretinography (PERG), which is significantly lower in the affected eye, and the pattern reversal visual evoked potential (PVEP), which showed a significantly longer latency in the affected eye (Maehara *et al.,* 2007).

10. Additional ERG modalities

(i) Pattern electroretinography

This test measures the retinal response to a contrast inversion pattern, usually using a checkerboard pattern. In humans, it provides information on macular function, as well as retinal ganglion cell function, and can be used to study diseases such as glaucoma (Bach *et al.,* 2013). In dogs with glaucoma, studies have shown reductions in pattern ERG function corresponding to increased intra-ocular pressure, despite scotopic and photopic ERG analysis being normal (Grozdanic *et al.,* 2010). Pattern ERG is rarely used in veterinary practice.

(ii) Multifocal ERG

This test provides better spatial resolution of retinal function than regular full-field flash ERG. Multifocal ERG creates a topographic map of the retina, allowing assessment of the local retinal activity in different areas. It is typically performed in photopic conditions and thus primarily measures cone responses. In humans, multifocal ERG can be used for inherited diseases to: (i) better localise and evaluate conditions which tend to preferentially affect certain areas of the retina, such as Stargardt macular dystrophy; (ii) better classify the effects of *retinitis pigmentosa*; and (iii) evaluate retinal damage after surgical treatment (Hood *et al.,* 2012). In dogs, multifocal ERG has been used to better understand the multifocal retinopathy in Dachshunds with CLN2, a form of neuronal ceroid lipofuscinosis. This condition is characterised by progressive vision loss culminating in blindness, cognitive and motor decline, neurodegeneration, and premature death (Whiting *et al.,* 2015).

(iii) Visual evoked potentials

Visual evoked potentials (VEP) can evaluate visual acuity objectively. They are useful for assessing post-retinal visual pathways and represent visual cortex waves following a light stimulus. Visual evoked potentials are classified into flash-stimulated VEP, which uses a white light, and pattern VEP, which uses a contrast-reversing black and white checkboard pattern-reversal (Maehara *et al.,* 2018).

Visual evoked potentials are representations of electroencephalographic activity of the visual cortex following light stimulation. They have been used as a diagnostic aid in several human disorders, including Alzheimer's disease and demyelinating disorders such as multiple sclerosis. They have also been used for intraoperative monitoring during procedures such as pituitary tumour resection (Chang *et al.,* 2022). One possible reason for the limited use of VEP in dogs is the apparent contamination of recordings from the electroencephalographic activity, possibly influenced by the choice of recording electrode placement (Chang *et al.,* 2022).

Visual evoked potentials can be recorded under sedation and general anaesthesia. Each recording corresponds to the average of 400 flashes of white light (1.5/sec) from a photostimulator held approximately 20cm from the eye while the contralateral eye is covered. The recording bandpass is generally set at 1-100Hz. Three subcutaneous needle electrodes are used to record the responses: the positive electrode is placed in the midline of the nuchal crest, the negative (recording) at the midline, just caudal to the eyes, and the reference ('ground') electrode at the vertex (Strain *et al.*, 1990). The pupils need not be dilated for the flash-stimulated VEP. Pattern VEP is typically recorded with pupils unaltered by mydriatic or miotic drugs, but mydriasis can increase amplitudes. (Maehara *et al.*, 2018; Odom *et al.*, 2016). Pattern VEP, is rarely used in veterinary practice, uses checkerboard light stimulus.

Flash-stimulated VEP is characterised by a series of five positive and negative peaks: P1, N1, P2, N2, and P3 (**Figure 12.10**), with peak P2 being the most prominent (Strain *et al.*, 1990). The earliest detectable component has a peak time of approximately 30ms post stimulus, and components are recordable with peak times of up to 300ms. Peaks are described as negative and positive in a numerical sequence. This nomenclature is recommended to differentiate the flash-stimulated VEP from the pattern VEP. The three main peaks of pattern VEP are positive (N75), negative (N100) and positive (N135), in accordance with previously published guidelines (Odom *et al.*, 2016). With flash-stimulated VEP, measurements consist of the implicit time to each of five peaks, identified as P1, N1, P2, N2, and P3, and the peak-to-peak amplitudes P1-N1, N1-P2, P2-N2, and N2-P3 **(Figure 12.10**) (Strain *et al.*, 1990). However, very few studies on VEP have been conducted in cats and dogs.

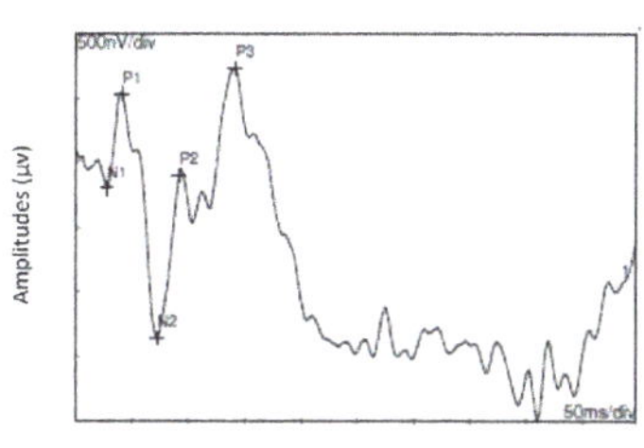

Figure 12.10. Normal flash-stimulated VEP in a healthy dog.

References

Acland GM. Diagnosis and differentiation of retinal diseases in small animals by electroretinography. Semin Vet Med Surg Small Anim. Feb 1988;3(1):15-27. PMID: 3283886.

Aguirre GD. Electroretinography in Veterinary Ophthalmology. Journal of the American Animal Hospital Association. 1973;9: 234-237.

Asanad S, Karanjia R. Full-Field Electroretinogram. StatPearls. StatPearls Publishing

Copyright © 2023, StatPearls Publishing LLC.; 2023. PMID: 32491415.

Auten CR, Thomasy SM, Kass PH, Good KL, Hollingsworth SR, Maggs DJ. Cofactors associated with Sudden Acquired Retinal Degeneration Syndrome: 151 dogs within a reference population. Vet Ophthalmol. May 2018;21(3):264-272. doi:10.1111/vop.12504. PMID: 28845542.

Bach M, Brigell MG, Hawlina M, *et al.* ISCEV standard for clinical pattern electroretinography (PERG): 2012 update. Doc Ophthalmol. Feb 2013;126(1):1-7. doi:10.1007/s10633-012-9353-y. PMID: 23073702.

Carter RT, Oliver JW, Stepien RL, Bentley E. Elevations in sex hormones in dogs with sudden acquired retinal degeneration syndrome (SARDS). J Am Anim Hosp Assoc. Sep-Oct 2009;45(5):207-14. doi:10.5326/0450207. PMID: 19723843.

Chang S, Zwueste D, Ambros B, Norton J, Leis ML. Comparison of the effect of sedation and general anaesthesia on pattern and flash visual evoked potentials in normal dogs. BMC Vet Res. Jul 13 2022;18(1):272. doi:10.1186/s12917-022-03375-5~. PMID: 35831819. PMCID: PMC9277965.

Ekesten B, Komáromy AM, Ofri R, Petersen-Jones SM, Narfström K. Guidelines for clinical electroretinography in the dog: 2012 update. Doc Ophthalmol. Oct 2013;127(2):79-87. doi:10.1007/s10633-013-9388-8. PMID: 23728902.

Freeman KS, Good KL, Kass PH, Park SA, Nestorowicz N, Ofri R. Effects of chemical restraint on electroretinograms recorded sequentially in awake, sedated, and anesthetized dogs. Am J Vet Res. Jul 2013;74(7):1036-42. doi:10.2460/ajvr.74.7.1036. PMID: 23802676.

Grozdanic SD, Lazic T, Kecova H, Mohan K, Adamus G, Kuehn MH. Presumed cancer-associated retinopathy (CAR) mimicking Sudden Acquired Retinal Degeneration Syndrome (SARDS) in canines. Vet Ophthalmol. Mar 2021;24(2):125-155. doi:10.1111/vop.12853. PMID: 33369040. PMCID: PMC8048582.

Grozdanic SD, Harper MM, Kecova H. Antibody-mediated retinopathies in canine patients: mechanism, diagnosis, and treatment modalities. Vet Clin North Am Small Anim Pract. Mar 2008;38(2):361-87, vii. doi:10.1016/j.cvsm.2007.12.003. PMID: 18299012.

Grozdanic SD, Kecova H, Harper MM, Nilaweera W, Kuehn MH, Kardon RH. Functional and structural changes in a canine model of hereditary primary angle-closure glaucoma. Invest Ophthalmol Vis Sci. Jan 2010;51(1):255-63. doi:10.1167/iovs.09-4081. PMID: 19661222. PMCID: 3258664.

Gum GG. Electrophysiology in Veterinary Ophthalmology. Vet Clin North Am Small Anim Pract. 1980/05/01/ 1980;10(2):437-454. doi: 10.1016/S0195-5616(80)50039-2. PMID: 6998098.

Hoffman A, Sisler S, Pappania M, Hsu K, Ross M, Ofri R. Electroretinography is a prognostic indicator for postoperative vision in dogs undergoing retinal reattachment surgery. Vet Ophthalmol. May 2018;21(3):273-280. doi:10.1111/vop.12505. PMID: 28952177.

Hood DC, Bach M, Brigell M, *et al.* ISCEV standard for clinical multifocal electroretinography (mfERG) (2011 edition). Doc Ophthalmol. Feb 2012;124(1):1-13. doi:10.1007/s10633-011-9296-8. PMID: 22038576. PMCID: PMC4466109.

Kelawala DN, Patil DB, Parikh PV, Sheth MJ, Joshi CG, Reddy B. Clinical studies on progressive retinal atrophy in 31 dogs. Iran J Vet Res. Spring 2017;18(2):119-123. PMID: 28775752. PMCID: PMC5534255.

Komáromy AM, Abrams KL, Heckenlively JR, *et al.* Sudden acquired retinal degeneration syndrome (SARDS) – a review and proposed strategies toward a better understanding of pathogenesis, early diagnosis, and therapy. Vet Ophthalmol. Jul 2016;19(4):319-31. doi:10.1111/vop.12291. PMID: 26096588.

Kommonen B. The DC-recorded dog electroretinogram in ketamine-medetomidine anaesthesia. Acta Vet Scand. 1988;29(1):35-41. doi:10.1186/bf03548389. PMID: 2904729. PMCID: PMC8152565.

Kommonen B, Karhunen U, Raitta C. Effects of thiopentone halothane-nitrous oxide anaesthesia compared to ketamine-xylazine anaesthesia on the DC recorded dog electroretinogram. Acta Vet Scand. 1988;29(1):23-33. doi:10.1186/bf03548388. PMID: 3202057. PMCID: PMC8152564.

Maehara S, Itoh N, Wakaiki S, Yamasaki A, Tsuzuki K, Izumisawa Y. The effects of cataract stage, lens-induced uveitis and cataract removal on ERG in dogs with cataract. *Vet Ophthalmol.* Sep-Oct 2007;10(5):308-12. doi:10.1111/j.1463-5224.2007.00559.x. PMID: 17760711.

Maehara S, Itoh Y, Ito Y, Hayashi M, Masuko A. Measurement of visual acuity in Beagle dog by visual evoked potential with pattern stimulation. J Vet Med Sci. Nov 23 2018;80(11):1758-1761. doi:10.1292/jvms.18-0334. PMID: 30282843. PMCID: PMC6261824.

Millichamp NJ. Retinal degeneration in the dog and cat. Vet Clin North Am Small Anim Pract. May 1990;20(3):799-835. doi:10.1016/s0195-5616(90)50063-7. PMID: 2194359.

Montgomery KW, van der Woerdt A, Cottrill NB. Acute blindness in dogs: sudden acquired retinal degeneration syndrome versus neurological disease (140 cases, 2000-2006). Vet Ophthalmol. Sep-Oct 2008;11(5):314-20. doi:10.1111/j.1463-5224.2008.00652.x. PMID: 19046291.

Odom JV, Bach M, Brigell M, *et al.* ISCEV standard for clinical visual evoked potentials: (2016 update). Doc Ophthalmol. Aug 2016;133(1):1-9. doi:10.1007/s10633-016-9553-y. PMID: 27443562.

Smith SM, Westermeyer HD, Mariani CL, Gilger BC, Davidson MG. Optic neuritis in dogs: 96 cases (1983-2016). Vet Ophthalmol. Sep 2018;21(5):442-451. doi:10.1111/vop.12528. PMID: 29251394.

Speros P, Price J. Oscillatory potentials. History, techniques and potential use in the evaluation of disturbances of retinal circulation. Surv Ophthalmol. Jan-Feb 1981;25(4):237-52. doi:10.1016/0039-6257(81)90093-x. PMID: 7010647.

Strain GM, Jackson RM, Tedford BL. Visual evoked potentials in the clinically normal dog. J Vet Intern Med. Jul-Aug 1990;4(4):222-5. doi:10.1111/j.1939-1676.1990.tb00901.x. PMID: 2401969.

Violette NP, Newbold GM, Chen C, Miller EJ, Gemensky-Metzler AJ. Effects of gabapentin and trazodone on electroretinographic responses in clinically normal dogs. Am J Vet Res. Jun 13 2022;83(8). doi:10.2460/ajvr.22.03.0047. PMID: 35895792.

Whiting RE, Pearce JW, Castaner LJ, *et al.* Multifocal retinopathy in Dachshunds with CLN2 neuronal ceroid lipofuscinosis. Exp Eye Res. May 2015;134:123-32. doi:10.1016/j.exer.2015.02.012. PMID: 25697710. PMCID: PMC4426040.

Yu HA, Jeong MB, Park SA, *et al.* The determination of dark adaptation time using electroretinography in conscious miniature Schnauzer dogs. *J Vet Sci.* Dec 2007;8(4):409-14. doi:10.4142/jvs.2007.8.4.409. PMID: 17993756. PMCID: PMC2868158.

SECTION 13

Tests of hearing

Ezio Bianchi

Key points:

- The propagation of sound waves from the external environment to the auditory cortex involves the external ear canal, the tympanic membrane, the middle ear, the oval window, the perilymphatic fluid of the inner ear, the organ of Corti and spiral ganglion, the cochlear nerve and central auditory pathway to the temporal cortex.
- Deafness (hypoacusia) can be divided into conductive deafness (disorders of the outer and/or middle ear) and sensorineural deafness, which may result from dysfunction of the cochlea, peripheral or central auditory pathways.
- The recording of brainstem auditory evoked responses is the most commonly used method to assess auditory function in animals. This is performed by sending click sounds of various intensities into the external ear canal and recording 5 main waves using three subcutaneous needles (two recording electrodes: a cathode and an anode, and a reference) placed at specific sites around the head. The presence/absence of the waves and their latencies allows assessment of the auditory pathway and hearing ability.

1. Introduction

Sound produces a conscious acoustic sensation through a four-step process (**Figure 13.1**):

- The first step is the collection and funnelling of sound waves in the outer ear, towards the tympanic membrane;
- Then, the middle ear transmits vibrations of the tympanic membrane to the oval window that compresses the perilymphatic fluid of the inner ear;
- The third step is the transduction of the waves in the perilymph into electrical impulses in the cochlear nerve through activation of the organ of Corti and spiral ganglion;
- The last step is the transmission of electric impulses along the central auditory pathway to the auditory cortex.

Figure 13.1. Anatomical diagram depicting the structures involved in the production of a conscious acoustic sensation. 1: outer ear; 2: tympanic membrane; 3: middle ear; 4: malleus, incus and stapes; 5: oval window; 6: cochlea (organ of Corti, spiral ganglion); 7: peripheral vestibular apparatus; 8: vestibulocochlear nerve.

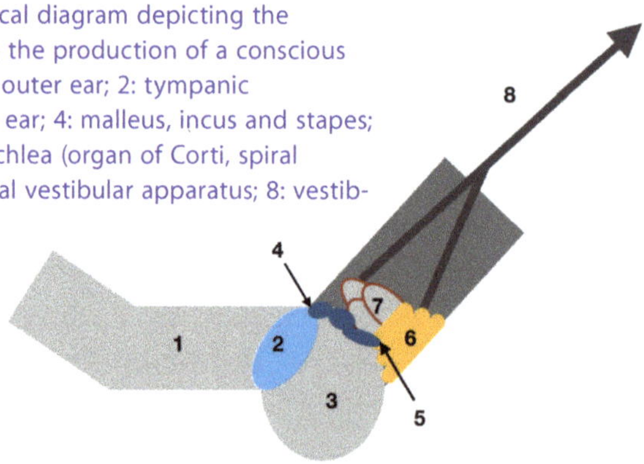

Deafness (hypoacusia) is the consequence of a structural or functional abnormality of this complex process and can be investigated in companion animals using specific diagnostic tests:

- Disorders affecting the outer and/or middle ear cause conductive deafness. Impedance audiometry tests (e.g., tympanometry, acoustic reflex, etc.), that directly evaluate the function of the tympanic membrane and structures of the middle ear, are used to diagnose conductive deafness.

- Disorders affecting the cochlea, peripheral or central auditory pathways cause sensorineural deafness. The tests used to investigate sensorineural deafness are brainstem auditory evoked responses (BAER – most commonly), otoacoustic emissions (OAE) and auditory steady-state responses (ASSR). Brainstem auditory evoked responses may also be used for diagnosis of conductive deafness.

2. Brainstem auditory evoked responses: definitions and methods

(i) Definitions

The recording of brainstem auditory evoked responses (BAER) (also known as brainstem auditory evoked potentials [BAEP] or auditory brainstem responses [ABR]) is the most commonly used method to assess auditory function in animals. Brainstem auditory evoked responses are far-field potentials evoked along the auditory pathway following acoustic stimulation. They are produced within 10ms of the stimulus and are defined as early latency potentials, because they reflect the activation of the cochlear nerve and neural structures of the brainstem (Sims and Moore, 1984).

Other auditory potentials recorded more than 10ms after the stimulus are classed as middle latency potentials (10-50ms) and long latency potentials (>50ms) (Farley and Starr, 1983). These potentials, originating at higher levels in the central auditory pathway, are affected by level of consciousness and anaesthesia and therefore less used in the diagnosis of hearing impairment in dogs and cats.

(ii) Equipment and type of stimulation

Brainstem auditory evoked responses recording can be performed with either dedicated stand-alone equipment, or by using electro-diagnostic systems designed for clinical neurophysiology that commonly contain many other functionalities and can generate the auditory stimulus needed for the test.

Stimulation of the auditory structures can be accomplished by using air-conducted or bone-conducted stimuli.

a. Air-conducted stimulation

The air-conducted click is the most widely used acoustic stimulus and is generated by a transducer delivering a square electrical pulse of 100μs. The click is a broadband stimulus that includes many frequencies and activates large portions of the cochlea. To investigate frequency specific hearing, more selective stimulation of the cochlea with pure tones is necessary. Tones are stimuli developed to produce a frequency specific BAER. The frequency of the tone, and consequently the area of the cochlea evaluated, can be chosen by the operator.

The transducers used to produce air-conducted acoustic stimuli can be headphones or insert earphones (**Figure 13.2**). The latter are usually preferred because they create less stimulus artefacts and allow a better acoustic insulation of the stimulated ear (Strain, 2011; Scheifele and Clark, 2012).

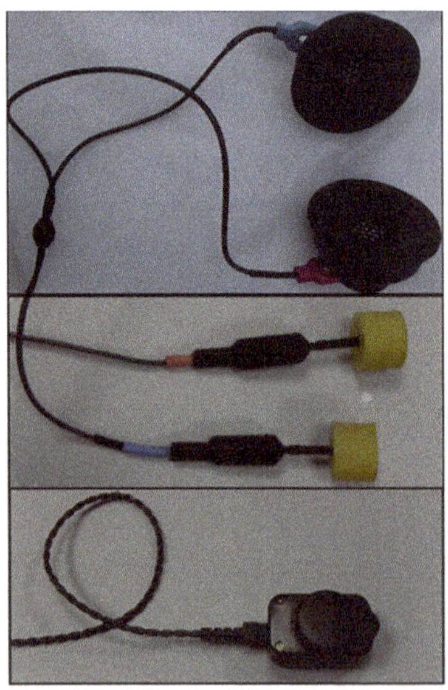

Figure 13.2. Transducers used for stimulation of auditory structures. Headphones (upper picture), insert earphones (middle picture), bone stimulator (lower picture).

b. Bone-conducted stimulation

Bone-conducted stimuli are produced by specific transducers creating vibrations applied to the ipsilateral mastoid process of the temporal bone. The vibratory stimulus bypasses the conductive structures of the outer and middle ear and directly activates the cochlea. Bone stimulation is therefore indicated to differentiate conductive from sensorineural deafness (Sims, 1988; Munro *et al.*, 1997).

(iii) Stimulation characteristics

a. Stimulus polarity

The stimulus polarity is dependent on the movement of the transducer membrane during acoustic stimulation. With rarefaction polarity, the membrane first moves outwards and then inwards.

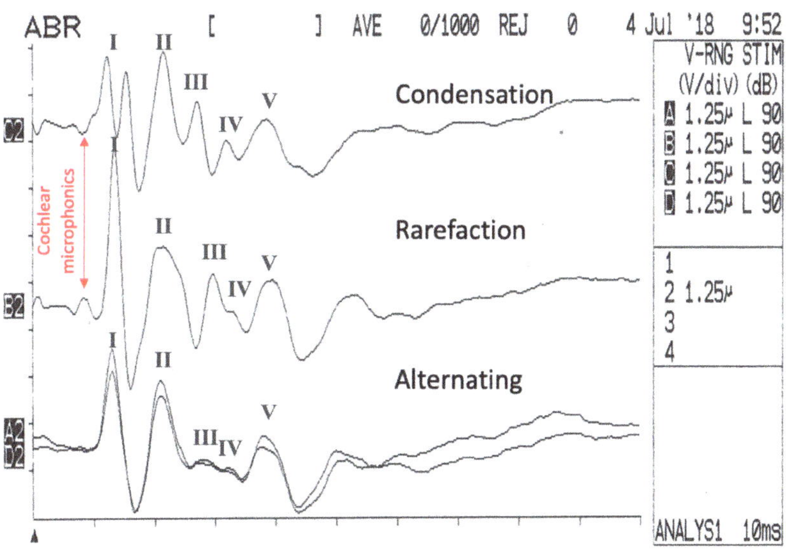

Figure 13.3. Effect of stimulus polarity on BAER waveform. Alternating polarity is the result of the summation of waveforms obtained with both rarefaction and condensation polarity. Therefore, alternating polarity eliminates cochlear microphonics but might induce partial phase cancellation of BAER waves, as happens for wave III and IV of this normal dog. 1 ms/division; 1.25 μV/division.

The opposite happens with condensation polarity. The operator can choose the polarity of the stimulus or decide to alternate between the two polarities (i.e., alternating polarity). Rarefaction and condensation polarity induce BAER of slightly different latencies and amplitudes (Sims, 1988). Because of the latency shift between the two polarities, summation of waves obtained with rarefaction and condensation makes BAER waveforms recorded with alternating polarity slightly less definite (Chiappa, 1997). However, recordings with rarefaction or condensation polarities may contain cochlear microphonics that are potentials produced by the outer hair cells of the cochlea in response to acoustic stimuli and precede the first wave (I) of the BAER. Their polarity is the same as the polarity of the stimulus used. Therefore, cochlear microphonics are cancelled out by using an alternating polarity and this may help when differentiation between cochlear microphonics and wave I is difficult (**Figure 13.3**).

b. Stimulation rate

The stimulation rate is the number of stimuli per second that are delivered to the patient (1 stimulus per second = 1Hz). The higher the stimulus rate, the shorter the duration of the test. A progressive reduction in resolution of BAER waveforms is expected with an increasing stimulation rate. However, rates up to 91Hz do not significantly affect waveform clarity in dogs (Wilson *et al.*, 2011).

c. Stimulus intensity

In practice, the stimulus intensity is usually expressed in decibels above normal hearing level (dB HL or dB nHL). Zero dB nHL represents the average hearing threshold of a group of normal-hearing people. The intensity of the stimulus directly influences the BAER waveform. With increasing intensity, the latencies of the waves decrease, and the amplitudes of the waves increase (Sims, 1988).

d. Masking sound

Each ear is tested separately. The non-tested, contralateral, ear receives white noise to prevent unwanted cross-stimulation from the tested ear (crossover effect). To reduce the risk of crossover effect, the intensity of the contralateral masking noise should be ~30-40dB below the intensity of the stimulus used for the tested ear (Strain, 2011).

(iv) Recording

Recording of BAER is usually performed using subdermal needle electrodes. In the most commonly used montage, called the mastoid-vertex montage, the anode electrode is placed at the vertex of the skull (midway between the eyes and nuchal crest along the midline) and the cathode just cranial to the base of the ear (mastoid area) of the stimulated ear (**Figure 13.4a**). Another possible montage uses the same position for the anode electrode, while the cathode is placed at the level of the dorsal spinous process of the T1 vertebra (the T1-vertex montage) (**Figure 13.4b**). The reference electrode can be inserted subcutaneously in various areas, such as the nuchal crest, base of the neck or contralateral mastoid area. The active electrode is connected to the amplifier so that the positive electrical activity detected at the vertex produces an upward deflection on the screen (non-inverting input – see 'Section 2.1 – Amplifier'). For optimal recording, the impedance of the electrodes must be below 10kΩ. The impedance difference between the cathode and the anode should be less than 3kΩ.

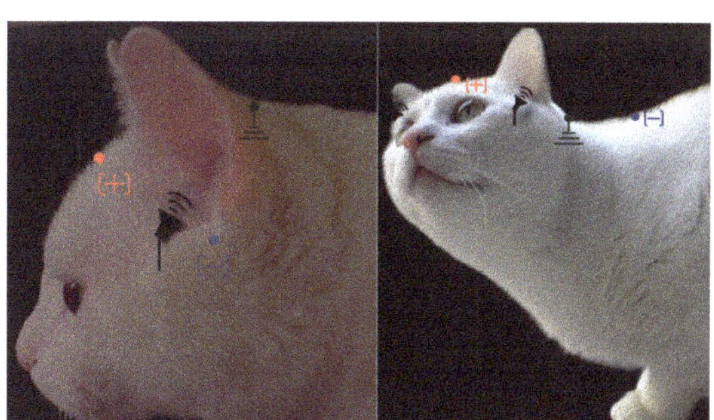

Figure 13.4. Position of recording needles in mastoid-vertex montage (a: left picture) and in T1-vertex montage (b: right picture). Anode electrode: red; cathode: blue; reference: green.

The amplifier of the equipment is often in a non-inverting configuration, and set to filter the recorded signal using a low cut-off/high pass filter (usually 15-150Hz) and a high cut-off/low pass filter (usually 1500-3000Hz). The low amplitude signal of BAER requires significant amplification, with an amplification factor of 100,000 to 200,000 usually applied in dogs and cats.

Despite amplification, the low voltage BAER still requires averaging the responses from several hundred stimuli to obtain a clear waveform. Averaging the signal allows the extraction of the potentials that are 'evoked' by each stimulus, and therefore replicated with a fixed latency and amplitude from the random background noise. An automatic artefact rejection system is also present in most amplifiers. Automatic artefact rejection excludes from the averaging process the traces that contain potentials of very high amplitudes that exceed a predetermined threshold, like muscle activity. The number of responses that need to be averaged depends on the background noise and amplitude of the waves. From 250 to 2000 stimulations may be necessary to obtain a sufficiently clear trace. At least one other trial, obtained with the same settings, should be performed and superimposed to the first recording, to verify waveform consistency (Sims, 1988; Chiappa, 1997; Strain, 2011; Scheifele and Clark, 2012).

3. Brainstem auditory evoked responses: normal waveform

(i) Morphology of the brainstem auditory evoked responses

The normal BAER waveform is composed of 6-7 vertex positive waves, which are usually labelled using Roman numerals (**Figure 13.5**). The latency of the waves is measured from the onset of the stimulus to the positive peak. The amplitude of the waves is measured from the top of the positive peak to the trough of the immediately following negative peak (**Figure 13.6**).

The BAER waveform completes maturation around day 40 after birth in dogs and day 20 in cats (Strain *et al.*, 1991; Poncelet *et al.*, 2002).

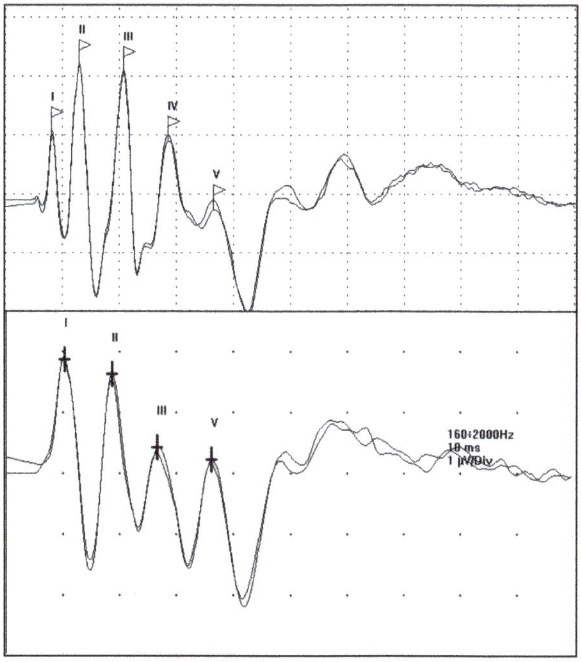

Figure 13.5. Normal BAER waveforms. Wave IV is often not visible because it can merge with wave III or V (lower picture). 1ms/division; 1µV/division.

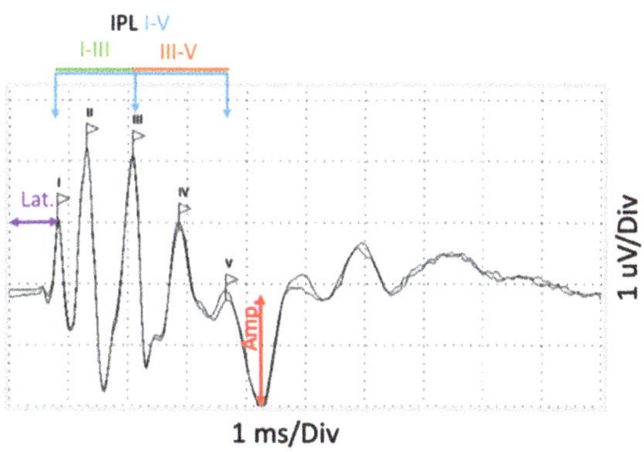

Figure 13.6. Examples of measurement of wave amplitude (Amp), peak latency (Lat) and inter-peak latencies (IPL).

Waves I and V are usually easy to identify in a normal subject. These two waves, together with wave III, are the most clinically relevant waves for interpretation of the test. Wave I is the first after the stimulus. Wave V has a large amplitude and duration because of its large and slow negative (downwards) deflection. Wave IV is often not clearly identifiable because it can partially or completely merge with wave III or wave V (**Figure 13.5**). The BAER waveform is also influenced by the montage of recording electrodes used; the mastoid-vertex montage improves the recognition of the first two waves, that have larger amplitudes. In contrast, with the T1-vertex montage waves IV and V have larger amplitudes, whilst waves I and II are usually smaller (Sims, 1988).

Anaesthetics and sedatives are typically used to reduce muscle artefacts and ease of testing for the patient and the clinician. These drugs have a very limited effect on the morphology of the BAER waveform, in particular on peak latencies.

(ii) Sources of the brainstem auditory evoked responses

Each of the BAER waves is produced by the activation of one or more neural structures of the auditory pathway. Despite being extensively investigated, the precise contribution of the different neural elements of the brainstem to the generation of specific BAER waves has yet to be completely elucidated. Wave I originate from the ipsilateral cochlear nerve. Wave II is produced by the ipsilateral cochlear nucleus/proximal cochlear nerve. The neural generator of wave III is the dorsal nucleus of the trapezoid body, and possibly other nuclei of the ipsilateral and/or contralateral superior olivary complex of the pons. Wave V is usually considered to originate from the ipsilateral and/or contralateral caudal colliculus, or structures in its close proximity. The origin of waves IV, VI and VII is uncertain (Achor and Starr, 1980; Strain, 2011).

4. Brainstem auditory evoked responses: interpretation of results

The initial analysis starts with an inspection of the BAER waveform: the morphology is examined in order to recognise at least wave I, II, III and V. To determine the auditory BAER threshold, the lowest stimulus intensity at which wave V can be identified needs to be found (**Figure 13.7**). This can be done by repeating the test with

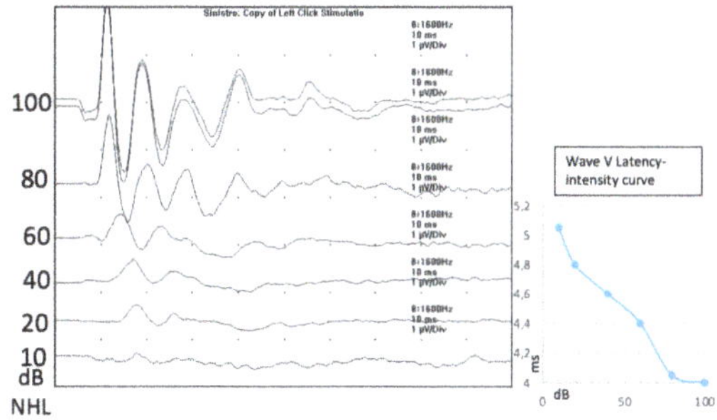

Figure 13.7. Measurement of BAER threshold in a normal dog. Decreasing the stimulus intensity from 100 to 10dB nHL induces a progressive reduction of wave amplitudes and increase of wave latencies. 1ms/division; 1μV/. The right picture is the wave V latency-intensity curve of the same subject. The auditory threshold for this dog is 20dB.

reducing stimulus intensity, for example using 90dB nHL initially, and 70, 50, 30, 10 and 0 dB nHL. Clicks or tones can be used for stimulation. In the latter case, the correlation between frequency of the tone and threshold can be reported on a graph (tone audiogram) (Poncelet *et al.*, 2002).

Other clinical evaluations are based on the values of amplitude and latency of the individual waves. Absolute amplitudes of the waves are very variable, even between normal subjects, meaning that they are of limited utility. Therefore, the ratio between waves (particularly between wave V and wave I amplitudes) is more useful. This parameter, that compares a wave produced in the midbrain (V) with a wave originating from the cochlear nerve (I), may *decrease* with disorders affecting the central portion of the auditory pathway (i.e., retro-cochlear lesions resulting in a smaller wave V amplitude, with an unaffected wave I amplitude).

Absolute latencies of the waves are influenced by both the method of stimulation, such as intensity and polarity of the stimulus, and the type of transducer (e.g., headphones or insert earphones). An increase of similar magnitude in the latencies of all peaks is often present with conductive deafness, meaning the interpeak latencies will remain the same. The absolute latency of wave V induced by different stimulus intensities can be used to create a latency-intensity function (**Figure 13.7 and 13.8**). The graphic representation of the function (wave V latency-intensity curve) is usually affected in hearing impairment, and a shift of the curve to the right is expected with conductive deafness. In sensorineural cochlear hypoacusia, the slope of the latency-intensity curve is usually steeper (**Figure 13.8**) (Poncelet *et al.*, 2000).

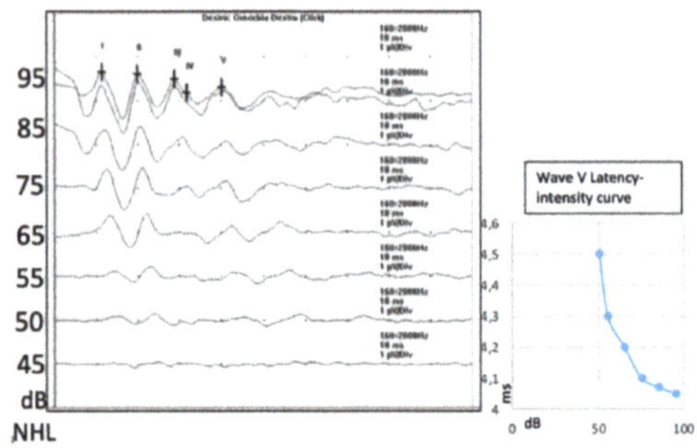

Figure 13.8. Measurement of BAER threshold in a dog with sensorineural cochlear hypoacusia. The threshold is approximately 50dB nHL. 1ms/division; 1μV/division. The wave V latency-intensity curve is steeper compared to normal dogs (compare to the curve shown in **Figure 13.7**).

Interpeak latencies are measured between wave I, III and V (i.e., interpeak latencies I-III, III-V, I-V) (**Figure 13.6**). A prolongation of the interpeak latency may reflect a conduction defect in the auditory pathway. Based on the putative neural generators of the waves, the increase of an interpeak latency may help in the localisation of the lesion (Sims, 1988; Chiappa, 1997; Strain, 2011; Scheifele and Clark, 2012).

5. Brainstem auditory evoked responses in deafness

The main use of BAER in dogs and cats is for screening animals for pigment-associated (congenital sensorineural) deafness, i.e., cochleo-saccular degeneration. In these subjects, the cochleo-saccular degeneration may affect one or both ears. The complete degeneration of the cochlea is associated with the absence of transduction of the air or bone-conducted stimulus into an electric impulse. In the affected ear, the BAER waveform is not identifiable at all, even with higher intensities of stimulus (**Figure 13.9**). A flat BAER tracing can also be recorded in other congenital

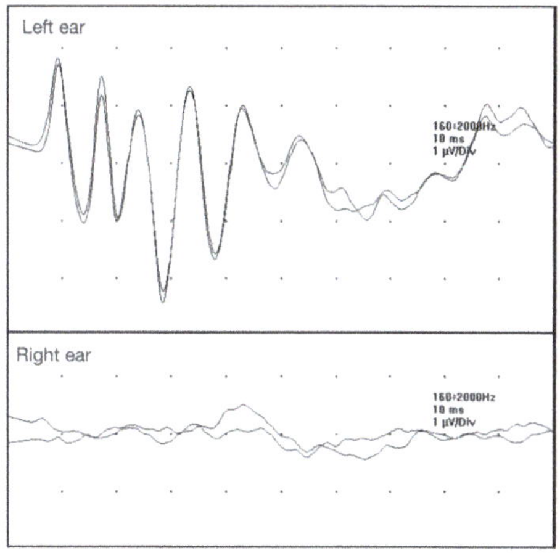

Figure 13.9. BAER from a 2-month-old dog with pigment-associated deafness caused by unilateral (right-sided) cochleo-saccular degeneration. The tracing of the right ear is flat despite the use of a high intensity stimulus (105dB nHL). The tracing of the left ear is normal. 1ms/division; 1μV/division.

(i.e., neuroepithelial degeneration) or acquired disorders causing a complete cochlear degeneration.

Occasionally, a negative potential with a latency between 2 and 3 ms can be recorded in ears affected by cochleo-saccular deafness using higher stimulus intensities (**Figure 13.10**). This acoustically evoked, short latency, negative response is thought to be the result of acoustic activation of vestibular end organs (Bianchi *et al.,* 2020).

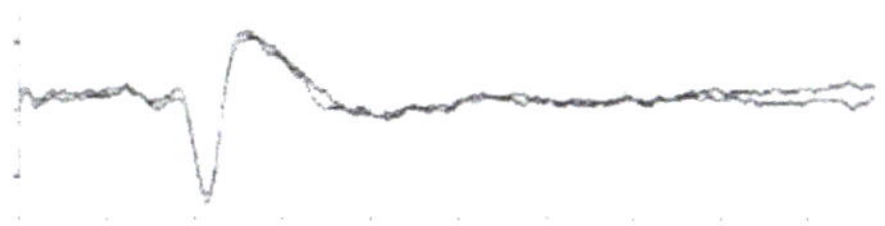

Figure 13.10. BAER from the left ear of a 1-year-old cat with pigment-associated deafness caused by cochleo-saccular degeneration. The abnormal waveform recorded using 105 dB nHL stimulus, termed an 'acoustically evoked short latency negative response', is thought to be the result of acoustic activation of vestibular end organs. 1ms/division; 0.62 μV/division.

Brainstem auditory evoked responses are also used as a diagnostic tool for acquired conductive or sensorineural deafness. The expected findings with conductive hearing loss and acoustic stimulation are:

- An increase of BAER threshold.
- A reduction of wave amplitudes and an increase of absolute peak latencies.
- A wave V latency-intensity curve with normal slope but shifted to the right.
- A normal waveform and threshold using bone stimulation (**Figure 13.11**).

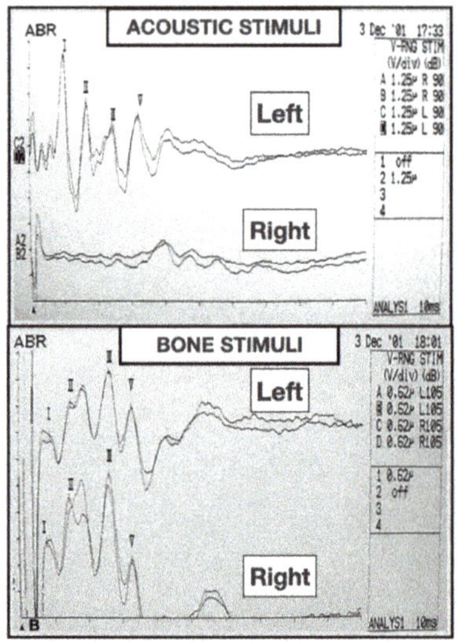

Figure 13.11. BAER from a cat with unilateral conductive deafness caused by an inflammatory polyp of the right middle ear. Acoustic stimulation with 90dB nHL clicks (upper picture) shows a severe reduction of wave amplitudes and prolongation of peak latencies in the right ear, with a normal BAER in the left ear. With bone stimulation of 105dB nHL, normal BAER waveforms are recorded in both ears (lower picture). Upper picture: 1ms/division; 1.25 μV/division. Lower picture: 1 ms/division; 0.62 μV/division

Cases of acquired sensorineural deafness that are referred for an audiological evaluation are most commonly associated with dysfunction of the cochlea and/or cochlear nerve. In these cases, BAER shows an increase of auditory threshold with both air and bone-conducted stimulation. As for puppies with cochleo-saccular degeneration, it may be impossible to obtain an identifiable BAER waveform in cases with acquired sensorineural hearing loss, even with loud stimuli. The wave V latency-intensity curve has a steeper slope, especially in the part of the graph corresponding to lower stimulus intensities (**Figure 13.8**).

As there is bilateral representation of the extensive central auditory pathways, brainstem (or hemispheric) lesions that are sufficient to induce significant auditory impairment will also be associated with severe neurologic deficits associated with damage to other structures or pathways in the near vicinity (e.g., reduced level of mentation, tetraparesis, proprioceptive deficits). Brainstem auditory evoked responses (BAER) of these subjects may reveal the absence of one or more waves, a decrease of wave V/wave I amplitude ratio and an increase of inter-peak latencies. Lesions affecting the auditory cortex, or other parts of the forebrain involved in auditory function, should not cause abnormalities of BAER (Poncelet *et al.*, 2000; Strain, 2011; Scheifele and Clark, 2012).

6. Other tests for sensorineural deafness

(i) Otoacoustic emissions

Otoacoustic emissions (OAE) are low intensity sounds originating from the outer hair cells of the organ of Corti. Otoacoustic emissions are classified as spontaneous if produced by the cochlea without stimulation, and evoked if recorded in response to a stimulation. Evoked OAE are obtained by stimulating the ear with an acoustic stimulus produced by a probe deeply inserted into the external ear canal. The evoked OAE are recorded by a microphone that is included in the probe.

Two types of evoked OAE testing are used in clinical settings: transient evoked OAE and distortion product OAE.

- Transient evoked OAE are recorded in response to a rapid-onset and short-duration click or tone. The acoustic waveform recorded is averaged and measured based on amplitude in dB, percentage reproducibility, and amplitude to noise ratio;
- Distortion product OAE are recorded in response to stimulation with two simultaneous tones of a given frequency and sound pressure level. The resulting pure tone propagated back from the cochlea (the distortion product) is recorded and analysed by the instrument.

Evoked OAE testing is a sensitive indicator of loss of cochlear function and has some advantages over other tests like BAER. In particular, evoked OAE testing is fast and non-invasive, and the result (pass or refer) is provided directly by the instrument without the need of interpretation from the operator. These advantages are especially useful when OAE testing is used for screening for deafness in puppies.

One disadvantage of transient evoked or distorsion product OAE is that the presence of a conductive deafness, and the associated increase of hearing threshold, may prevent a correct and precise evaluation of cochlear function. Furthermore, these tests only assess the function of the outer hair cells of the organ of Corti. Disorders that selectively affect inner hair cells, the cochlear nerve and/or other parts of the auditory pathway are not detected by evoked OAE testing (Strain, 2011; Scheifele and Clark, 2012; Sims *et al.*, 2017).

(ii) Steady-state responses

Steady-state responses are evoked, oscillatory, electrical cerebral responses that are entrained to the frequency and phase of temporally modulated stimuli. The auditory steady state response (ASSR) is a response produced by the cortex and brainstem to rapid auditory stimuli. During ASSR testing, acoustic stimulation is provided through insert earphones and auditory potentials are recorded with electrodes positioned with a montage similar to BAER testing. The ASSR is evoked by presenting trains of sound stimuli at a high repetition rate to the stimulated ears (often binaurally). Analysis of ASSR provides the amplitude and phases in the frequency spectrum and, by using a sophisticated statistics-based algorithm, detects the hearing threshold of both ears at various frequencies. These ASSR-based audiograms are more objective and accurate than BAER-based tone audiograms. Scientific reports of ASSR in dogs and cats are still scarce (Markessis *et al.*, 2006; Scheifele and Clark, 2012).

References

Achor LJ, Starr A. Auditory brain stem responses in the cat. I. Intracranial and extracranial recordings. Electroencephalogr Clin Neurophysiol. 1980 Feb;48(2):154-73. doi: 10.1016/0013-4694(80)90301-6. PMID: 6153332.

Bianchi E, Cantoni AM, Poncelet L. The acoustically evoked short latency negative response (ASNR) in a unilaterally deaf cat with histologically-confirmed cochleosaccular degeneration. BMC Vet Res. 2020 Jun 26;16(1):215. doi: 10.1186/s12917-020-02426-z. PMID: 32586340; PMCID: PMC7318522.

Chiappa KH. Brain Stem Auditory Evoked Potentials: Methodology. In: Chiappa KH (ed.) Evoked Potentials in Clinical Medicine 3rd ed. Lippincott-Raven; Philadelphia, 1997, p.157-197

Farley GR, Starr A. Middle and long latency auditory evoked potentials in cat. I. Component definition and dependence on behavioral factors. Hear Res. 1983 May;10(2):117-38. doi: 10.1016/0378-5955(83)90049-7. PMID: 6863152.

Markessis E, Poncelet L, Colin C, Coppens A, Hoonhorst I, Deggouj N, Deltenre P. Auditory steady-state evoked potentials (ASSEPs): a study of optimal stimulation parameters for frequency-specific threshold measurement in dogs. Clin Neurophysiol. 2006 Aug;117(8):1760-71. doi: 10.1016/j.clinph.2006.03.023. Epub 2006 Jun 22. PMID: 16798083.

Munro KJ, Paul B, Cox CL. Normative auditory brainstem response data for bone conduction in the dog. J Small Anim Pract. 1997 Aug;38(8):353-6. doi: 10.1111/j.1748-5827.1997.tb03484.x. PMID: 9282342.

Poncelet LC, Coppens AG, Deltenre PF. Audiograms estimated from brainstem tone-evoked potentials in dogs from 10 days to 1.5 months of age. J Vet Intern Med. 2002 Nov-Dec;16(6):674-9. doi: 10.1892/0891-6640(2002)016<0674:aefbtp>2.3.co;2. PMID: 12465764.

Poncelet L, Coppens A, Deltenre P. Brainstem auditory evoked potential wave V latency-intensity function in normal Dalmatian and Beagle puppies. J Vet Intern Med. 2000 Jul-Aug;14(4):424-8. doi: 10.1892/0891-6640(2000)014<0424:baepwv>2.3.co;2. PMID: 10935893.

Scheifele PM, Clark JG. Electrodiagnostic evaluation of auditory function in the dog. Vet Clin North Am Small Anim Pract. 2012 Nov;42(6):1241-57. doi: 10.1016/j.cvsm.2012.08.012. PMID: 23122179.

Sims MH. Electrodiagnostic evaluation of auditory function. Vet Clin North Am Small Anim Pract. 1988 Jul;18(4):913-44. doi: 10.1016/s0195-5616(88)50090-6. PMID: 3264964.

Sims MH, Moore RE. Auditory-evoked response in the clinically normal dog: early latency components. Am J Vet Res. 1984 Oct;45(10):2019-27. PMID: 6497099.

Sims MH, Plyler E, Harkrider A, McLucas K. Detection of Deafness in Puppies Using a Hand-Held Otoacoustic Emission Screener. J Am Anim Hosp Assoc. 2017 Jul/Aug;53(4):198-205. doi: 10.5326/JAAHA-MS-6528. Epub 2017 May 23. PMID: 28535131.

Strain G M. Deafness in dogs and cats. CABI; Cambridge: MA, 2011

Strain GM, Tedford BL, Jackson RM. Postnatal development of the brain stem auditory-evoked potential in dogs. Am J Vet Res. 1991 Mar;52(3):410-5. PMID: 2035914.

Wilson WJ, Mills PC, Bradley AP, Petoe MA, Smith AW, Dzulkarnain AA. Fast assessment of canine hearing using high click-rate BAER. Vet J. 2011 Jan;187(1):136-8. doi: 10.1016/j.tvjl.2009.10.009. Epub 2009 Nov 8. PMID: 19900825.

SECTION 14

Electroencephalography

Thomas Parmentier, Fiona James

Key points

- Electroencephalography (EEG) represents the electrical potential difference between cerebral locations over time, generated mainly by neuronal activity and influenced by glial cells.
- EEG is crucial for distinguishing between epileptic and non-epileptic paroxysmal episodes in dogs and cats, enhancing diagnosis and treatment accuracy.
- Accurate EEG interpretation relies on correct identification of a cortical signal and localisation, and distinguishing physiological from pathological patterns.
- Common EEG findings include normal background rhythms, interictal epileptiform discharges, and ictal patterns. Recognising these patterns is key to accurate diagnosis.
- EEG artefacts are common and should not be mistaken for cortical patterns.
- Drugs and mentation states significantly influence EEG readings. Understanding these effects is crucial for interpreting EEG results accurately.
- Coupling EEG with video recordings enhances the ability to correlate electrical activity with observed clinical signs, improving diagnostic confidence.

1. Physiological principles of EEG – source of EEG signal

Understanding how the EEG signal is generated and its correlation to the neuronal activity responsible for its generation is crucial for accurate interpretation.

(i) What is an electroencephalogram?

It is the graphic representation of the difference in electrical potentials between two cerebral locations, plotted over time. The electrical potential is the extracellular electrical potential (also called local field potential) around neurons and glial cells in the area of the cortex underneath the scalp electrodes used to record it. Neurons are the main generators of this electrical potential due to their selective permeability to certain ions. However, glial cells may participate directly or indirectly through modulation of neuronal activity.

The extracellular electrical potential around neurons is mainly generated by the summation of all synaptic currents created during neuronal activity. Pre-synaptic neurons release neurotransmitters that will bind to receptors on post-synaptic neurons and modulate their permeability to specific ions. Binding of neurotransmitters to their receptors causes shifts of these ions between the extracellular and intra-cellular space which are called post-synaptic potentials. Post-synaptic potentials can be excitatory (leading to a depolarisation of the post-synaptic neuron) or inhibitory (leading to the hyperpolarisation of the post-synaptic neuron) depending on the neurotransmitters released and their receptors. In the case of excitatory post-synaptic potentials in dendrites, Na^+ ions enter at dendrites causing a local extracellular deficit in positive ions, called an 'active sink' (or a relative excess of negative ions, red arrows in **Figure 14.1**) and the depolarisation of the neuron. The extracellular space therefore becomes more negatively charged in the cortex that is active compared to less active cortex. This difference in extracellular ions will be picked up by scalp electrodes as the difference in electrical potential of the areas of the cortex underlying the electrodes (measured in µV). The opposite happens with inhibitory post-synaptic potentials as negative Cl^- ions enter and K^+ ions exit neurons, causing an excess of positive charges extracellularly. The ions that actively entered the neurons during the stimuli will exit away from the sink creating 'passive sources' (blue arrows in **Figure 14.1**). Sinks and sources effectively turn neurons into a dipole with an extremity that is more negative and one more positive to compensate (or vice-versa). **Figure 14.1** recapitulates the effect of excitatory and inhibitory post-synaptic potentials depending if the synapse is located on the dendrites close to the electrodes or the neuronal cell body away from the electrode. In this regard, the EEG signal does not differentiate between an excitatory post-synaptic potential at the dendrites and an inhibitory post-synaptic potential at the cell bodies (and vice-versa).

Typically, a scalp electrode records the sum of the activity of the neurons contained in approximately 6-7cm^2 of cortex which amounts to tens or hundreds of thousands of neurons. The neurons mainly responsible for generating EEG signals are located in layers 3, 5 and 6 of the cerebral cortex. If these neurons fire simultaneously, a spike will be picked up by scalp electrodes. The amplitude of the spike depends on the density of these neurons, their synchronisation and their distance to the electrode. Note that action potentials do not contribute significantly to the EEG. This is because of their short duration (around 1ms) and their small field as they spread rapidly along axons.

Not all cortical neurons however contribute equally to the EEG. Neurons that contribute the most to the EEG signal are radially oriented with regards to the skull with dendrites (where Na^+ ions enter) being more superficial (closer to the scalp and therefore the scalp electrode) than their cell bodies (where K^+ ions exit). This creates the relatively more negative extracellular potentials during an excitatory stimulus at the dendrites. Radially oriented neurons are in the cortical gyri. In comparison, neurons located

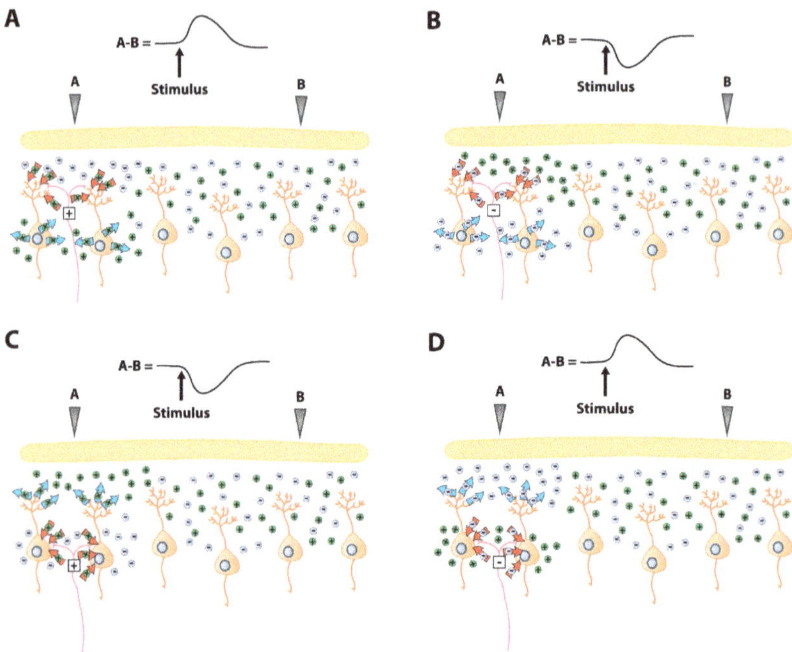

Figure 14.1. Effect of post-synaptic potentials on the EEG signal. A. Excitatory post-synaptic potential at the dendrites. B. Inhibitory post-synaptic potential at the dendrites. C. Excitatory potential at the cell body. D. Inhibitory potential at the cell body. A and B represent scalp electrodes. Red arrows represent the active sinks provoked by the excitatory/inhibitory stimuli and blue arrows represent passive sources. By convention, a negative deflection is represented upward on the EEG.

in the cortical sulci have their dendrites and cell bodies located at the same distance in regard to the skull and therefore no negative potential is detected by the scalp electrode upon neuronal depolarisation. Therefore, mostly neurons located in the cortical gyri contribute to the EEG. The activity of tangentially oriented neurons in the sulci can still be recorded however if the signal is strong enough (see tangential dipole).

Neurons located deeper in subcortical structures and the thalamus only contribute indirectly to the EEG. Indeed, these neurons are located too far away from the scalp for the electrodes to pick up changes in local field potential surrounding these neurons. However, as they send projections to cortical neurons and modulate their activity, activity of the subcortical and thalamic neurons will have an important effect on the EEG.

At the level of an individual neuron, the cellular correlate of an epileptic seizure is called a paroxysmal depolarising shift. This is a prolonged depolarisation of the neuron caused by an excitatory stimulus that induces the opening of NMDA and voltage-gated calcium channels provoking an influx of calcium inside the neuron. This prolonged depolarisation is then followed by a sustained hyperpolarisation due to the opening of potassium channels (**Figure 14.2**). An extracellular electrode would record

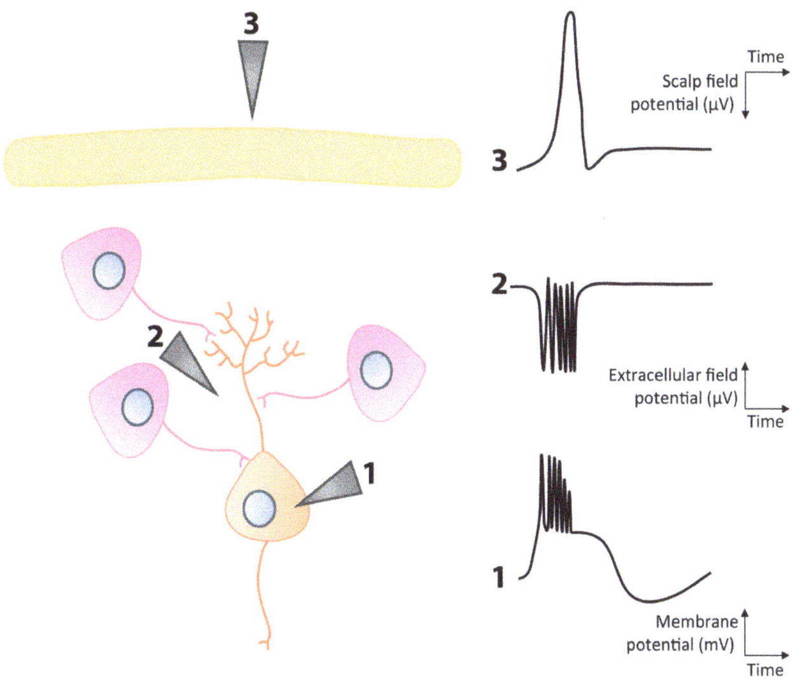

Figure 14.2. Cellular basis of the EEG interictal spike. 1. Intracellular electrode. The epileptiform discharge is a paroxysmal depolarising shift. 2. Extracellular electrode. The epileptiform discharge is a burst of negative extracellular potentials. 3. Scalp electrode. The epileptiform discharge is a spike. Note the reverse polarity for scalp EEG.

the paroxysmal depolarising shift as a burst of negative potentials. If several thousand neighbouring neurons undergo synchronised depolarising shifts, as it is the case when an epileptic focus is active, the shift in electrical potential that they will provoke will be recorded by a scalp electrode as a spike (**Figure 14.2**).

2. EEG recording technique

(i) Electrode types

Different types of electrodes are used in veterinary medicine. Subdermal electrodes such as wires (**Figure 14.3**, left) or monopolar needles (**Figure 14.3**, center) are the most common types of EEG electrodes used with animals. These are inserted under the patient's skin and secured with tape and bandages. To allow long-term recording on awake patients, subdermal wires are preferred to needles as they are more comfortable. Contrary to

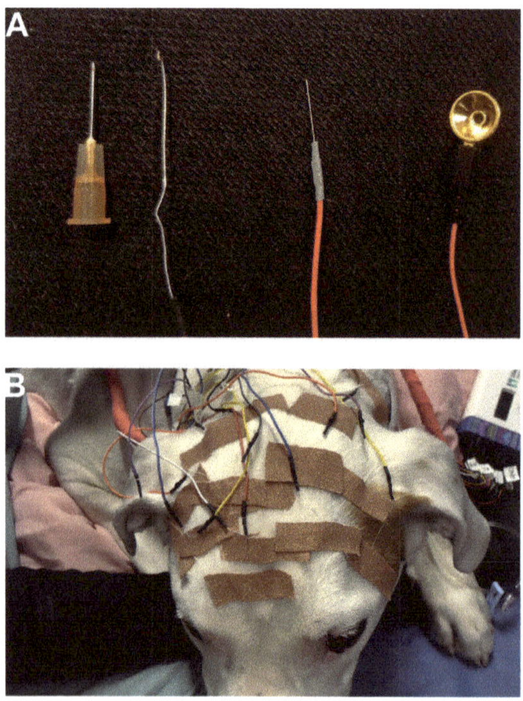

Figure 14.3. EEG electrodes. A. Subdermal wire electrode (left, with associated needle to insert it), subdermal needle (middle) and gold cup surface electrode (right). The electrodes are then connected to the amplifier through the electrical wire (red). B. Subdermal electrodes placed subcutaneously in a patient. Electrodes are secured with tape and then with a self-adhesive bandage (not shown) to prevent unwanted removal.

EEG in humans, surface electrodes (**Figure 14.3**, right) are rarely used in veterinary patients due to the difficulty of making them stay on the patients' head during awake recordings.

(ii) Electrode placement and impedance

No consensus exists on the correct electrode placement in veterinary EEG and several have been proposed (Holliday and Williams, 1998; Pellegrino and Sica, 2004; Hasegawa, 2016; James *et al.*, 2017). Because of brain and skull shape variation between dogs, the underlying cortex recorded by a specific electrode is quite variable which can complicate accurate localisation of a signal to a precise brain region as well as comparison of EEGs between patients (Rogers *et al.*, 2024). Ideally, recording (active) electrodes should be evenly spaced and allow the recording of all the different regions of the cortex. In human EEG, the consensus placement relies on the 10-20 system which uses 19 active electrodes that are placed at 10 and 20% intervals across the skull (**Figure 14.4**). A reference electrode is placed over a region of the head not contaminated by electrical signals from the brain such as the nasion, the mastoid regions or the ear lobes. A ground electrode also needs to be placed on the patient but its location does not matter. The ground electrode is used for safety by preventing aberrant electrical current coming from the EEG equipment to leak through the patient potentially causing burns or more serious adverse effects. A ground electrode is also used to reject large changes in electrical potential due to instrumentation that affect both active and reference electrodes such as power line noise (causing 50-60Hz interference). This filter is called common mode rejection.

Electrode nomenclature used in veterinary EEG is the same as for human EEG. The letter refers to the area of the skull underlying the electrode (Fp: pre-frontal, F: frontal, C: central, T: temporal, P: parietal, O: occipital) and odd numbers are used for left hemisphere while even numbers are used for the right hemisphere. The z index refers to midline electrodes.

Figure 14.4 depicts the equivalent of the 10-20 system for dogs. However, because of differences in the shape of the skull and the use of subdermal electrodes, electrodes Fp1 and Fp2 located just above the medial canthus of the eyes are not well tolerated in dogs. Similarly, electrodes P5 and P6 are difficult to place in some dogs as they are located where the ears are. Therefore, these 4 electrodes are not commonly used in dogs. The distance between the nasion and occipital protuberance is measured and Cz is placed in the middle which is usually at the vertex. Fz and Pz are placed at 20% interval from Cz. F7 and F8 are placed just above the lateral canthus of the eyes and T3/T4 at the base of the ears. F3/F4 are placed in the middle of the distance from F7/F8 to Fz. C3/C4 are located in the middle of the distance from T3/T4 to Cz. P3/P4 and O1/O2 are aligned with F3/C3 and F4/C4 (**Figure 14.4**). The reference electrode is easily placed on the nasion, and a ground electrode is placed in the cervical area. If an electrode has to be moved to another position, it is important to move the corresponding electrode on the other side of the scalp in a symmetrical position to be able to compare the signal from the left and right hemispheres.

Impedance is the equivalent of resistance for alternating currents. Electrode impedance should ideally be kept between 0,1-5 kΩ, although up to 10 kΩ is acceptable for continuous recording. More importantly, electrodes should have their respective impedance in a similar range, otherwise a 50-60Hz interference is observed.

(iii) Montages

The EEG montage represents the arrangement of the signals from electrodes into different channels. The most common types of montages used are referential and bipolar montages. In referential montages, every channel is composed of the difference in potential between an active electrode and a common reference electrode. In bipolar montages, channels are composed of the difference between two adjacent active electrodes, organised in chains so that one electrode is common between two subsequent

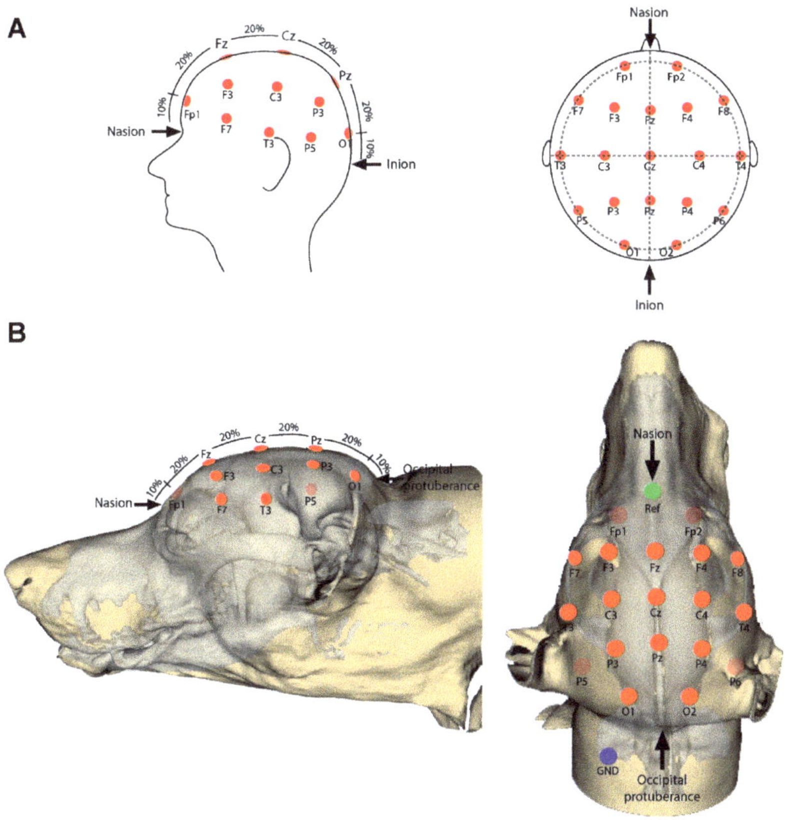

Figure 14.4. 10-20 electrode placement system in humans and dogs. A. 10-20 system in humans. B. Corresponding 10-20 system in dogs. Electrodes Fp1/Fp2 and P5/P6 are not commonly used as they can be difficult to place and are less tolerated in dogs. Ref: reference electrode. GND: ground electrode

channels (**Figure 14.5**). In each montage, the different channels can be arranged in a longitudinal (e.g. front to back of the head) or transverse fashion (e.g. left to right). Thanks to digital recording used nowadays, the signal from each electrode is recorded compared to a common machine reference in the amplifier so that the recording can be reformatted easily into different montages after the recording is finished. Other montages exist such as common average montages (where the signal of each active electrode is compared to the average of all electrodes) or Laplacian montages (where the signal for each active electrode is compared to the average signal of its surrounding electrodes).

Each montage has advantages and inconveniences so that multiple montages should be used for accurate source localisation. Referential montages accurately display the shape and amplitude

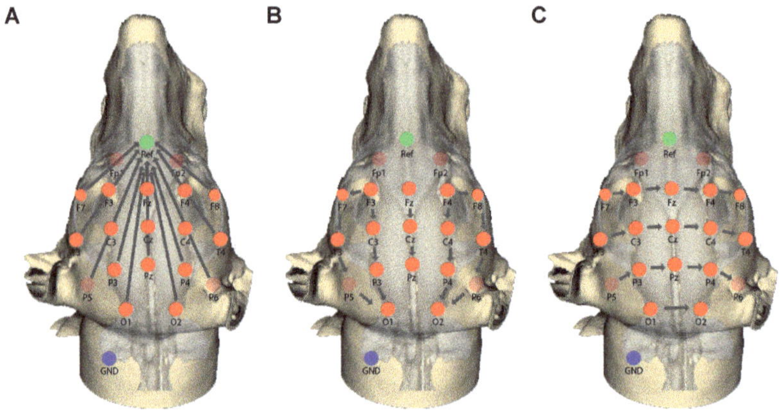

Figure 14.5. Examples of different montages used in veterinary EEG. A. Referential montage. B. Longitudinal bipolar montage. C. Transverse bipolar montage. The grey arrows represent the electrode signal compared in each channel

of the waveforms. However, the reference electrode can be affected by artefacts or actually record some electrical activity from the brain which will contaminate all the channels. On the contrary, bipolar montages do not rely on a single reference electrode and therefore display less artefacts than referential montages. Bipolar montages are also useful for localising discharges. However, the shape and amplitude of discharges is distorted in bipolar montages which makes these montages less useful for recognising specific patterns. Moreover, if both electrodes of one channel are equally distant from the discharge source, the signals from each channel will cancel out and the channel will not display any waveform (see *principles of source localisation*).

(iv) Amplifiers

EEG electrodes are connected to an amplifier in order to magnify the signal as the difference of electrical potentials between two electrodes is only in the order of microvolts. The amplifier also allows common mode rejection to filter out electrical signals that are common to both active and reference electrodes. Modern amplifiers digitalise the EEG signal by sampling the continuous changes in potential at regular intervals. The sampling frequency needs to be at least twice faster than the highest frequency to be recorded in order to avoid aliasing. Many digital EEG devices are also now capable of storing the data directly in an internal memory or transmitting wirelessly to a computer, allowing EEG recording in awake and ambulatory patients. These amplifiers are particularly helpful to record specific paroxysmal episodes that may be visible only when the patient is not sedated or anesthetised.

(v) Frequency filters

Frequency filters are signal processing techniques used to isolate or eliminate EEG signals of specific frequencies. Filters are now digital which means that they are applied through the EEG software and can be modified during or after recording. As most interesting EEG signals are between 0.5 and 30Hz, a 0.5–70Hz band-pass filter is commonly used to eliminate signals with frequencies outside this range. Moreover, a 50/60Hz notch filter (to eliminate signals of 50 or 60Hz) can also be used to eliminate the artefact caused by the alternating current (see the *artefacts* section). It is important to minimise the use of frequency filters and to carefully evaluate their impact on the EEG as filters can distort or sometimes eliminate important EEG signals, preventing correct EEG interpretation.

(vi) Video-synchronisation

By coupling EEG recording with video-synchronisation, the investigator is able to interrogate the epileptic nature of certain paroxysmal episodes. This is most interesting when the recording is performed on awake patients capable of behaving normally to show the behaviour of interest. The observation of the paroxysmal episode synchronised with epileptiform discharges on the EEG allows the diagnosis of epilepsy with a high certainty or on the contrary can rule out that the paroxysmal episodes are epileptic seizures.

(vii) Effect of anaesthesia/sedation and other drugs on the EEG

Most EEG devices used initially in veterinary patients could not store the EEG data or transmit it wirelessly to a computer and therefore needed to be wired directly to a computer preventing their use in awake, ambulatory patients. Sedation and/or anaesthesia was therefore routinely used to record EEG. This may have contributed to the low sensitivity of EEG to detect epileptiform discharges in some studies as several drugs used for sedation or general anaesthesia, such as benzodiazepines and propofol, are also used as anti-convulsants. By recording EEG on sedated or anesthetised patients, the investigator also only relies on interictal discharges for the diagnosis of epilepsy as the patient may not display the clinical manifestation of a seizure. Although wireless, ambulatory EEG can record EEG on awake patients, sedation or general anaesthesia are also routinely used for convenience during electrode placement. However, no significant decrease was detected in one study in the diagnostic capability of ambulatory EEG by using sedation and or general anaesthesia for patient instrumentation, provided that EEG recording was continued when patients were awake and behaving normally (Parmentier *et al.*, 2020).

Drugs also have specific effects on EEG which should be considered during EEG interpretation. These effects are summarised in **Table 14.1**.

Drug	Effect on EEG
Alpha-2 agonists	Increase in sleep spindles, K-complexes and vertex waves
Baclofen, serotoninergic syndrome	Tri-phasic waves
Cannabis	Little to no effect on the EEG. However, THC can provoke an increase in alpha activity and decrease in beta and theta activity.
Cyclosporine	Diffuse and local slowing, epileptiform discharges
GABA agonists (barbiturates, benzodi-azepines, tri-cyclic antidepressant, CNS stimulant	Increase in beta activity (especially during acute use and predominantly in frontal region), waxing and waning amplitude. Spindle-like activity and burst-suppression patterns at toxic levels
Halogenated gases and propofol	At induction: alpha frequency similar to sleep spindles, K-complexes, vertex waves and positive occipital sharp transients of sleep. As the dosage increase, an increase in beta activity, then generalised slowing, then burst suppression pattern
Ketamine	Loss of alpha rhythm, increase in beta activity and amplitude
Opioids	Loss of beta activity and slowing of alpha activity. With higher doses, diffuse theta activity is seen and then some delta activity as dose increases
Phenytoin	Generalised theta activity and increase in delta activity at toxic levels.
Specific serotoninergic reuptake inhibitors	Increased theta activity, polyspikes

Table 14.1: Effect of specific drugs on EEG.

(viii) Activation procedures

Activation procedures are meant to trigger epileptiform discharges in susceptible patients in order to increase the diagnostic yield of EEG. The main activation procedures in human and veterinary patients are hyperventilation and intermittent photic stimulation.

Hyperventilation consists in provoking deep breathing for 3-5 minutes at a frequency of 20 respirations/minute. A bilateral diffuse increase in delta and theta activity as well as a slowing of alpha and beta rhythms are normally seen. However, epileptic patients may show epileptiform discharges as well as lateralised or focal slowing. In human EEG, it is most useful to trigger epileptiform discharges from lesions in the temporal region. Hyperventilation has been evaluated briefly in cats and dogs under anaesthesia with propofol and showed no added value for the diagnosis of epilepsy (Brauer *et al.*, 2011, 2012). However, the small size of the cohorts and limited coverage by a small number of electrodes may have influenced these results. Moreover, no changes in the background activity was seen with hyperventilation in cats- (Brauer *et al.*, 2012). This may be due to the influence of general anaesthesia as many cats experienced a burst-suppression pattern typical of deep anaesthesia which would preclude the observation of background changes due to hyperventilation. In conclusion, as hyperventilation can only be used in anesthetised and intubated veterinary patients which may interfere with the EEG as explained above, this procedure is not practical and may be of limited value in veterinary EEG.

Intermittent photic stimulation consists in delivering flashes of light 30cm away from the patient. Flashes should be given for 5-7 seconds while the eyes are open and closed at increasing frequency going from 1 to 60Hz. Once an induced seizure is observed, the stimulation is stopped and then resumed at a decreasing frequency starting at 60Hz. Intermittent photic stimulation can induce several types of responses. In normal individuals, a physiological response called the photic driving response is elicited and consists in a bilateral symmetrical rhythmic activity in the occipital region time-locked with the flashes. A physiological photomyogenic response may also be seen, which is a muscle artefact time-locked with the flashes and due to eyelid and extra-ocular muscle activity. In epileptic patients, a photoparoxysmal response can be triggered by photic stimulation. It consists in spikes, spike-and-wave, polyspikes or multiple spike-and-wave activity that are not time-locked to the flashes. These epileptiform patterns are mostly generalised and can happen over the occipital, parietal or fronto-central regions. Intermittent photic stimulation has also been used in dogs and cats. While it showed no added value in patients under general anaesthesia, photic stimulation can trigger epileptiform activity in awake patients (Brauer *et al.*, 2011; Wielaender *et al.*, 2017). As it is easily performed on awake patients, this activation procedure should be used when available. Contra-indications to photic stimulation include patients that experience status epilepticus and use of drugs that dilate the pupils.

3. EEG interpretation

EEG interpretation relies on answering two main questions for correct analysis:

1. For any specific pattern, is it artefactual or is it originating from the cerebral cortex?
2. If it is a cortical pattern, is it physiological or pathological?

The answer to the first question relies on correct source localisation and knowledge about artefacts that are frequently observed in EEG. Answering the second questions relies on pattern recognition, knowledge of which patterns are normal or abnormal in different contexts as well as the association between different patterns and epilepsy.

(i) Artefacts

EEG commonly has a low signal to noise ratio with frequent artefacts. It is therefore very important to recognise the different artefacts and avoid recording them if possible. Artefacts are categorised into two groups: physiological artefacts originating from the patient and external artefacts originating from the equipment or the environment.

Physiological artefacts are generated by the electrical activity of other organs than the brain such as the muscles, the heart or movements of the tongue and eyes.

- Muscle artefacts (**Figure 14.6A**) are low amplitude, high frequency waveforms. These are common artefacts especially with subdermal needles and are not reduced with topical lidocaine (Ward, James and Monteith, 2016). To minimise these artefacts, care should be taken to place the electrodes just under the skin and not in the subcutaneous muscles of the head.
- Other artefacts such as blinking **(Figure 14.6B**) and eye movement are also frequent and are characterised by large amplitude, low frequency waveforms more pronounced over frontal electrodes.
- ECG artefact (**Figure 14.6C**) is easily recognised from its frequency that matches the heart rate. Coupling ECG recording with the EEG also helps in identifying this artefact.
- Other physiological artefacts are triggered by movements of the animal such as swallowing, panting, coughing, tremoring, walking… Video-synchronisation can be particularly helpful to distinguish these movement artefacts from epileptic seizures.

External artefacts are signals coming from outside of the patient. 'Electrode pop' (**Figure 14.7A**) is characterised by a brief, very large amplitude signal affecting only one electrode and is associated with disconnection of an electrode. The 50/60Hz alternating current artefact (**Figure 14.7B and 7C**) is also common when an electrode has a significantly higher impedance than other electrodes. This turns the ground electrode into an active electrode which allows the recording of this artefact. It can be resolved by replacing the electrode with high impedance, replacing the ground electrode or applying a 50/60Hz notch filter. Other instrumental artefacts are created when the electrodes or cables are manipulated or

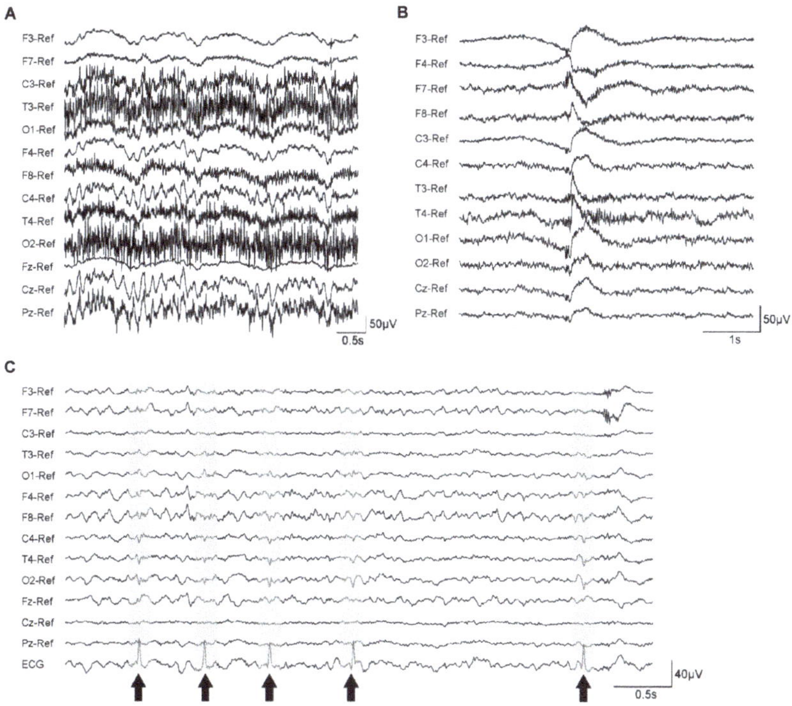

Figure 14.6. Examples of physiological artefacts. A. Muscle artefact most prominent in channels C3-Ref, T3-Ref, T4-Ref and O2-Ref. This artefact is characterised by high frequency, low amplitude waveforms superimposed to the background. B. Blinking artefact identified as waveforms of large amplitude, most prominent in the frontal channels located near the eyes. C. ECG artefact. Several waveforms with a spike-like morphology are seen in several channels (shaded areas) and are time-locked with the ECG signal (arrows). The µV scale is for the EEG channels and does not apply to the ECG channel.

by other electrical devices connected to the patients (ventilator, continuous rate infusion devices, etc..., **Figure 14.7D**).

As a general guide, patterns that are seen on a single channel, have atypical waveforms, have frequencies < 1Hz or > 70Hz and/or appear precisely periodic, are more likely to be artefacts than cortical signals. Some artefacts such as eye movement artefacts are helpful to characterise the sleep stage of the patient.

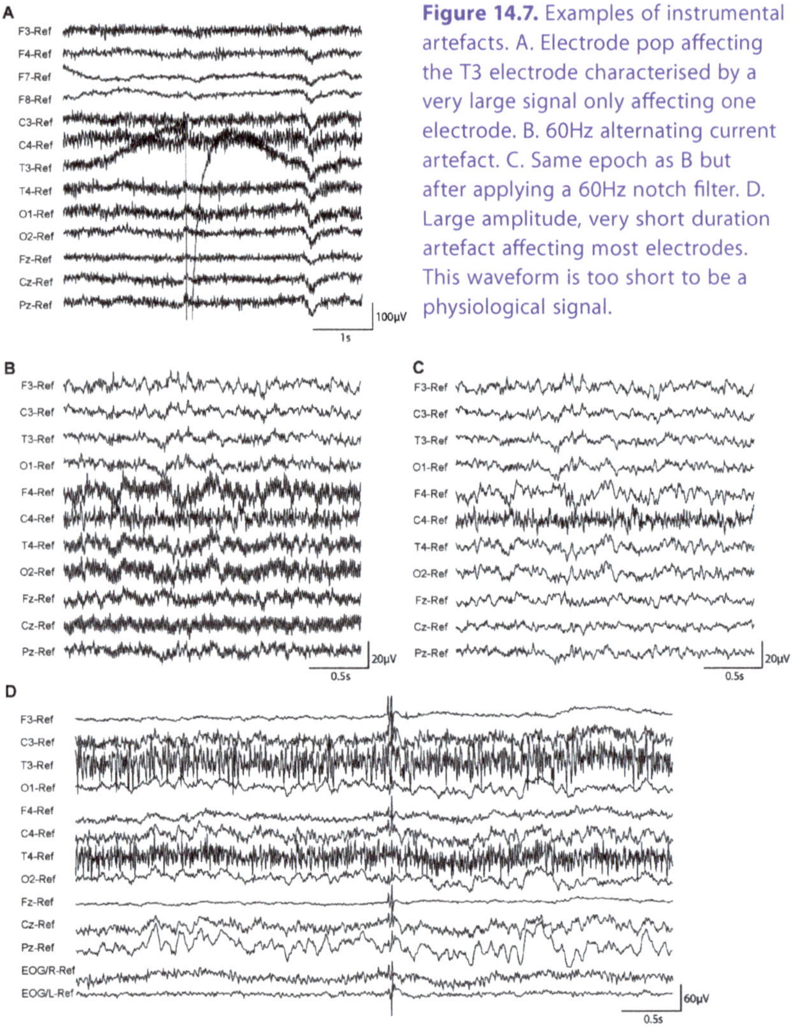

Figure 14.7. Examples of instrumental artefacts. A. Electrode pop affecting the T3 electrode characterised by a very large signal only affecting one electrode. B. 60Hz alternating current artefact. C. Same epoch as B but after applying a 60Hz notch filter. D. Large amplitude, very short duration artefact affecting most electrodes. This waveform is too short to be a physiological signal.

(ii) Principles of source localisation – is the signal of cortical origin?

To be identified as a signal originating from the cortex, a specific wave of interest on the EEG should meet these criteria:

1- Field: a cortical signal is often recorded by multiple electrodes.

2- Lag: the electrode closest to the cortical source will record the signal first and there is an increase in latency the further the electrode is from the cortical source of the signal
3- Gradient: the electrode closest to the cortical source will record the signal with the highest amplitude and there is a decrease in amplitude the further the electrode is from the cortical source.

It is often necessary to switch between the referential and bipolar montage to correctly identify the cortical origin of a signal. On referential montages, localisation is made mainly by analyzing the amplitude of the wave form with the electrode closest to the source showing the maximum amplitude. The phase of the signal (upward or downward deflection) depends on the polarity (positive or negative) of the recorded potential which cannot be known (see **Figure 14.1**). However, in the case of epileptic foci, the extracellular potential is mainly the result of cortical excitation and therefore is negative and represented as an upward deflection on the EEG (**Figure 14.8A**). If the reference electrode is contaminated, the waveform is seen in all channels and may also change phase (**Figure 14.8B**). As a general rule, if a field potential has a single polarity (negative or positive, hence not a tangential dipole), the phase of the signal on EEG should not change between channels unless the reference is contaminated. Two phase reversals seen on a referential montage is almost always an indicator of reference electrode contamination. However, a phase reversal on referential montage without reference contamination indicates the presence of a tangential dipole (see below, **Figure 14.9**). To confirm or rule out reference electrode contamination, a new reference spatially located further away from the previous reference should be used. This reformatting can be done in the EEG software after recording with digital EEG.

In bipolar montages, localisation mainly relies on instrumental phase reversal: the phase changes from upward and downward in two adjacent channels sharing a common electrode. If an instrumental phase reversal is observed, the common electrode

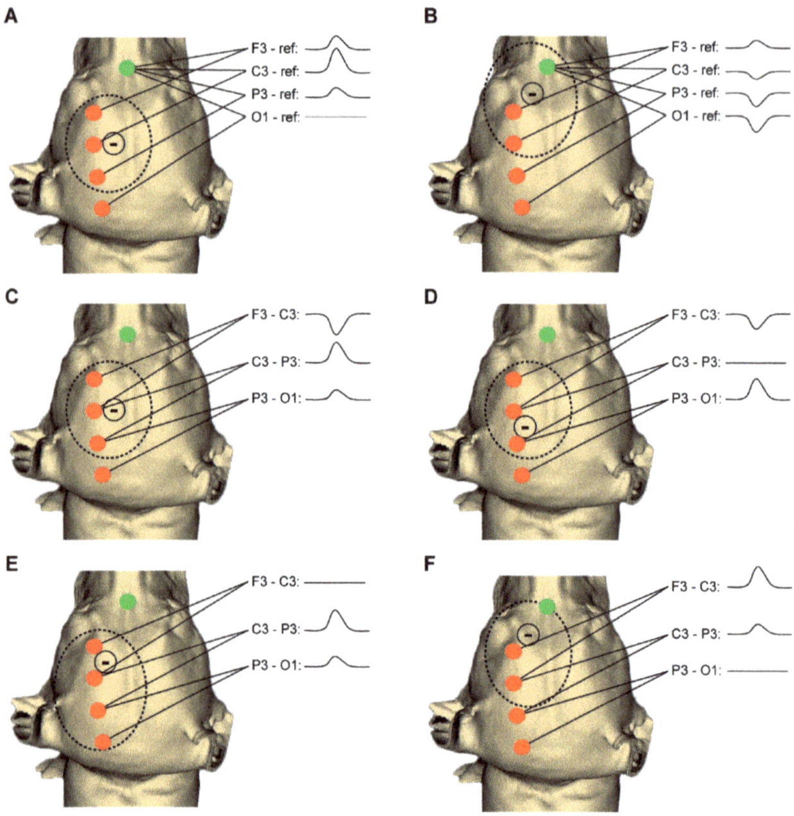

Figure 14.8. Examples of source localisation on the EEG. The "-" sign represents the polarity and localisation of the cortical signal. The dashed circle represents the field of the signal. A negative signal is represented by convention by an upward deflection. A. Longitudinal referential montage. Highest amplitude noted on the channel with the electrode closest to the source of the signal. B. Longitudinal referential montage. Note the phase reversal between the first and second channels. All channels also record the signal. These features suggest a contamination of the reference electrode. To resolve this, a new reference located away from the previous reference (e.g. O1) should be chosen. C. Longitudinal bipolar montage. Instrumental phase reversal between the channels sharing the electrode closest to the source of the signal (C3). D. Longitudinal bipolar montage. Instrumental phase reversal with phase cancellation (C3-P3). This indicates that the signal is recorded similarly by C3 and P3. E. Longitudinal bipolar montage. End-of-chain phenomenon with phase cancellation. The signal is recorded similarly by F3 and C3. As F3 is not shared by other channels, no phase reversal is noted. F. Longitudinal bipolar montage. End-of-chain phenomenon without phase cancellation. The absence of recorded signal in the P3-O1 channel is not due to a phase cancellation but because these electrodes are outside of the field of this signal.

is closest to the source of the signal (**Figure 14.8C**). In the case where two electrodes are as close to the source, a phase cancellation is observed (**Figure 14.8D**). If the source of the signal is closer to an electrode that is not shared by two different channels, an end-of-chain phenomenon is observed which is an absence

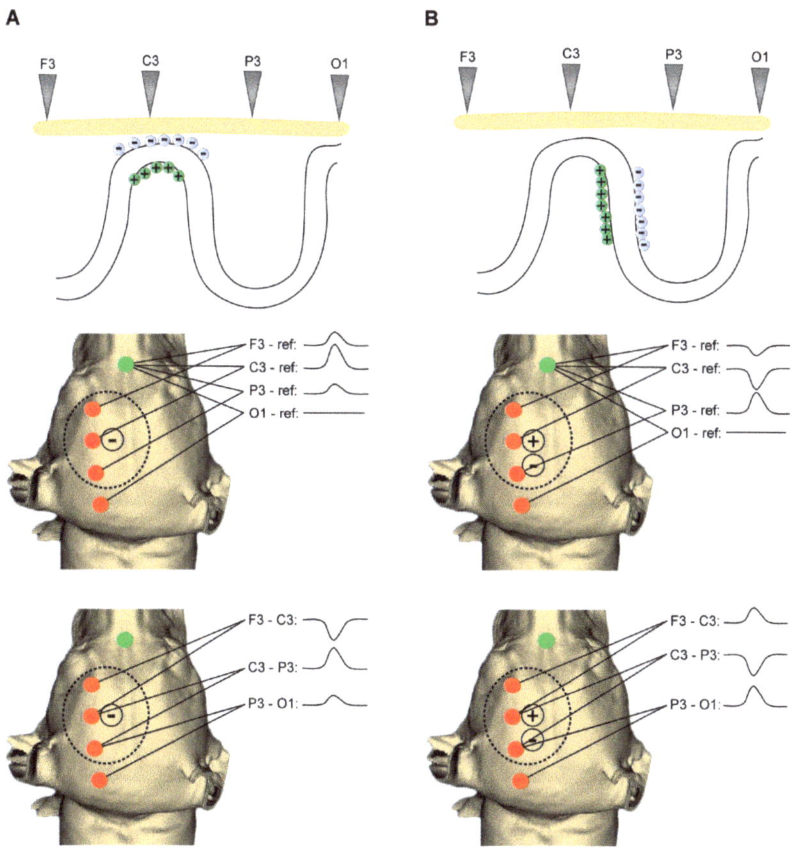

Figure 14.9. Recording differences between radial and tangential dipoles. A. Example of recording of a negative radial dipole, similar to examples presented in **Figure 14.6** with maximal negativity closest to C3. The highest amplitude is seen over the C3-ref channel on the longitudinal referential montage and an instrumental phase reversal is noted between the F3-C3 and C3-P3 channels on the longitudinal bipolar montage. B. Example of a recording of a tangential dipole with maximum positivity over C3 and maximum negativity over P3. A true phase reversal is noted between the C3-ref and P3-ref channel on the referential montage. Two phase reversals are noted on the bipolar montage.

of instrumental phase reversal on a bipolar montage (**Figure 14.8E and Figure 14.8F**). As a common reference electrode is not used, reference electrode contamination is not an issue in bipolar montages.

These principles are valid when the source is originating from radially organised neurons located in a gyrus, which is most often the case. However, if the signal originates from tangentially

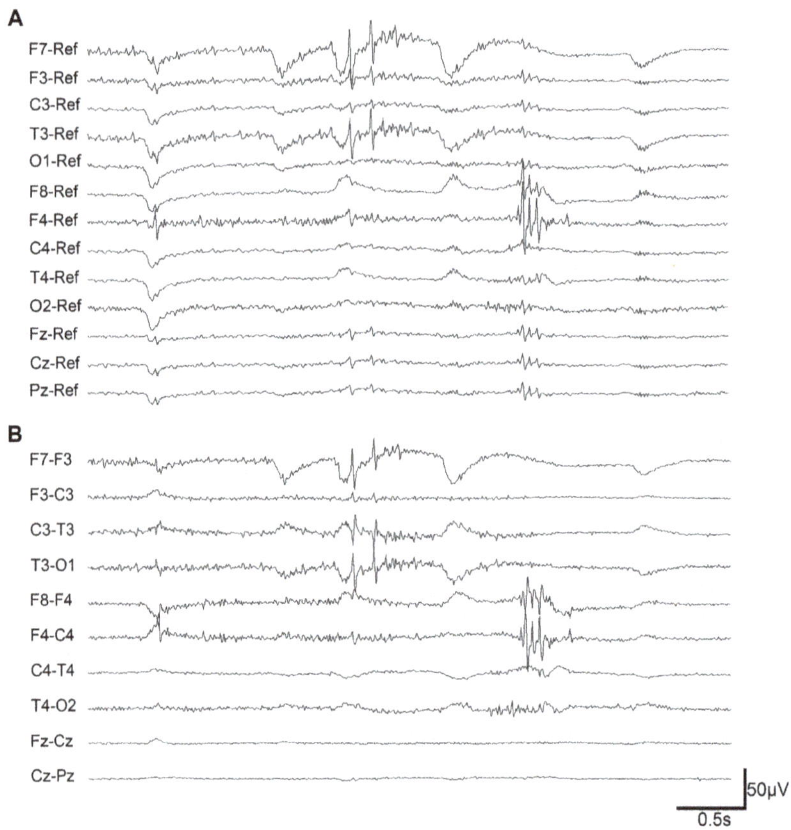

Figure 14.10. Discharge localisation using different montages. Example of an epileptiform discharge representation in referential (A) and bipolar montages (B). Several spikes are noted with maximal amplitude at F4 and F7 on the referential montage. Note the instrumental phase reversal between the F8-F4 and F4-C4 channels in the bipolar montage confirming the localisation over the F4 electrode. Another instrumental phase reversal is observed between C3-T3 and T3-O1.

organised neurons located in a sulcus or if the cortical anatomy is abnormal (e.g. cortical dysplasia), a tangential dipole is created and can be recorded on the EEG. In these cases, a true phase reversal is observed on the referential montage (**Figure 14.9**).

An example of epileptiform spikes in referential and bipolar montages is shown in **Figure 14.10**.

(iii) Physiological signals of the EEG

Apart from the case of brain death, the EEG will record physiological signals that are either classified as part of the background (background activity) or transient physiological signals. It is important to recognise physiological signals for two main reasons: 1) Background activity is tightly linked to the awake/sleep stages and informs us on the mental states of the patient (awake, drowsy, light/deep sleep) and can be altered in some pathological conditions and 2) Physiological transients should not be mistaken for epileptiform activity.

Of note, the EEG patterns presented here are extrapolated from the human literature. Although several of them have been recorded in animals, it is unclear if all those patterns are present in veterinary EEG.

EEG signals that are of clinical interest have a frequency that lies between 0.1-100Hz and especially in the 0.5-70Hz explaining the band-filters used for EEG recording. Higher frequency signals have been more recently discovered (High-frequency and very-high-frequency oscillations) but require recording EEG with a sample frequency at least twice as high as the highest frequency of interest (e.g. recording at 200Hz if interested in signals up to 100Hz). This is to avoid an artefactual reduction in frequency of the EEG signal if the sample frequency is too low ('aliasing' effect). Ripples (80-250Hz) and fast ripples (250-500Hz) are high frequency oscillations best recorded with intracranial EEG due to the higher muscle artefacts of scalp EEG.

Frequency of signals are categorised into different bands based on their neurophysiological basis. The main EEG bands are summarised in **Table 14.2**.

Band	Frequency range
Delta	< 4Hz
Theta	4–8Hz
Alpha	8–13Hz
Beta	14–30Hz
Gamma	30–80Hz

Table 14.2: Main EEG frequency bands.

We will describe the main physiological EEG signals recorded in the adult, mature brain and then consider the effect of age on EEG.

Delta activity (0–<4Hz)

Delta waves are slow, polymorphic waves (**Figure 14.11A**). They are thought to arise from two different sources: thalamocortical neurons that generate spontaneous burst of activity at 1–2Hz and the interaction between excitatory pyramidal neurons and inhibitory interneurons in the cortex.

Delta waves are normally only observed during sleep or general anaesthesia and should not be seen in patients outside the slow-wave stage of sleep. Delta waves are generalised and more prominent over the rostral region of the head.

Theta activity (4–<8Hz)

Theta waves are thought to be generated mainly by neurons in the limbic system, especially the hippocampus. Theta waves are normally seen only during drowsiness and sleep, are bilateral, symmetrical and of maximal amplitude over the rostral electrodes (**Figure 14.11B**).

Alpha activity (8–<13Hz)

Alpha waves are generated by cortical neurons, mainly in the visual cortex although other generators of waves of the same frequencies are located in the somatosensory cortex (mu activity). Neurons generating alpha waves are located in all layers of the cortex. Alpha activity is therefore seen predominantly in the occipital channels and should be bilaterally symmetrical (less than 50% difference in amplitude between both hemispheres). The amplitude of alpha waves is larger when the animal is relaxed with their eyes closed and attenuates when the animal opens their eyes, a phenomenon called 'reactivity' which illustrates the synchronisation of neurons when the visual cortex is not stimulated by visual inputs and their desynchronisation when eyes are open and visual inputs are present (**Figure 14.11C**).

In humans, the alpha rhythm appears around 4 months of age at approximately 4Hz and the frequency progressively increases with age to reach 8–13Hz but the generalisation to veterinary patient is unknown. Variation in the alpha wave frequency has been reported in humans without an underlying pathology. For example, a transient decrease in alpha frequency below 8Hz (alpha drop-out) is seen when the patient transitions from wakefulness to drowsiness. Moreover, a transient increase (around 1Hz) in the frequency of alpha activity is observed in the first second after eye closure ('Alpha squeak'). Some fast (twice the alpha frequency) and slow (1/2 the alpha frequency) alpha variants can be observed but should be always concomitant with alpha activity in the normal range in healthy patients.

Mu activity (7–11Hz)

Mu activity is often in the same frequency range as the alpha rhythm but is more predominant over the central and centro-parietal channels during wakefulness as it is generated by neurons in the somatosensory cortex. It is considered the resting rhythm of the motor and sensory cortex. Mu activity is not blocked by eye opening but by contralateral movement. Mu waves are generally spiky in their positive phase (usually downwards) and round in their negative phase (upward).

Beta activity (13–<30Hz)

Beta waves are bilateral, symmetrical waves of low amplitude, predominant over the fronto-central channels. Beta activity is observed during wakefulness and is associated with increased level of alertness. Neurons generating beta activity are also located in the cerebral cortex.

Beta waves amplitude is frequently increased with anti-seizure medications (benzodiazepines, barbiturates) but the increase in amplitude should be bilateral and symmetrical (**Figure 14.11D**).

Gamma activity (30–80Hz)

Gamma waves are also generated in the cerebral cortex and predominantly seen in awake, alert individuals. Gamma waves however are not easily observed with routine scalp EEG due to the use of 70Hz low-pass filters, their low amplitude and similar frequencies to muscle artefacts.

Lambda waves

Lambda waves are di- or triphasic, bilateral, synchronous waves that occur predominantly in the occipital area during visual exploration in awake individuals. They are linked to saccadic eye movements. They are more common between 2 and 15 years old in humans but their prevalence is unknown in animals as visual exploration is rarely provoked in these patients.

(iv) Effect of sleep

The EEG is very dependent on the mental status of the patient as different frequency bands will be predominant in different

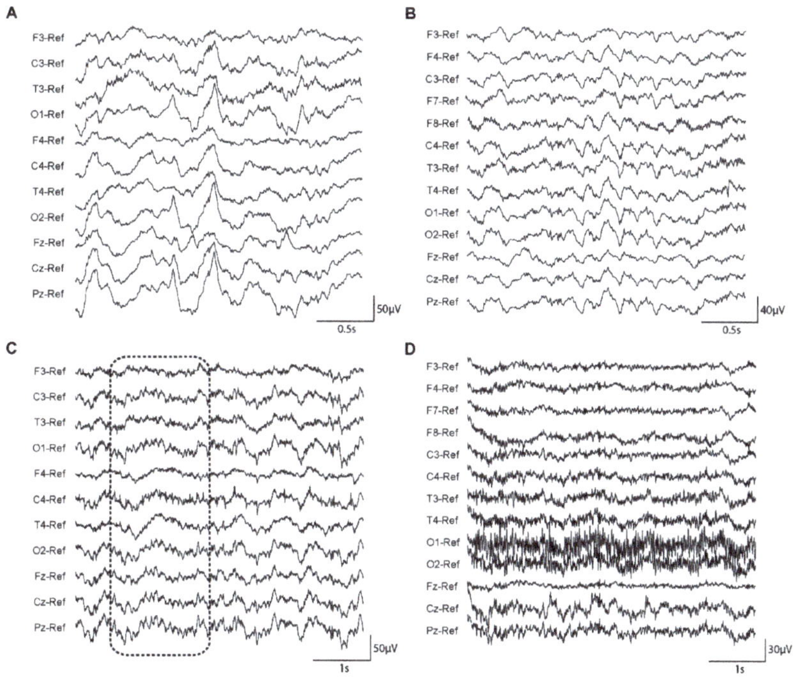

Figure 14.11. Physiological EEG background rhythms. A. Waves of delta frequency. B. Waves of theta frequency. C. Alpha activity more prominently in the caudal electrodes during eyes closure in a patient (dashed lines). D. Beta activity in an awake patient. Note the muscle artefact contaminating electrodes O1 and O2.

stages: wakefulness, drowsiness, sleep, rapid-eye movement (REM) sleep… Conversely, it is possible to deduct the mental state of the patient by analyzing the background activity of the EEG. Knowing the effect of sleep on the EEG is important as the background of the EEG should match the mental state of the patient. Moreover, certain patients exhibit an increase in seizure probability during drowsiness or sleep so including natural sleep during the EEG of these patients may increase the sensitivity of EEG. It may also be necessary to record EEG during natural sleep to differentiate an epileptic disorder from sleep disorders which have been reported in veterinary patients (Bush *et al.*, 2004; Schubert, Chidester and Chrisman, 2011; Barker *et al.*, 2016; Shea *et al.*, 2018; Mondino *et al.*, 2021). In human epileptology, sleep deprivation is used as an activation procedure to enhance the sensitivity of EEG by increasing the probability of recording natural sleep during which interictal epileptiform discharges (ED) may appear as well as by increasing the probability of observing interictal ED or ictal ED by decreasing the seizure threshold in epileptic individuals. The effect of sleep deprivation on the EEG has been briefly evaluated in dogs and cats and an increase in slow-wave sleep is observed in both species after preventing individuals to sleep completely during the day (around 14 hours), similarly to what is observed in humans (Tobler and Scherschlicht, 1990; Kis *et al.*, 2014; Reicher *et al.*, 2021). However, the effect of sleep deprivation on the appearance and frequency of epileptiform discharges in veterinary patients has not been evaluated yet.

Sleep stages

Sleep stages in veterinary patients and humans are mostly comparable and a summary of the sleep-staging guidelines used in human polysomnography is presented here (American Academy of Sleep Medicine Scoring Manual). Sleep-staging should be made by examining 30-seconds epochs (portions) of the EEG.

- Stage W (wakefulness):
    - >50% of the epoch has alpha rhythm over the posterior region
    - Or if no alpha rhythm is present but frequent eye movements and normal or high muscle tone
- Stage N1 (drowsiness): It is a stage at the interface between wakefulness and sleep.
    - Predominant (>50%) activity is in the 4–7Hz range (theta activity)
    - Vertex sharp waves
    - Slow eye movements
    - Possible reduction in the frequency of alpha activity (alpha drop-out)

- Stage N2:
  - o one or more K-complexes unassociated with arousal or one or more trains of sleep spindles
  - o > 50% of epoch consists in theta activity
- Stage N3 (slow-wave sleep):
  - o > 20% of the epoch consists in slow wave activity (0.5–2Hz)
- Stage R (REM sleep. **Figure 14.12A**):
  - o Rapid eye movements
  - o Low amplitude, mixed frequencies
  - o Low muscle tone
  - o Absence of K-complexes or sleep spindles

Sleep transients

Several physiological EEG patterns happen only during certain stages of sleep and help differentiate the distinct stages. These patterns should not be confounded with epileptiform discharges.

- Vertex waves: these are sharp potentials with maximum amplitude at the vertex (Cz). It is often represented as a small positive spike followed by a larger sharp transient of negative polarity (**Figure 14.12B**). Vertex waves are present in sleep stage N1.
- Positive occipital sharp transient of sleep (POSTS): sharp transients of maximal amplitude over the occipital region. They are bilaterally synchronous and often displayed as a reverse checkmark pattern on the EEG of positive polarity. POSTS are more commonly seen in humans in stage N2 and N3 in adolescent and young adults and are absent in blind individuals. They have not been described yet in veterinary patients.
- Sleep spindles: bursts of 11–15Hz activity predominantly seen over the central region. They are generated by synchronous cortical and thalamic activity. Sleep spindles are seen in stage N2 and N3 (**Figure 14.12C**).

- K-complexes: bi- or triphasic transient that consists of a large amplitude wave of negative polarity followed by a smaller wave of positive polarity. The amplitude is maximal over the frontal region. K-complexes can be superimposed with sleep spindles. Prevalence of K-complexes is higher in stage N2 and N3 (**Figure 14.12C**).
- Benign sporadic sleep spikes: mono or biphasic spikes < 50μV and < 50ms in duration. They are seen uni- or bilaterally over the temporal electrodes during stage N1 and N2. They do not disturb the background.

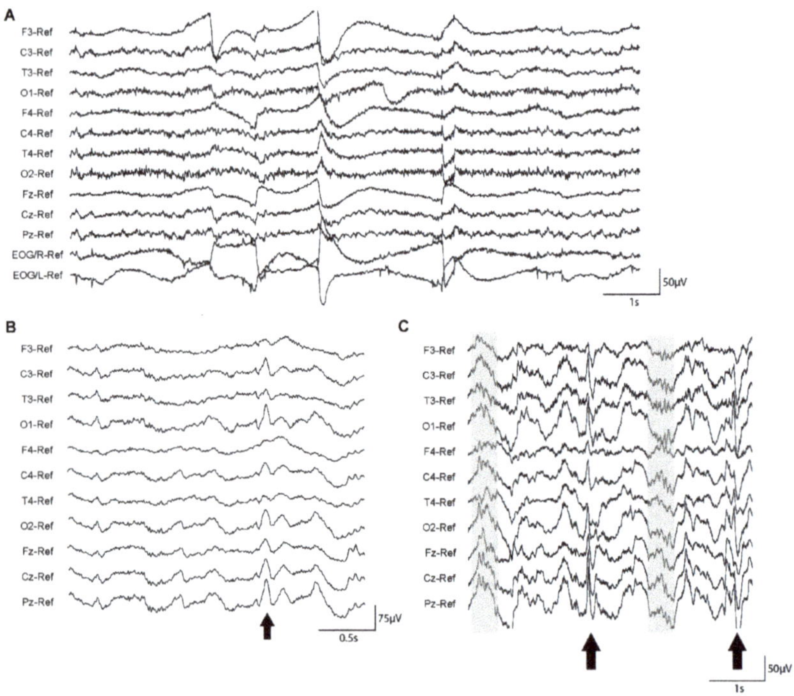

Figure 14.12. Effect of sleep on the EEG. A. Characteristic EEG during REM sleep. Note the fast frequency, low amplitude background similar to what is normally seen in wakefulness. However, frequent eye movements are seen, characterised by large amplitude waves, more prominent in the frontal electrodes and of opposite polarity in the electrooculogram channels (EOG/R-Ref and EOG/L-Ref) located close to the right and left eyes respectively. B. Vertex wave (arrow). C. K-complexes (arrows) and sleep spindles (shaded areas) on a delta activity background during stage N3 sleep.

(v) REM sleep disorders

REM-sleep disorders are non-epileptiform disorders characterised by increased muscle tone and movements happening during REM sleep which on the contrary is characterised by muscle atony apart from the extra-ocular muscles. Diagnosis of REM-sleep disorders in a patient exhibiting abnormal movements during sleep can be made by recording the EEG during sleep and observing if the abnormal movements are occurring during REM sleep and are associated with epileptiform discharges or not (**Figure 14.13**).

Narcoleptic patients may exhibit stage R at the onset of sleep, but this is a non-specific finding also present during certain drug withdrawal or sleep deprivation.

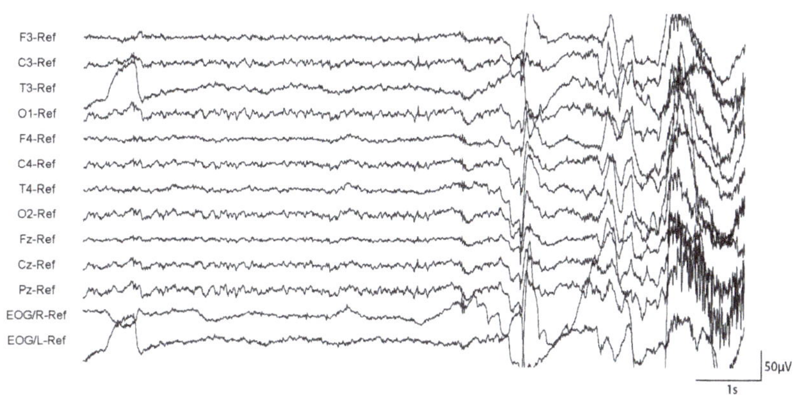

Figure 14.13. Example EEG of REM sleep disorder. This epoch shows a fast frequency, low amplitude background with eye movement (beginning of epoch) characteristic of REM sleep. Marked movement artefacts are seen abruptly at the end of the epoch and confirmed with synchronised video recording. No epileptiform discharges were seen throughout the entire recording.

(vi) Effect of age on the EEG

The characteristics of EEG depending on the age of the patient has been very well described in humans which allows the correct interpretation of the EEG in premature, infants, adolescents and adults. Changes in the EEG with age correlate with the progressive maturation of the brain that occurs after birth. Research on the age-dependent features of the EEG in dogs and cats is scarce although some features are shared between humans and dogs. However, it is unknown if most of the same age-dependent characteristics seen in humans are seen in veterinary patients.

In humans, occipital alpha activity appears around 4 months of age and initially has a frequency around 4Hz that increases with time to reach the alpha range around 3 years old. Some characteristic patterns like a theta-delta rhythm juxtaposed with the alpha rhythm (called the posterior slow wave of youth) is observed in individuals aged 8-22 years old and normally not present in adults. Similarly, POSTS are more common in adolescent and young adults. Changes in EEG characteristics are also seen in the elderly when a mild decrease in alpha wave frequency is observed.

In dogs, EEG recordings in postnatal individuals shows a progressive increase in amplitude with all frequency bands being observed after 5 weeks of age and a mature awake EEG similar to adults is observed around 3-4 months old (Morgan, Steadman and Lambert, 1973; Iotchev *et al.*, 2019). However, analysis of EEG activity during sleep suggests that a fully mature EEG occurs around 14-month-old as the age-related differences stabilise around this age. Similar to what is observed in humans, the proportion of time spent in REM sleep stage is larger in younger dogs and decreases with age. Moreover, younger dogs exhibit more delta activity than adults and less alpha and theta activity during sleep (Reicher *et al.*, 2021).

4. Abnormal patterns on the EEG

(i) *Abnormal background activity*

Background activity should correlate with the mental state of the individual (see *effect of sleep*). In awake patients, the background is mainly composed of low amplitude, high frequency activity in the beta range as well as EMG artefacts consistent with increased muscle tone. A posterior dominant alpha rhythm may be noticed upon eye closure. As the patient gets drowsy and then falls asleep, the background will be mainly composed of theta and then delta activity, except in REM-sleep.

Background slowing

Slowing refers to the presence of waves of slower frequency (delta or theta) than expected for the mental status of the patient. Although theta and delta waves are normal during drowsiness and sleep, background slowing localised to one region or generalised slowing in awake patients are abnormal findings.

Localised background slowing is usually due to a focal cortical or white matter lesion localised underneath the affected electrodes.

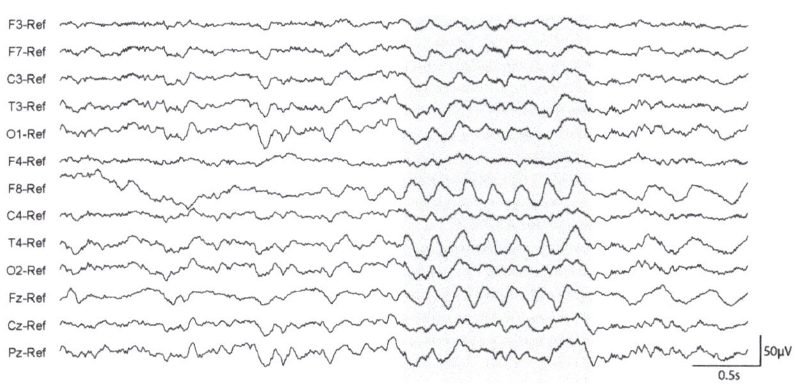

Figure 14.14. Localised background slowing. Waves of 5Hz frequency observed over F8, T4 and Fz (shaded area). Compare with the 6Hz waves of lower amplitude in the contralateral electrodes.

It occurs when there is a decrease >1Hz between a region and the contralateral region (asymmetry in frequency, **Figure 14.14**). Generalised background slowing is more often associated to a diffuse lesion of the subcortical white matter but is not specific for a particular disease.

Amplitude abnormalities

Localised amplitude abnormalities are also called amplitude asymmetry and happen when a decrease of more than 50% (alpha rhythm) or 35% (beta rhythm) is observed in a particular region compared to the other side. If the amplitude remains over 10μV it is called attenuation. If the amplitude is <10μV then it is described as suppression.

The side with the reduced amplitude is usually the affected side except in the case of skull defect where the amplitude is increased over the defect. Causes of decreased amplitude include unilateral cortical lesion and change in conduction medium such as in the case of a subdural hematoma, abscess...

Discontinuity

Continuity: the EEG background is described as continuous if the epoch examined does not contain any period of attenuation or suppression. It is described as nearly continuous if periods of attenuation/suppression occur is 1-9% of the recording and discontinuous if it occurs in 10-49% of the recording (**Figure 14.15**). If attenuation/suppression occurs in 50-99% of the recording, the activity is described as a burst-suppression pattern. The background is described as attenuated/suppressed if the attenuation/suppression occurs over >99% of the recording.

Burst-suppression/attenuation pattern is more commonly seen in comatose patients or in response to the administration of anesthetic drugs. In comatose patient, the evolution of burst-suppression patterns can be used as a prognostic marker. An

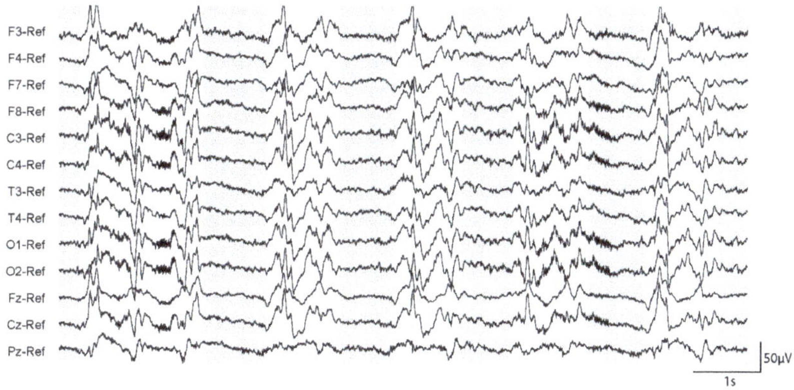

Figure 14.15. Discontinuity. Periods of suppression (shaded areas) occurring in around 40% of the recording. This EEG is therefore classified as discontinuous

increase in the length of the suppression over time is associated with poorer prognosis than a decrease of the suppression period and evolution of the EEG toward continuity (Ruijter *et al.*, 2018).

Highly epileptiform bursts in burst-suppression patterns are bursts that contain epileptiform discharges or potentially ictal rhythmic discharges with a frequency > 1Hz (**Figure 14.16**). The presence of these epileptiform patterns in > 50% of the bursts may be predictive of seizure recurrence in patients with medically-induced

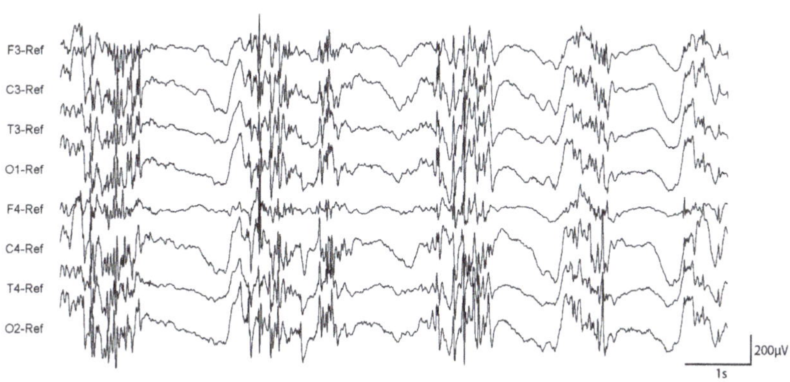

Figure 14.16. Highly epileptiform bursts. Epoch shows a burst-suppression pattern. Within the bursts, polyspikes and spike-and-waves patterns >1Hz in frequency are observed.

burst-suppression pattern for the treatment of status epilepticus (Johnson, Martinez and Ritzl, 2016; Thompson and Hantus, 2016) this has not been shown to improve outcome. We examined EEG characteristics in patients treated with IV anesthetic therapy (IVAT.

(ii) Interictal patterns: sporadic epileptiform discharges

Once a specific waveform has been established not to be an artefact or a physiological transient, EEG interpretation should try to determine the pathological significance of the discharge. One of the main clinical questions behind performing an EEG is if the patient is experiencing epileptic seizures. EEG is the most specific test to answer that question by recording discharges that are associated with epileptic conditions. In between seizures, abnormal interictal activity can be recorded in the brain of epileptic patients. These interictal epileptiform discharges are called sporadic epileptiform discharges (SED). SED are di- or triphasic waveforms of cortical origin (usually of negative polarity and displaying a field, gradient and lag). They also stand out from background activity by either disrupting the background activity or being of different duration than waveforms from the background activity.

SED are non-rhythmic, non-periodic discharges that happen in between seizures so they are not associated with any clinical manifestation. However, their recording is highly associated with an epileptic condition occurring in the patient. SED are thought to represent inhibiting mechanisms from the brain that manage to contain an epileptic seizure from being generated. SED can take three main forms:

- Spikes if the duration is between 20-70ms (**Figure 14.17**)
- Sharp waves if the duration is between 70-200ms
- Spike-and-slow waves if a spike is associated with a wave with a duration larger than 200ms. The spike of one spike-and-slow wave complex (SWC) can be superimposed with the wave of the previous complex (**Figure 14.18**).

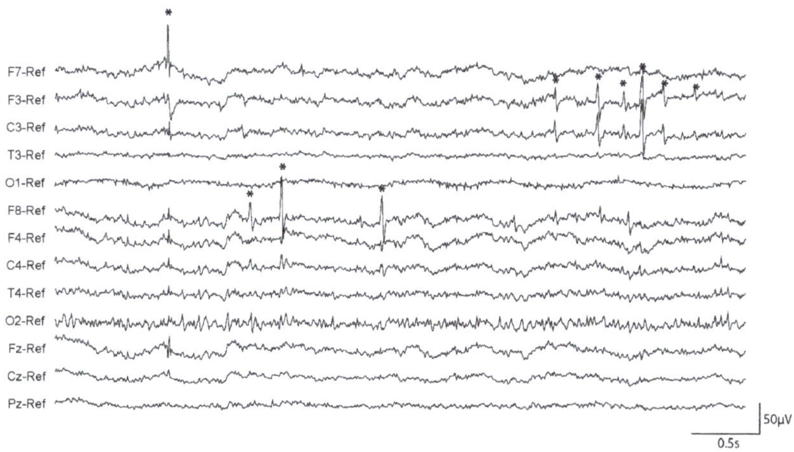

Figure 14.17. Interictal spikes. EEG of a dog with epileptic seizures showing multiple, independent spikes of di-phasic morphology over F7, F8 and F3-C3. These discharges were not associated with clinical manifestations.

SED may repeat briefly (no more than a few seconds) but have little to no variation in shape. SED can be focal or generalised depending on if they happen in one or both hemispheres. They may also be generated by multiple dependent or independent foci. In case of independent foci, SED are observed over different electrode areas without any timing correlation.

Figure 14.18. Spike-and-slow waves. Burst of discharges of generalised spike-and-slow wave morphology most prominent over the temporal regions bilaterally. Asterisks show the spike components and arrows show the slow wave components of the discharges

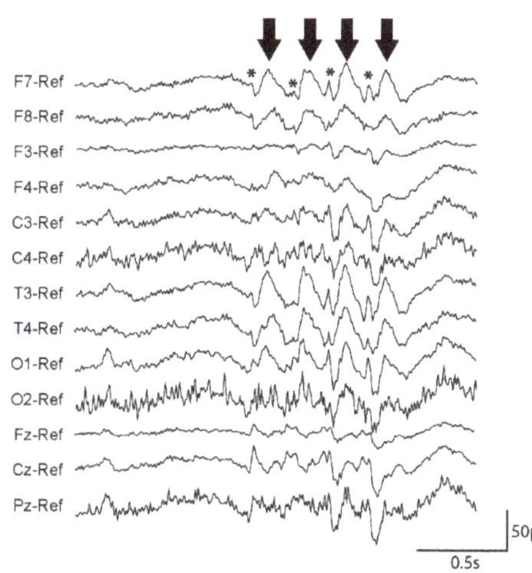

(iii) Ictal patterns: electrographic/electroclinical seizures

Abnormal epileptiform activity can also be recorded during an epileptic seizure or status epilepticus. Any pattern lasting longer than 10 seconds and consisting of repeated epileptiform discharges (spike, sharp wave or spike-and-wave) with a frequency >2.5Hz or with evolution of its morphology, frequency and/or amplitude is considered an electrographic seizure. If the pattern lasts more than 10 continuous minutes or is present in at least 20% of any

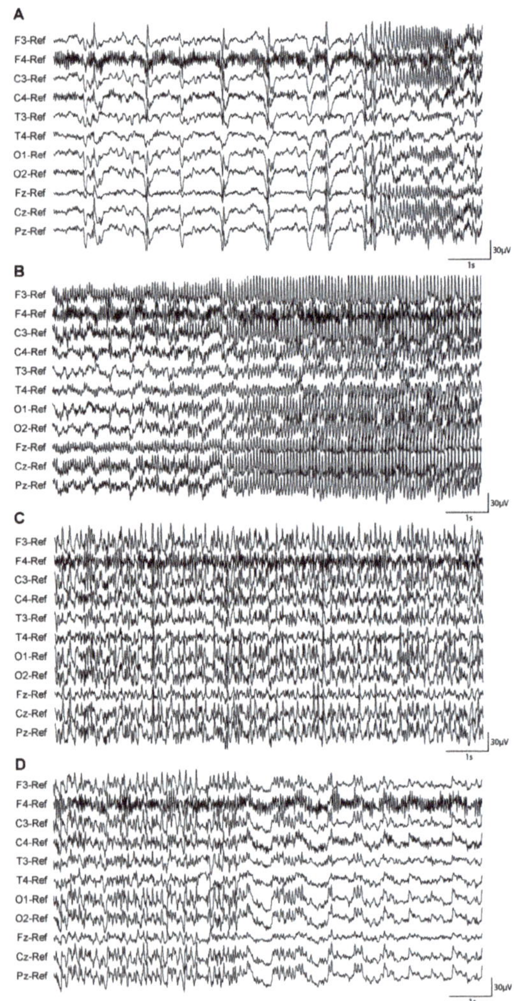

Figure 14.19: Example of ictal pattern evolution. Epochs of an EEG during an electrographic seizure initiation (A), after 30 seconds (B), after 1 minute (C) and at seizure termination (D). A. Before seizure initiation, note the generalised periodic discharges occurring at a 1Hz frequency (asterisks). The electrographic seizure begins with generalised polyspikes occurring at a 12Hz frequency. B. During the seizure, an increase in amplitude of the spikes is noted C. Evolution of the morphology toward a spike-and-sharp-wave pattern with a decrease in frequency to 8Hz. D. Electrographic seizure termination with cessation of the epileptiform pattern.

60-minute recording, it is considered an electrographic status epilepticus (Hirsch *et al.*, 2021). **Figure 14.19** shows the evolution of an epileptiform pattern throughout an electrographic seizure.

If clinical manifestations are time-locked with a pattern of repeated epileptiform discharges, it is considered an electroclinical seizure, regardless of its duration (**Figure 14.20**). However, these manifestations may be subtle and not always recognised by external observers, such as during an absence seizure. Video synchronisation during EEG may help discriminating interictal from ictal ED by being able to look for clinical manifestations time-locked the pattern of interest. An electroclinical seizure should also be suspected if there is improvement of the clinical manifestations and the EEG after parenteral administration of anti-seizure medications.

Electrographic/electroclinical seizures consist in repeated spikes, sharp waves or SWC that usually change in morphology, frequency and amplitude throughout the seizure. They are also characterised by an abrupt end followed by resuming background activity of normal or decreased frequency. Interictal ED may be seen at a higher frequency after a focal electrographic/electroclinical

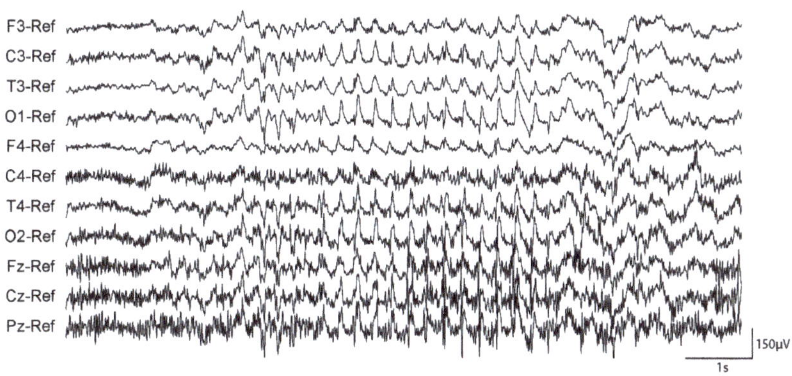

Figure 14.20. EEG recording of an absence seizure in a dog. Generalised 4Hz spike-and-slow-wave pattern lasting 5 seconds. Because an interruption of behaviour and staring into space (consistent with clinical manifestations of an absence seizure) was noticed time-locked to the EEG pattern, this episode be classified as a an electroclinical seizure.

seizure. If an electroclinical seizure lasts for more than 5 minutes (convulsive seizure) or 10 minutes (non-convulsive seizure) or if an electroclinical seizure is present on at least 20% of any 60-minute recording, then it is called an electroclinical status epilepticus.

Similarly to SED, electrographic/electroclinical seizures can be either focal, primarily generalised or focal with secondary generalisation depending on their hemispheric distribution. Focal epileptiform patterns are more commonly associated with a focal irritative cortical lesion such as a tumour, an inflammatory focus, a stroke, etc. On the contrary, generalised epileptiform patterns are more commonly observed in idiopathic epilepsy or diffuse cortical disorders such as toxic, metabolic, electrolytic disturbances, global anoxia, etc. The EEG is often obscured by muscle and movement artefacts during a convulsive seizure which can prevent the visualisation of epileptiform discharges during the event (**Figure 14.21**).

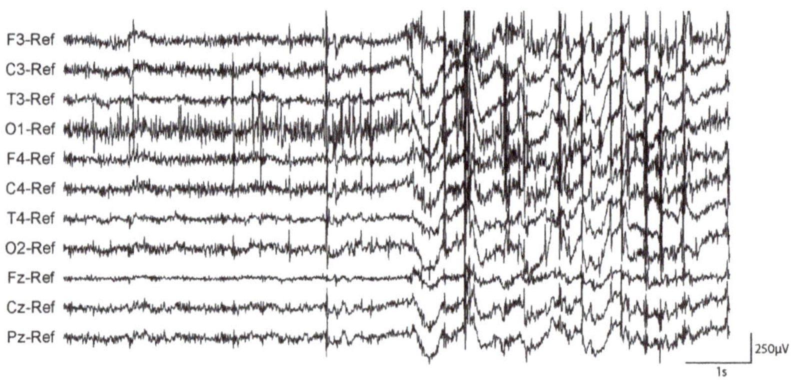

Figure 14.21. Example of a myoclonic seizure in a 10-year-old miniature smooth-haired Dachshund. Muscle artefacts time-locked with myoclonic jerks recorded through video-synchronised EEG. Some spikes can be visualised in between artefacts. The rest of the EEG showed spikes as well as spike-and waves. This patient experienced myoclonic seizures as well as a generalised tonic-clonic seizure.

Different patterns of electrographic seizures are associated with different type of clinical seizures (**Table 14.3**).

Ictal ED pattern	Seizure type
3-4Hz spike-and waves, frontal maximum	Absence seizures
4-6Hz spike-and-waves, antero-dominant	Myoclonic seizures
>10Hz fast waves + occasional spike and wave	Clonic seizures
>10Hz wave of increasing amplitude and decreasing frequency	Tonic seizures
>10Hz wave of increasing amplitude, decreasing frequency and interrupted by slow waves	Tonic-clonic seizures

Table 14.3. Ictal epileptiform discharge pattern and their associated seizure type.

(iv) Rhythmic and periodic patterns

Rhythmic and periodic patterns are described by using a main term referring to their localisation and a main term describing the pattern (see **Table 14.4**). This description is based from the ACNS critical care EEG terminology (Hirsch *et al.*, 2021). Modifiers terms are used to further describe the pattern including prevalence, frequency, duration, number of phases, sharpness, voltage, evolution, if it is stimulus-induced and if they are other distinct morphological features ('plus'). The plus modifier can be used if one ore more features are associated with the rhythmic and periodic patterns:

- + F: superimposed fast activity (theta or faster) on periodic discharges or rhythmic delta activity
- + R: superimposed rhythmic delta activity on periodic discharges
- + S: superimposed spike/sharp waves on rhythmic delta activity
- +FR (periodic discharges) or +FS (rhythmic delta activity) if both features are present.

To apply the plus modifier, it is important to distinguish if the features are associated with the periodic/rhythmic pattern or simply part of the background, in which case the plus modifier does not apply. For more information, the reader is directed to the ACNS critical care EEG terminology guidelines (Hirsch *et al.*, 2021). **Figure 14.22** shows an example of generalised rhythmic delta activity recorded in a dog. Other examples have been described in veterinary electroencephalography (Knipe *et al.*, 2023).

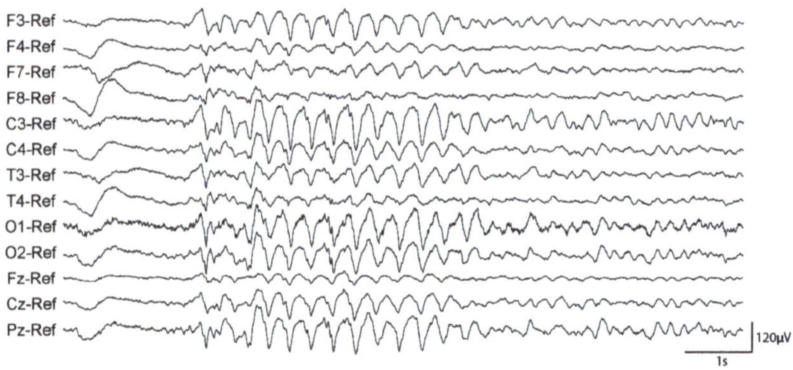

Figure 14.22. Rhythmic delta activity. Five second burst of generalised rhythmic delta activity of 3.5Hz, more prominent in the centro-occipital region with some occasional superimposed spikes.

EEG terminology

Main term #1 (localisation)	Main term #2 (pattern)
Generalised: bilateral, synchronous and symmetric	Periodic discharges
Lateralised: unilateral or bilateral asymmetric	Rhythmic delta activity
Bilateral independent: bilateral but not synchronous between the two hemispheres	Spike-and-wave/sharp-and-wave
Unilateral independent: two non-synchronous patterns observed in the same hemisphere	
Multifocal: at least three independent patterns with at least one in each hemisphere	

Table 14.4 : Main terms for describing rhythmic and periodic patterns. ACNS critical care**.**

Lateralised periodic discharges (LPDs)

LPDs (formerly termed periodic lateralised epileptiform discharges, PLEDs) are bi-, tri- or multiphasic focal spikes or sharp waves occurring periodically at the rate of 0.5-2Hz. They are usually confined to one hemisphere (**Figure 14.23**). LPDs are highly associated with epileptic seizures so that their recording raises the suspicion for epilepsy in the patient (Lin and Drislane, 2018).

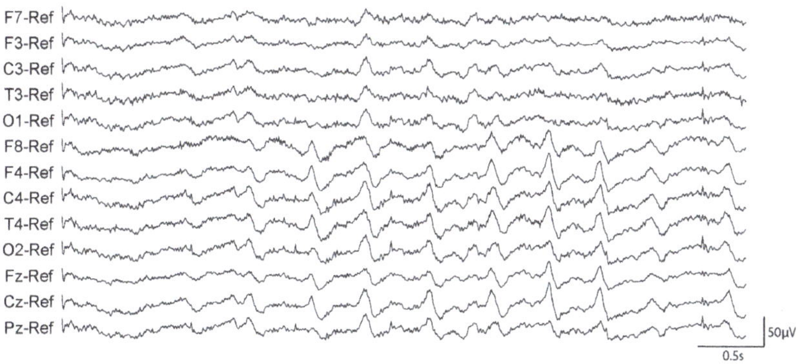

Figure 14.23. Lateralised periodic discharges. Periodic sharp waves, most prominent over the right hemisphere and frontal region occurring at a 2Hz frequency.

Generalised periodic discharges with triphasic wave morphology (GPDTW)

GPDTW, previously called triphasic waves are sharply contoured discharges characterised by an initial upward deflection followed by a larger downward deflection and then a slower rising upward deflection. Typical GPDTW last around 300-600ms and are bilateral, symmetric and synchronous discharges occurring periodically. A fronto-occipital lag can also be observed. Atypical GPDTW have also been described and although they share a triphasic morphology, their maximum amplitude may not be over the fronto-central regions, may have inverse polarity or be asymmetric or asynchronous (**Figure 14.24**).

GPDTW are abnormal discharges associated with several conditions. They are frequently observed in patients with metabolic or toxic encephalopathy such as hepatic or renal encephalopathy, intoxications, electrolyte disturbances, etc. (Wrzosek *et al.*, 2017).

GPDTW are not pathognomonic for metabolic encephalopathy and can also be observed in diseases affecting the subcortical white matter tracts.

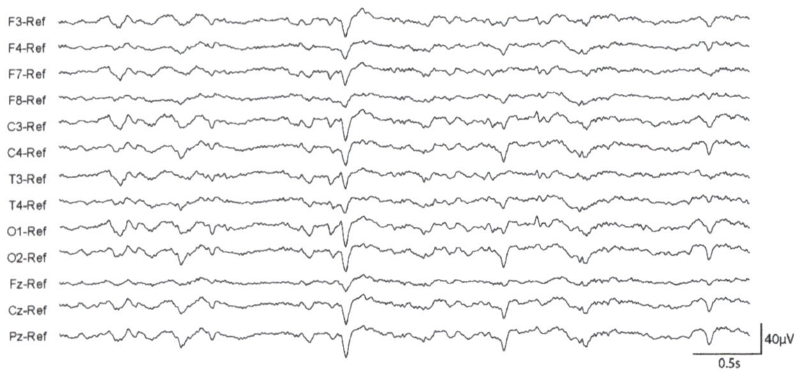

Figure 14.24. Generalised periodic discharges with triphasic morphology. Generalised periodic discharges with a triphasic morphology occurring at a frequency of approximately 1Hz and with maximal amplitude over the centro-occipital regions.

(v) Possible ictal patterns: the ictal-interictal continuum

Some patterns do not fit the definitions of ictal discharges but may potentially represent ictal activity as they may be associated with impaired responsiveness of the patient when the recording is performed on awake, behaviour animals. Their observation in a patient should raise the suspicion of epilepsy.

Possible electrographic seizures – These patterns include:

- Periodic discharges or spike-and-wave patterns between 1-2Hz over at least 10 seconds
- Periodic discharges or spike-and-wave patterns between 0.5-1Hz over at least 10 seconds and with plus modifiers or fluctuation in frequency
- Lateralised rhythmic delta activity > 1Hz, over at least 10 seconds and with a plus modifier or fluctuating frequency.

Brief potentially ictal rhythmic discharges (BIRD): If a pattern consists of rhythmic activity > 4Hz, lasts for less than 10 seconds with a similar morphology and location as SED or with an evolving amplitude or frequency, it is described as a brief potentially ictal rhythmic discharge (BIRD). BIRD are therefore electrographic seizure-like patterns that do not reach the 10-second criteria.

(vi) Deviation from normal patterns

Deviation from delta activity

Delta activity is abnormal if:

- Localised to only a few channels (localised slowing). This is usually associated with a cortical or white matter lesion.
- More prominent in the caudal regions: this is usually associated with the post-ictal phase.
- Present in awake, drowsy patients or during light sleep (generalised slowing). This is a sign of a diffuse encephalopathy, a thalamic or a midbrain lesion. The significance of intermittent rhythmic delta activity in awake patients depends on its localisation:
    - o Frontal intermittent rhythmic delta activity: 2-3Hz bisynchronous burst of high amplitude lasting at least 2 seconds. It is abnormal except during hyperventilation or hypnagogic hypersynchrony (the brief transition between drowsiness and sleep, sometimes associated with a jerk and the sensation of falling). This pattern is associated with a focal structural brain lesion or is a nonspecific sign of encephalopathy.
    - o Temporal intermittent rhythmic delta activity. This pattern can be seen during drowsiness and light sleep. It usually has a frequency of 1–4Hz and lasts at least 3 seconds. It has been associated with temporal lobe epilepsy and hippocampal sclerosis in humans although it is not sure if it is present in animals.

- o Occipital intermittent rhythmic delta activity. This pattern is observed in children < 15 years old so it is unclear if it is present in young animals. It is associated with primarily generalised epilepsy especially absence seizures.

Deviation from theta activity

Theta activity is abnormal if:

- Maximal amplitude is observed over the caudal electrodes. This is a nonspecific sign of encephalopathy.
- Localised to only a few channels (localised slowing). This is usually associated with a cortical or white matter lesion.
- It happens in intermittent bursts of asymmetrical theta activity during wakefulness (generalised slowing). This is associated with subcortical dysfunction.

Unilateral blocking of alpha rhythm

Unilateral blocking of alpha rhythm when both eyes are opened (called Bancaud's phenomenon) leads to paradoxical alpha rhythms on the side where it is not attenuated by eyes opening. This side is abnormal and is seen predominantly in patients with a lesion in the occipital lobe but can also be less commonly observed with lesions of the parietal and temporal lobes.

Unilateral mu rhythm

A strictly unilateral mu rhythm may indicate a lesion in the cortex underlying the centro-parietal electrodes on the same side.

Deviation from beta activity

Beta activity is abnormal if there is an asymmetry of more than 35% in amplitude between both hemispheres or if it is only present focally.

(vii) Patterns of unknown significance

The prevalence of these patterns in veterinary patient has not been reported. If they occur, they may easily be confounded with epileptiform patterns. One of the distinguishing features between epileptiform patterns and patterns of unknown significance is that the latter do not evolve in their morphology, amplitude and frequency compared to epileptiform patterns.

Fast/slow alpha variants

These are rhythmic activity of twice or half the frequency of the alpha activity. They always occur concurrently with alpha activity within the alpha frequency range and have the highest amplitude in the posterior region.

Rhythmic midtemporal theta bursts of drowsiness

This pattern is a burst of 5-7Hz rhythmic activity with maximum amplitude in the temporal leads. It occurs during drowsiness and light sleep. The bursts are bilaterally synchronous or independent.

Midline theta rhythm (Ciganek rhythm)

4-7Hz rhythm with a sinusoidal appearance and maximum amplitude over the midline electrodes. This pattern is seen during wakefulness or drowsiness.

14 and 6Hz positive bursts

Rhythmic activity consisting of 6Hz and 14Hz bursts of activity predominantly over the temporal region. These patterns are more often observed during light sleep or drowsiness in children and adolescent humans. They are thought to be a developmental pattern.

6Hz spike and wave bursts

Bilateral, synchronous bursts of 6Hz SWC lasting 1-2 seconds and of maximum amplitude over the midline electrodes. The spike may not always be clearly distinguishable. They happen more commonly in wakefulness and drowsiness

Wicket spikes

Short runs of 6-11Hz monophasic spikes with maximum amplitude over the anterior/temporal region. They do not disrupt the background or are followed by slow waves. Wicket spikes are usually unilateral but shift sides during the recording. They are more commonly seen during drowsiness and light sleep.

5. Practical applications of EEG

(i) Determining the epileptic nature of paroxysmal episodes

Paroxysmal episodes are repeated intermittent clinical manifestations occurring at a variable frequency in patients. This encompasses epileptic seizures as well as other movement disorders (dyskinesia) or behavioural episodes. The diagnosis of epilepsy with EEG relies on the recording of interictal or ictal epileptiform discharges whereas ruling out an epileptic nature of the paroxysmal episodes requires recording the EEG during the episode of interest and not observing any epileptiform discharges associated with the episode of interest. EEG is the most specific tool to confirm that a patient with paroxysmal episode is suffering from epilepsy. During interictal EEG recording in humans, the presence of epileptiform discharges is seen in approximately 1-4% of non-epileptic individuals while they are observed in around 50% of patients with epilepsy (Goodin and Aminoff, 1984; Geut *et al.*, 2017). Therefore, the odds ratio of having epilepsy if interictal epileptiform discharges are observed is around 24. This specificity might be even more increased with continuous EEG as it allows to record not only interictal discharges but ictal discharges as well.

The sensitivity of EEG however is rather low as only around 50% of human patients with epilepsy will show epileptiform discharges on their first interictal EEG (Goodin and Aminoff, 1984). The absence of interictal epileptiform discharges therefore cannot rule out epilepsy in a patient. The sensitivity of EEG may be increased with repeated or continuous recordings as well as adding video-synchronization. Video recordings help determine the epileptic or non-epileptic nature of an episode by assessing the presence/absence of epileptiform discharges time-locked with the episode of interest.

The use of interictal EEG in veterinary medicine has shown sensitivity ranging from 20 to 86%. The diagnostic accuracy of EEG depends on the paroxysmal episode frequency in dogs with weekly episodes allowing a probability of confirming/excluding epilepsy around 50% using continuous ambulatory EEG (James *et al.*, 2017).

Moreover, in continuous, ambulatory EEG, a 30-minute recording showed at least one abnormality in only 50% of the cases, similar to what is found in human EEG. On the contrary, 95% of EEG showed at least one abnormality within 4.5 hours arguing for a minimum recording time of several hours (Parmentier *et al.*, 2020). Other studies have shown that electrographic seizures (without clinical manifestations) are relatively common in dogs suggesting that clinical observation alone underestimates epileptic seizure prevalence (Granum *et al.*, 2019; Ukai *et al.*, 2021).

(ii) Status epilepticus monitoring

Status epilepticus (SE) is defined clinically as a prolonged epileptic seizure resulting from the failure of the mechanisms responsible for seizure termination or activation of mechanisms leading to prolonged seizure activity. In humans, dogs and cats, most generalised tonic-clonic seizures last less than 5 minutes and therefore, a practical definition of SE is a prolonged seizure lasting more than 5 minutes (Trinka *et al.*, 2015). After 30 minutes of continuous generalised tonic-clonic seizure, irreversible neuronal damage is likely. For focal or non-convulsive seizures, a SE is defined when the seizure lasts more than 10 minutes with irreversible neuronal damage after 60 minutes of prolonged focal seizure activity. Non-convulsive SE can happen on its own or following a convulsive seizure. Non-convulsive SE should therefore be suspected in patients that do not recover consciousness within the expected timeframe after a convulsive seizure. Some drugs such as baclofen can also induce non-convulsive SE.

Similar definitions are used to define SE on the EEG. An electrographical SE is defined by a continuous epileptiform pattern lasting more than 5 minutes (convulsive seizure) or 10 minutes (non-convulsive seizure) or if a continuous epileptiform pattern is present on at least 20% of any 60-minute recording (Hirsch *et al.*, 2021).

The EEG of convulsive status epilepticus has the same ictal patterns than shorter seizures and can be obscured by muscle and movement artefacts. At the end of the status epilepticus, a generalised slow-wave (delta and theta) activity or suppressed background is usually observed. Some focal status epilepticus (*epilepsia partialis continua*) may however have no changes on the EEG, possibly because a small region of the cortex in involved or because the epileptic focus is located too deeply.

EEG is even more important for the diagnosis of non-convulsive SE which can be missed in a clinical setting following a convulsive status and misinterpreted for non-specific signs of encephalopathy. The EEG of non-convulsive status contains continuous or frequent, recurrent or rhythmic spikes, polyspikes and SWC as well as rhythmic delta activity. Epileptiform activity occurs usually in the 3-4Hz frequency range. Changes can be focal (focal non-convulsive status epilepticus) or generalised (absence status epilepticus).

EEG is an important tool for the management of status epilepticus to assess the efficacy of the treatment. In humans, the presence of electrographic seizures on EEG is associated with a relapse of clinical seizure and recurrence of status epilepticus upon tapering of intravenous anti-seizure. Recommendations are to adjust the treatment to completely suppress electrographic seizures for around 12-24 hours before attempting to taper the drugs. The presence of sporadic epileptiform discharges does not seem to be associated with status epilepticus treatment failure and it is unclear if a medically-induced discontinuous EEG pattern (burst-suppression or complete suppression) provides greater survival (Krishnamurthy and Drislane, 1999; Neurocritical Care Society Status Epilepticus Guideline Writing Committee *et al.*, 2012). It is also unknown if these guidelines apply similarly in veterinary patients but should be considered especially in the treatment of refractory status epilepticus.

When treating a patient for SE, placing an EEG can therefore guide the clinician to adjust the doses of drugs, confirm disappearance or recurrence of electrographic seizures and detect non-convulsive SE. It can also help to distinguish non-convulsive SE from post-ictal or medically-induced encephalopathy as the patient may perform repetitive movements that can be misinterpreted for convulsive activity (Cuff *et al.*, 2014). In the case of post-ictal or medically-induced encephalopathy, no epileptiform discharge is seen and the EEG consists in disorganised slow- wave (delta or theta) activity without rhythmicity.

(iii) Coma monitoring and brain death

EEG can be very useful to monitor patients in coma as specific patterns will be seen in during coma (Young *et al.*, 1997):

- Alpha coma: alpha rhythm may be predominant in the frontal or posterior region. Frontally predominant alpha rhythm is observed in post-anoxic coma while posteriorly predominant alpha rhythm is observed in coma caused by brainstem lesions caudal to the ponto-mesencephalic junction.

- Spindle coma: presence of sleep spindles, vertex waves and K-complexes in comatose patients.
- Beta coma: presence of diffuse 12-16Hz beta activity. This pattern is often associated with barbiturate or benzodiazepine intoxication.

EEG can be used to grade and monitor the severity of encephalopathy in hospitalised patients. EEG of encephalopathic patients will originally show a predominance of waves in the alpha frequency (grade 1), then theta frequency (grade 2) and then delta frequency (grade 3) as the severity increases. During grade 3, spindle coma pattern can be observed. As the severity progresses, the EEG can evolve into a burst-suppression pattern (grade 4) with or without the presence of epileptiform discharges or an alpha coma pattern during the bursts. Finally, an isoelectric EEG can be observed in the most severe encephalopathies (grade 5).

An important prognostic factor is the reactivity of the EEG in comatose patients. Reactivity of the EEG is a change in EEG activity is induced by stimulation. This change can be a change in the background frequency or amplitude. However, muscle activity detected by the EEG, such as in the case of an eye blink secondary to tactile stimulation of the face (palpebral reflex) does not represent reactivity. Preservation of reactivity, even if it is to noxious stimuli, is a positive prognostic indicator while loss of reactivity is associated with a poorer outcome in comatose patients (Juan *et al.*, 2015).

Finally, EEG can also serve to confirm brain death in a patient that may be mechanically ventilated or spontaneously breathing. To assess brain death, several criteria have been established in humans (Stecker *et al.*, 2016):

- At least 8 electrodes should be used
- Electrode impedance should be between 0.1 and 10,000 ohms
- Sensitivity should be at least 2μV
- Recording should be performed for at least 30 minutes
- High-frequency filter should be set above 30Hz and low frequency filter should be below 1Hz
- EEG should show a lack of reactivity to intense somatosensory or audiovisual stimuli.

The absence of EEG activity while recording using these criteria allows the diagnosis of brain death.

(iv) EEG in anaesthesia monitoring

Anesthetic drugs have a significant dose-dependent effect on mentation as well as EEG activity. Signals recorded on the EEG will change depending on the dose of anesthetics used and the depth of anaesthesia. Proprietary EEG indices such as the bispectral index have been developed for assessing anaesthesia depth (Myles *et al.*, 2004). Their use in human medicine is controversial while they have not been clinically validated in dogs and cats yet.

Anesthetics drugs that mainly act through GABA receptor activation such as halogenated inhalants, propofol, barbiturates, benzodiazepines and etomidate initially induce frontally dominant activity in the alpha and low-beta range. Then, theta and delta activity become more prominent, followed by a burst-suppression pattern and finally an isoelectric EEG as the dose and the depth of anaesthesia increase. Burst-suppression is not seen with benzodiazepines in humans.

Ketamine and dexmedetomidine do not induce the same effects on the EEG. Low doses of ketamine will induce beta and low gamma activity while higher doses induce beta and delta activity. Dexmedetomidine induces a pattern similar to sleep stage N2 (predominant theta activity with sleep spindles, vertex waves and K-complexes) at low doses and N3 (theta and delta activity) at higher doses.

Often used during anaesthesia, opioids produce a dose dependent increase in theta and delta activity.

The ideal EEG pattern during anaesthesia is not known. However, EEG monitoring during anaesthesia may help assessing the depth of anaesthesia objectively and in real-time.

(v) Non-epileptic disorders

Ruling out epileptic seizures with EEG can be a difficult task due to the low sensitivity of short, interictal EEG and may require continuous EEG recording in awake patients for several hours in order to record the EEG during an episode of interest. However, if a non-epileptic episode is recorded, the EEG is typically normal. Some non-epileptic disorders can however present changes in the EEG such as during a syncope. At the beginning of the syncope, generalised theta activity is observed followed by high-amplitude, generalised delta activity. At the patient recovers, delta activity reverses back to theta activity and then alpha activity predominantly in the occipital region (Brenner, 1997).

(vi) Quantitative EEG

New analysis tools have been developed in recent years to allow the extraction of EEG data and represent it graphically. This constitutes an important help for the screening and interpretation of EEG, especially long EEG recordings as it can be used as a screening tool to direct the electroencephalographer to periods of interest. These techniques are grouped under the term quantitative electroencephalography (qEEG). Briefly, qEEG relies on the decomposition of the EEG signal using various mathematical algorithms. Frequency-domain analysis, also known as power spectral analysis, is a type of qEEG analysis that breaks down the

EEG signal into its different frequency components. The most commonly used algorithm for that purpose is the fast Fourier transform. The power spectrum is then represented as a plot of frequency vs amplitude. Time-frequency analysis incorporates the time component to display how the power spectrum changes over time. Commonly used algorithms for that purpose are the short-time Fourier transform and the wavelet transform. The signal is displayed as a 3-dimensional array with time in the x-axis, frequency in the y-axis and power as a color-coded scale on the z-axis. These graphical representations help quickly localise events of interest that are associated with transient increase in the power of certain frequencies. qEEG can also be helpful in monitoring burst-suppression patterns for example in a comatose or anesthetised patient.

Other algorithms aim to aid in signal source localisation or evaluating connectivity between regions by analyzing the correlation between EEG signal recorded by separate electrodes. We direct the reader to specific articles for more information (Sansevere, Hahn and Abend, 2019; Kaleem and Swisher, 2022).

(vii) The EEG report

Guidelines have been proposed for EEG reports (Tatum *et al.*, 2016). The EEG report should contain comments about specific features of the EEG and provide an overall interpretation of the EEG findings. To increase interobserver agreement, the EEG report should use the specific terms from the consensus glossary. Four main sections have been proposed for EEG reporting:

History

This section should contain patient identification and signalment, a brief history including the purpose of the EEG as well as any other relevant clinical information such as current treatments or concurrent diseases.

Technical description

This section should include the date and location of the EEG, the type of electrodes and electrode placement system as well as the filter used. The report should also indicate if sedation or general anaesthesia was used including the drugs and doses. Any other information that may affect EEG interpretation should be reported such as the use of activation methods, video-synchronisation, ambulatory EEG, etc. Finally, information about the mental status of the patient (alert, sleeping, comatose, etc.) should also be included to correlate mental status with background activity.

EEG description

First, a description of the EEG background activity and reactivity should be performed including the predominant frequency, location, rhythmicity and symmetry. State changes of the patient and associated changes in background rhythm should be reported as well as sleep staging if recorded.

The report should then state if specific features of the background activity such as amplitude/frequency asymmetry, periodic or rhythmic discharges are present. For any feature, the morphology, frequency, amplitude, symmetry, rhythmicity and location should be described as objectively as possible. The presence of sporadic epileptiform discharges or electrographic/electroclinical seizures should be described similarly (morphology, frequency, duration, amplitude, symmetry, rhythmicity and location). For seizures, the EEG reader should describe the onset and evolution of the discharges as well as the field of propagation and post-ictal EEG changes. An overall frequency of epileptiform discharges or electrographic seizures should be calculated on the entire length of the recording. If possible, clinical manifestations during the epileptiform discharges should be described based on direct observation or video-synchronisation.

For any abnormal features, it is important to describe the concurrent mental status of the patient and background activity during which these abnormal features happen.

If performed, changes in the EEG triggered by hyperventilation, photic stimulation or other activation methods should be described.

Lastly, any external or physiological artefacts should be described if present.

EEG interpretation

This section should provide the referring veterinarian with the conclusion of the EEG by stating if the EEG is normal or abnormal and the reasons for such interpretation. Abnormal findings should be summarised by order of importance to support the conclusion. It is important to interpret the findings in the light of the clinical manifestation of the patient and address directly the clinical question that motivated the EEG in the first place. However, apart from suggestions for further testing, suggestions on management are not recommended in the EEG report and should be left to the patient's clinician.

Electroclinical syndromes in dogs and cats

Syndrome	Clinical characteristics	Seizure type	Interictal EEG	Ictal EEG
Familial spontaneous feline epilepsy (Kuwabara *et al.*, 2010)	Obtained for research purposes by inbreeding Onset: 4-12 months Seizures induced by vestibular stimulation Hippocampal asymmetry on MRI volumetry	Head turning, unilateral facial twitching, salivation and circling with secondary generalised tonic-clonic convulsions	Spikes, multiple spikes, spike-and-waves, sharp waves over temporal region bilaterally	
Feline VGKC-complex/ LGI1 antibody-associated limbic encephalitis (Pakozdy *et al.*, 2014)	Bilateral T2 hyperintensity and CE in temporal cortex and hippocampus.	Orofacial automatisms, such as salivation, facial twitching, lip smacking, chewing, licking, staring, tremor, disorientation, panting, and unusual vocalisation		8Hz repetitive positive spikes. Greater in occipital region

Table 14.5 : Electroclinical syndromes in cats

Syndrome	Clinical characteristics	Seizure type	Interictal EEG	Ictal EEG
Juvenile myoclonic epilepsy of Rhodesian ridgeback (Wielaender *et al.*, 2017, 2018)	Onset: 6 weeks-18 months (median: 3.5 months) 4bp deletion in DIRAS1 gene	Initially: myoclonic jerks during drowsiness (trunk, limb, neck, face). Occasionally when alert. Generalised tonic-clonic seizures in 38% of dogs within 6 months. Absence seizures: staring episodes. Seizures triggered by photostimulation (35%) or noise	4–5Hz rhythmical slowing and 4 – 5Hz generalised SWC	4–5Hz SWC or polyspike-wave complexes with fronto-central maximum. biphasic spikes and paroxysmal bursts of 7–8Hz Photoconvulsive: 4/6 dogs
Genetic epilepsy of Belgian Shepherd dogs (Berendt *et al.*, 2008)	Mean onset: 3.3-years Polygenic transmission Associated with specific haplotype in ADAM23 gene Prevalence: 9.5% in breed, up to 33% in certain family	• 7-25% focal seizures: ataxia, crawling, swaying, fearful behavior, salivation, excessive attention seeking and disorientation • 18% primarily generalised tonic-clonic • 37-53% focal with secondary generalisation • Autonomic signs common	Sharp waves, spikes, and SWC complexes in variable derivations SED in 7/17 dogs	
Polymicrogyria in poodles (Jurney *et al.*, 2009)	Age of onset: 7 weeks – 5-years Clinical signs: blindness, behavior changes, hypermetria, delayed hopping, decreased PLR, resting nystagmus	• Circling and lip smacking	Spike and SWC centered on Cz and Pz recorded in one patient	

Syndrome	Clinical characteristics	Seizure type	Interictal EEG	Ictal EEG
Genetic epilepsy of Finnish Spitz (Jeserevics *et al.*, 2007)	Median age onset: 1.8-3 years (0.6-10 years) Prevalence in breed: 5.36% Male predisposed Most likely polygenic Controlled by ASD in 78.9% Lower FDG uptake in occipital cortex on PET-MRI	• Focal: 31% • Focal with secondary generalisation: 54% • Signs: tremors, weakness, tonic-clonic, autonomous signs • Median time: 11 minutes • 18.8% have multiple seizure type	Spikes, polyspikes, SWC in posterior-occipital Derivations IED in 20%	
Neonatal encephalopathy with seizures in Standard Poodles (Chen *et al.*, 2008)	Age of onset of seizures: 4-6 weeks Death by 7 weeks Cerebellar signs with dysplastic cerebellum ATF-2 mutation	• Focal: 31% • Focal with secondary generalisation: 54% • Signs: tremors, weakness, tonic-clonic, autonomous signs • Median time: 11 minutes • 18.8% have multiple seizure type	SWC in occipital derivations.	
Benign familial juvenile epilepsy of Lagotto Romagnolo (Jokinen *et al.*, 2007)	Mean age onset: 6.3 weeks Spontaneous remission by 8-13 weeks Histopathology: Purkinje cell inclusion bodies and vacuolation Associated with LGI2 mutation causing protein truncation. Some adults experience seizures and do not carry the LGI2 mutation. Interictal hypometabolism in occipital, temporal, parietal cortex (PET-MRI)	• Episodic stiffness, generalised tremor with preserved consciousness • Interictal ataxia and hypermetria	Focal sharp waves and spikes in occipital, temporal and parietal derivations (84% of dogs)	

Syndrome	Clinical characteristics	Seizure type	Interictal EEG	Ictal EEG
Familial frontal lobe epilepsy of Shetland Sheepdogs (Morita *et al.*, 2002)	Age of onset: 1-1.5 years Female predisposed (79%) Associated with increased glutamate in CSF and extracellular glutamate and aspartate in brain parenchyma + glutamate granules in perineuronal space. Reduced density of glutamate receptors in lateral nucleus of thalamus	• During sleep or drowsiness • Mostly generalised tonic-clonic contraction of muscles, excessive salivation, urination, repetitive jaw movements, opening and closing of the mouth, and staring.	Spikes and sharp waves initially only in frontal derivations. All derivations affected later in disease course	
Cavalier King Charles Spaniel (Driver *et al.*, 2013)	No association between seizures and ventriculomegaly/caudal fossa overcrowding	• 39 % primarily generalised • Tonic-clonic, tonic, atonic • 36 % focal epileptic seizures • Simple or complex • 25 % focal with secondary generalisation	Generalised SWC predominant over fronto-temporal region Sharp waves	
Idiopathic epilepsy in Golden retrievers (Srenk and Jaggy, 1996)	Age of onset: 24.9-27.5 months Male predisposed Mean survival time after diagnosis: 46 months No impact of castration on seizure frequency Better outcome with earlier treatment	• Generalised seizure: 83-92%	Generalised 12Hz spindles in epileptic dogs (n=5) vs control	

Syndrome	Clinical characteristics	Seizure type	Interictal EEG	Ictal EEG
Progressive myoclonic epilepsy – Lafora disease (Hajek *et al.*, 2016; Swain *et al.*, 2017; Demeny *et al.*, 2020; Flegel *et al.*, 2021)	• Miniature wirehaired Dachshund (Epm2b mutation): • Age of onset: 6.94 years (3.5-12) • Later on: Dementia, blindness aggression, deafness, incontinence (loss of training) • Beagles (NHRLC1 mutation): age of onset: 6.5 – 8 years • Basset hounds, Poodles, Pointer, Corgi	• Reflex/spontaneous myoclonus (77.8%) • Hypnic myoclonus • Jaw smacking/fly catching • Generalised tonic-clonic seizures • Progression in frequency and severity over time	Spikes, polyspikes, spike-and-waves.	Spikes, polyspikes, spike-and-wave. Myoclonus not necessarily correlated with EEG.
Absence seizures with myoclonus in a juvenile Chihuahua (Poma, Ochi and Cortez, 2010)	Onset at 4 months	• Absence seizure with myoclonus: Staring episodes with cessation of voluntary motor activity, head and nose twitching, pelvic limb jerking especially when drowsy.		4Hz SWC, generalised, bilaterally synchronous

Table 14.6 : Electroclinical syndromes in dogs

References

Barker, E.N. *et al.* (2016) Degenerative Encephalopathy in Nova Scotia Duck Tolling Retrievers Presenting with a Rapid Eye Movement Sleep Behavior Disorder *Journal of Veterinary Internal Medicine*, 30(5), pp. 1681–1689. doi: 10.1111/jvim.14575. PMID: 27717189. PMCID: PMC5032881.

Berendt, M. *et al.* (2008) Prevalence and characteristics of epilepsy in the Belgian shepherd variants Groenendael and Tervueren born in Denmark 1995–2004 *Acta Veterinaria Scandinavica*, 50(1), p. 51. doi: 10.1186/1751-0147-50-51. PMID: 19102738. PMCID: PMC2633289.

Brauer, C. *et al.* (2011) Electroencephalographic recordings in dogs: Prevention of muscle artifacts and evaluation of two activation techniques in healthy individuals *Research in Veterinary Science*, 90(2), pp. 306–311. doi: 10.1016/j.rvsc.2010.06.004. PMID: 20591453.

Brauer, C. *et al.* (2012) Activation procedures in the electroencephalograms of healthy and epileptic cats under propofol anaesthesia *Veterinary Record*, 170(14), pp. 360–360. doi: 10.1136/vr.100113. PMID: 22447460.

Brenner, R.P. (1997) Electroencephalography in Syncope *Journal of Clinical Neurophysiology*, 14(3). https://journals.lww.com/clinicalneurophys/Fulltext/1997/05000/Electroencephalography_in_Syncope.4.aspx. doi: 10.1097/00004691-199705000-00004. PMID: 9244159.

Bush, W.W. *et al.* (2004) Diagnosis of Rapid Eye Movement Sleep Disorder With Electroencephalography and Treatment With Tricyclic Antidepressants in a Dog *Journal of the American Animal Hospital Association*, 40(6), pp. 495–500. doi: 10.5326/0400495. PMID: 15533971.

Chen, X. *et al.* (2008) A neonatal encephalopathy with seizures in standard poodle dogs with a missense mutation in the canine ortholog of ATF2 *Neurogenetics*, 9(1), pp. 41–49. doi: 10.1007/s10048-007-0112-2. PMID: 18074159.

Cuff, D.E. *et al.* (2014) Use of continuous electroencephalography for diagnosis and monitoring of treatment of nonconvulsive status epilepticus in a cat *Journal of the American Veterinary Medical Association*, 244(6), pp. 708–714. doi: 10.2460/javma.244.6.708. PMID: 24568113.

Demeny, H. *et al.* (2020) EEG Patterns Orienting to Lafora Disease Diagnosis—A Case Report in Two Beagles *Frontiers in Veterinary Science*, 7, p. 589430. doi: 10.3389/fvets.2020.589430. PMID: 33251270. PMCID: PMC7674959.

Driver, C.J. *et al.* (2013) The association between Chiari-like malformation, ventriculomegaly and seizures in cavalier King Charles spaniels *The Veterinary Journal*, 195(2), pp. 235–237. doi: 10.1016/j.tvjl.2012.05.014. PMID: 22749114.

Flegel, T. *et al.* (2021) A retrospective case series of clinical signs in 28 Beagles with Lafora disease *Journal of Veterinary Internal Medicine*, 35(5), pp. 2359–2365. doi: 10.1111/jvim.16255. PMID: 34486182. PMCID: PMC8478043.0

Geut, I. *et al.* (2017) Detecting interictal discharges in first seizure patients: ambulatory EEG or EEG after sleep deprivation? *Seizure*, 51, pp. 52–54. doi: 10.1016/j.seizure.2017.07.019. PMID: 28797915.

Goodin, D.S. and Aminoff, Mi.J. (1984) DOES THE INTERICTAL EEG HAVE A ROLE IN THE DIAGNOSIS OF EPILEPSY? *The Lancet*, 323(8381), pp. 837–839. doi: 10.1016/S0140-6736(84)92281-5. PMID: 6143148.

Granum, L.K. *et al.* (2019) Prevalence of electrographic seizure in dogs and cats undergoing electroencephalography and clinical characteristics and outcome for dogs and cats with and without electrographic seizure: 104 cases (2009–2015) *Journal of the American Veterinary Medical Association*, 254(8), pp. 967–973. doi: 10.2460/javma.254.8.967. PMID: 30938610.

Hajek, I. *et al.* (2016) *NHLRC1* repeat expansion in two beagles with Lafora disease: Genetics in beagles with Lafora disease *Journal of Small Animal Practice*, 57(11), pp. 650–652. doi: 10.1111/jsap.12593. PMID: 27747878. PMCID: PMC5658008.

Hasegawa, D. (2016) Diagnostic techniques to detect the epileptogenic zone: Pathophysiological and presurgical analysis of epilepsy in dogs and cats *The Veterinary Journal*, 215, pp. 64–75. doi: 10.1016/j.tvjl.2016.03.005. PMID: 27052436.

Hirsch, L.J. *et al.* (2021) American Clinical Neurophysiology Society's Standardized Critical Care EEG Terminology: 2021 Version *Journal of Clinical Neurophysiology*, 38(1), pp. 1–29. doi: 10.1097/WNP.0000000000000806. PMID: 33475321. PMCID: PMC8135051.

Holliday, T.A. and Williams, D.C. (1998) Interictal paroxysmal discharges in the electroencephalograms of epileptic dogs *Seizure Disorders*, 13(3), pp. 132–143. doi: 10.1016/S1096-2867(98)80034-0. PMID: 9775503.

Iotchev, I.B. *et al.* (2019) Age-related differences and sexual dimorphism in canine sleep spindles *Scientific Reports*, 9(1), p. 10092. doi: 10.1038/s41598-019-46434-y. PMID: 31300672. PMCID: PMC6626048.

James, F.M.K. *et al.* (2017) Diagnostic Utility of Wireless Video-Electroencephalography in Unsedated Dogs *Journal of Veterinary Internal Medicine*, 31(5), pp. 1469–1476. doi: 10.1111/jvim.14789. PMID: 28758239. PMCID: PMC5598905.

Jeserevics, J. *et al.* (2007) Electroencephalography findings in healthy and Finnish Spitz dogs with epilepsy: visual and background quantitative analysis *Journal of veterinary internal medicine*, 21(6), pp. 1299–1306. doi: 10.1892/06-285.1. PMID: 18196740

Johnson, E.L., Martinez, N.C. and Ritzl, E.K. (2016) EEG Characteristics of Successful Burst Suppression for Refractory Status Epilepticus *Neurocritical Care*, 25(3), pp. 407–414. doi: 10.1007/s12028-016-0294-2. PMID: 27406818.

Jokinen, T. s. *et al.* (2007) Benign Familial Juvenile Epilepsy in Lagotto Romagnolo Dogs *Journal of Veterinary Internal Medicine*, 21(3), pp. 464–471. doi: 10.1111/j.1939-1676.2007.tb02991.x.

Juan, E. *et al.* (2015) EEG as an Indicator of Cerebral Functioning in Postanoxic Coma *Journal of Clinical Neurophysiology*, 32(6), pp. 465–471. doi: 10.1097/WNP.0000000000000199. PMID: 26629756.

Jurney, C. *et al.* (2009) Polymicrogyria in Standard Poodles *Journal of Veterinary Internal Medicine*, 23(4), pp. 871–874. doi: 10.1111/j.1939-1676.2009.0338.x. PMID: 19566852.

Kaleem, S. and Swisher, C.B. (2022) Utility of Quantitative EEG for Seizure Detection in Adults *Journal of Clinical Neurophysiology*, 39(3), pp. 184–194. doi: 10.1097/WNP.0000000000000768. PMID: 32810003.

Kis, A. *et al.* (2014) Development of a non-invasive polysomnography technique for dogs (Canis familiaris) *Physiology & Behavior*, 130, pp. 149–156. doi: 10.1016/j.physbeh.2014.04.004. PMID: 24726397.

Knipe, M.F. *et al.* (2023) Periodic discharges in veterinary electroencephalography—A visual review *Frontiers in Veterinary Science*, 10, p. 1037404. doi: 10.3389/fvets.2023.1037404. PMID: 36777678. PMCID: PMC9909489.

Krishnamurthy, K.B. and Drislane, F.W. (1999) Depth of EEG Suppression and Outcome in Barbiturate Anesthetic Treatment for Refractory Status Epilepticus *Epilepsia*, 40(6), pp. 759–762. doi: 10.1111/j.1528-1157.1999.tb00775.x. PMID: 10368075.

Kuwabara, T. *et al.* (2010) A familial spontaneous epileptic feline strain: A novel model of idiopathic/genetic epilepsy *Epilepsy Research*, 92(1), pp. 85–88. doi: 10.1016/j.eplepsyres.2010.08.010. PMID: 20850949.

Lin, L. and Drislane, F.W. (2018) Lateralized Periodic Discharges: A Literature Review *Journal of Clinical Neurophysiology*, 35(3), pp. 189–198. doi: 10.1097/WNP.0000000000000448. PMID: 29718828.

Mondino, A. *et al.* (2021) Sleep Disorders in dogs: A Pathophysiological and Clinical Review *Topics in Companion Animal Medicine*, 43, p. 100516. doi: 10.1016/j.tcam.2021.100516. PMID: 33556640.

Morgan, R.J., Steadman, J.W. and Lambert, P.D. (1973) Measurement of the change in the normal canine EEG with age *Electroencephalography and Clinical Neurophysiology*, 34(4), pp. 409–418. doi: 10.1016/0013-4694(73)90092-8. PMID: 4120315.

Morita, T. *et al.* (2002) Cliniconeuropathologic findings of familial frontal lobe epilepsy in Shetland sheepdogs *Canadian Journal of Veterinary Research*, 66(1), pp. 35–41. PMID: 11858647. PMCID: PMC226980.

Myles, P. *et al.* (2004) Bispectral index monitoring to prevent awareness during anaesthesia: the B-Aware randomised controlled trial *The Lancet*, 363(9423), pp. 1757–1763. doi: 10.1016/S0140-6736(04)16300-9. PMID: 15172773.

Neurocritical Care Society Status Epilepticus Guideline Writing Committee *et al.* (2012) Guidelines for the Evaluation and Management of Status Epilepticus *Neurocritical Care*, 17(1), pp. 3–23. doi: 10.1007/s12028-012-9695-z. PMID: 22528274.

Noachtar, S. and Rémi, J. (2009) The role of EEG in epilepsy: A critical review *Epilepsy & Behavior*, 15(1), pp. 22–33. doi: 10.1016/j.yebeh.2009.02.035. PMID: 19248841.

Packer, R. *et al.* (2015) Inter-observer agreement of canine and feline paroxysmal event semiology and classification by veterinary neurology specialists and non-specialists *BMC Veterinary Research*, 11(1), p. 39. doi: 10.1186/s12917-015-0356-2. PMID: 25881213. PMCID: PMC4337258.

Pakozdy, A. *et al.* (2014) EEG-confirmed epileptic activity in a cat with VGKC-complex/LGI1 antibody-associated limbic encephalitis *Epileptic Disorders*, 16(1), pp. 116–120. doi: 10.1684/epd.2014.0635. PMID: 24667692.

Parmentier, T. *et al.* (2020) Effect of prior general anaesthesia or sedation and antiseizure drugs on the diagnostic utility of wireless video electroencephalography in dogs *Journal of Veterinary Internal Medicine*, 34(5), pp. 1967–1974. doi: 10.1111/jvim.15856. PMID: 33463773. PMCID: PMC7517491.

Pellegrino, F. and Sica, R. (2004) Canine electroencephalographic recording technique: findings in normal and epileptic dogs *Clinical Neurophysiology*, 115(2), pp. 477–487. doi: 10.1016/S1388-2457(03)00347-X. PMID: 14744591.

Poma, R., Ochi, A. and Cortez, M.A. (2010) Absence seizures with myoclonic features in a juvenile Chihuahua dog *Epileptic disorders*, 12(2), pp. 138–141. Epub 2010 May 20. doi: 10.1684/epd.2010.0312. PMID: 20483714.

Reicher, V. *et al.* (2021) Developmental features of sleep electrophysiology in family dogs *Scientific Reports*, 11(1), p. 22760. doi: 10.1038/s41598-021-02117-1. PMID: 34815446. PMCID: PMC8611005.

Rogers, C.B. *et al.* (2024) Canine Electroencephalography Electrode Positioning Using a Neuronavigation System *Animals*, 14(11), p. 1539. doi: 10.3390/ani14111539. PMID: 38891586. PMCID: PMC11171057.

Ruijter, B.J. *et al.* (2018) The prognostic value of discontinuous EEG patterns in postanoxic coma *Clinical Neurophysiology*, 129(8), pp. 1534–1543. doi: 10.1016/j.clinph.2018.04.745. PMID: 29807232.

Sansevere, A.J., Hahn, C.D. and Abend, N.S. (2019) Conventional and quantitative EEG in status epilepticus *Seizure*, 68, pp. 38–45. doi: 10.1016/j.seizure.2018.09.011. PMID: 30528098.

Schubert, T.A., Chidester, R.M. and Chrisman, C.L. (2011) Clinical characteristics, management and long-term outcome of suspected rapid eye movement sleep behaviour disorder in 14 dogs *Journal of Small Animal Practice*, 52(2), pp. 93–100. doi: 10.1111/j.1748-5827.2010.01026.x. PMID: 21265848.

Shea, A. *et al.* (2018) Association between clinically probable REM sleep behavior disorder and tetanus in dogs *Journal of Veterinary Internal Medicine*, 32(6), pp. 2029–2036. doi: 10.1111/jvim.15320. PMID: 30315605. PMCID: PMC6272037.

Srenk, P. and Jaggy, A. (1996) Interictal electroencephalographic findings in a family of golden retrievers with idiopathic epilepsy *Journal of small animal practice*, 37(7), pp. 317–321. doi: 10.1111/j.1748-5827.1996.tb02398.x. PMID: 8840251.

Stecker, M.M. *et al.* (2016) American Clinical Neurophysiology Society Guideline 6: Minimum Technical Standards for EEG Recording in Suspected Cerebral Death *The Neurodiagnostic Journal*, 56(4), pp. 276–284. doi: 10.1080/21646821.2016.1245575. PMID: 28436789.

Swain, L. *et al.* (2017) Lafora disease in miniature Wirehaired Dachshunds *PLOS ONE*. Edited by F. Palau, 12(8), p. e0182024. doi: 10.1371/journal.pone.0182024. PMID: 28767715. PMCID: PMC5540395.

Tatum, W.O. *et al.* (2016) American Clinical Neurophysiology Society Guideline 7: Guidelines for EEG Reporting *The Neurodiagnostic Journal*, 56(4), pp. 285–293. doi: 10.1080/21646821.2016.1245576. PMID: 28436792.

Thompson, S.A. and Hantus, S. (2016) Highly Epileptiform Bursts Are Associated With Seizure Recurrence *Journal of Clinical Neurophysiology*, 33(1). https://journals.lww.com/clinicalneurophys/Fulltext/2016/02000/Highly_Epileptiform_Bursts_Are_Associated_With.12.aspx. doi: 10.1097/WNP.0000000000000232. PMID: 26844972.

Tobler, I. and Scherschlicht, R. (1990) Sleep and EEG slow-wave activity in the domestic cat: Effect of sleep deprivation *Behavioural Brain Research*, 37(2), pp. 109–118. doi: 10.1016/0166-4328(90)90086-T. PMID: 2322413.

Trinka, E. *et al.* (2015) A definition and classification of status epilepticus – Report of the ILAE Task Force on Classification of Status Epilepticus *Epilepsia*, 56(10), pp. 1515–1523. doi: 10.1111/epi.13121. PMID: 26336950.

Ukai, M. *et al.* (2021) Seizure frequency discrepancy between subjective and objective ictal electroencephalography data in dogs *Journal of Veterinary Internal Medicine*, 35(4), pp. 1819–1825. doi: 10.1111/jvim.16158. PMID: 34002887. PMCID: PMC8295668.

Ward, J., James, F. and Monteith, G. (2016) The effect of topical lidocaine on muscle artefacts in awake canine electroencephalogram recordings *The Veterinary Journal*, 213, pp. 6–8. doi: 10.1016/j.tvjl.2016.03.025. PMID: 27240906.

Wielaender, F. *et al.* (2017) Generalized myoclonic epilepsy with photosensitivity in juvenile dogs caused by a defective DIRAS family GTPase 1 *Proceedings of the National Academy of Sciences*, 114(10), pp. 2669–2674. doi: 10.1073/pnas.1614478114. PMID: 28223533. PMCID: PMC5347561.

Wielaender, F. *et al.* (2018) Absence Seizures as a Feature of Juvenile Myoclonic Epilepsy in Rhodesian Ridgeback Dogs *Journal of Veterinary Internal Medicine*, 32(1), pp. 428–432. doi: 10.1111/jvim.14892. PMID: 29194766. PMCID: PMC5787207.

Wrzosek, M. *et al.* (2017) The relationship between epileptiform discharges and background activity in the visual analysis of electroencephalographic examinations in dogs with seizures of different etiologies *The Veterinary Journal*, 222, pp. 41–51. doi: 10.1016/j.tvjl.2017.03.003. PMID: 28410675.

Young, G.B. *et al.* (1997) An Electroencephalographic Classification for Coma *Canadian Journal of Neurological Sciences/Journal Canadien des Sciences Neurologiques*, 24(04), pp. 320–325. doi: 10.1017/S0317167100032996. PMID: 9398979.

APPENDIX I

Useful definitions in electrodiagnosis and neuromuscular syndromes

Largely extracted from Kimura, Electrodiagnosis in Diseases of Nerve and Muscle: Principles and Practice, 4th Edition, Oxford University Press; (September 9, 2013).

Action potential: an electric potential that propagates along a single axon or muscle fibre membrane.

Active electrode: synonymous with exploring/recording electrode.

Afferent nerve: nerve carrying impulses from sensory receptors or sense organs toward the central nervous system.

Anode: the positive terminal of an electric current source.

Antidromic: propagation of a nerve impulse in the direction opposite to the physiologic conduction.

Amplitude (of an action potential): maximum voltage difference recorded between two points (usually peak to peak or baseline to peak).

Arrhythmic activity: a sequence of waves with inconstant period

Asymmetry: measured on referential recording

Asynchrony: non-simultaneous occurrence of EEG activity over regions on the same or opposite side of the brain. This is seen for example with epileptiform discharges with independent foci.

Axon (nerve fibre): projection of a nerve cell which conducts the electrical impulses (action potentials) away from the cell body.

Axonotmesis: nerve injury characterised by axon and myelin sheath disruption without disruption of the supporting connective tissue (endoneurium).

Backfiring: discharge of a motor neuron that travels antidromically.

Burst: pattern lasting more than 0.5 seconds and with at least 4 phases

Cathode: the negative terminal of an electric current source.

Chorea: an abrupt, unsustained contraction of different muscle groups.

Compound muscle action potential: a waveform representing the summation of multiple individual axon or muscle fibre action potentials recorded from a muscle.

Compound sensory nerve action potential: compound nerve action potential recorded from a sensory nerve or a mixed nerve.

Conduction block: failure of an action potential to propagate past a particular point in the nervous system, whereas conduction below that point remains possible.

Conduction velocity: speed of propagation of an action potential along a nerve, calculated in meters per second (m/s).

Cord dorsum potential: a field potential generated where the dorsal root axons synapse with the lower motor neurons and interneurons; this is also sometimes referred to as 'root entry zone potential'.

Cramp: a sudden, severe, and involuntary muscle contraction or over-shortening that is generally temporary and benign.

Decrement: reduction in the amplitude or area of the compound muscle action potential following repetitive nerve stimulation.

Demyelination: consequence of a disorder involving the myelin sheath, resulting in decreased conduction velocities and/or in a conduction block.

Depolarisation: change of an excitable cell's membrane potential to a more positive value. An action potential is generated when the cell is depolarised from its resting potential to a threshold.

Dermatome: area of skin which is supplied by afferent fibres from the dorsal root of a specific spinal nerve/specific spinal nerve ganglion.

Discharge: wave of <0.5s in duration or >0.5s and less than 3 phases.

Discontinuous: alternating periods of evident cerebral activity with marked attenuation of EEG signals.

Disorganisation: gross alteration of frequency, topography or quantity of EEG rhythms relative to previous records or homologous regions

Efferent nerve: nerve conducting signals from the central nervous system along motor axons to muscles and glands.

Electro decremental event: sudden reduction of EEG amplitude in large areas of brain, generally following epileptiform paroxysm.

Electromyography (EMG): recording and study of insertion, spontaneous and voluntary activity of muscle with a recording electrode (either a needle electrode for invasive EMG or a surface electrode for kinesiologic studies). The EMG is the recording of electrical activity in the muscle between a cathode and an anode in a small volume just as an ECG is the recording of the myocardium electrical activity between a negative and a positive surface electrodes/leads placed on the skin at a large distance (distal part of the limbs).

Electroneurography: recording and study of action potentials in peripheral nerves (= nerve conduction studies).

End-plate activity: spontaneous electrical activity recorded with a needle electrode inserted close to the muscle end-plate.

Epileptiform: may or may not be associated with epilepsy

Episodic: a set or group of waves that reoccur at variable intervals

Epoch: a period of time in an EEG record

Fasciculation: random, spontaneous contraction (twitching) of a group of muscle fibres belonging to single motor units. The twitch may be visible on the overlying skin but deeper fasciculation in a muscle is not visible. This produces fasciculation potentials.

Far-field potential: electrical potential that is recorded instantly away from its source.

Fibrillation potential: action potential from a single muscle fibre that occurs spontaneously or following movement of a needle electrode.

Frequency: number of cycles of a repetitive waveform recorded in one second, measured in hertz (Hz).

F-wave: action potential recorded from a muscle following a supramaximal stimulus to a motor nerve secondary to antidromic activation of motor neurons.

Gain: the factor by which power or voltage is increased in an amplifier.

'Ground' electrode: the common reference point for an electrical circuit reflecting background electrical activity, also called the reference electrode.

H-wave: compound muscle action potential recorded following submaximal stimulation of peripheral sensory fibres and monosynaptic activation of alpha motor neurons in the spinal cord.

Hyperpolarisation: change in the existing membrane potential to a more negative value.

Hypsarrhythmia: abnormal EEG pattern consisting in high amplitude bilateral independent polymorphic spikes and waves occurring in a disorganised background. It is considered an interictal pattern.

- Marked: decrease > 50% in amplitude or >1Hz in frequency
- Mild: decrease of less than 50% in the amplitude or of 0.5-1Hz in frequency of the activity in a region compared to another

Impedance: the measure of the opposition that a circuit presents to a current when a voltage is applied.

Insertion activity: electrical activity induced by the insertion or movement of an electrode within the muscle.

Jitter: variability of consecutive discharges of the interpotential interval between two muscle fibre action potentials belonging to the same motor unit.

Latency: time lapse between a stimulus and a response.

Miniature end-plate potential: muscle fibre potential resulting from the spontaneous release of individual acetylcholine quanta from the pre-synaptic axon terminal.

Mixed nerve: nerve that contains both afferent and efferent axons and as a consequence conducts both sensory and motor information.

Motor nerve: nerve that transmit motor information from the central nervous system to the muscles via efferent fibres.

Motor unit: the anatomic element consisting of a ventral horn cell, its axon, the neuromuscular junction, and all the muscle fibres innervated by the axon.

Motor unit action potential: electrical potential that is the sum of potentials generated by muscle fibres from a motor unit located within the area of recording of the EMG needle.

Motor point/determining the motor point location: the motor point of a muscle is the location of the skin area above the muscle in which an electrical stimulation applied transcutaneously evokes a muscle twitch with the least current. It needs to be electrophysiologically identified and is different from the location of the motor entry point, which is the point where the motor branch enters the muscle belly. Stimulation pen-electrodes can be used in humans to quickly and efficiently 'scan' the skin and determine the location of the motor point. Location of motor points in specific muscles has been published in dogs.

Myelin sheath: lipidic insulating layer surrounding the axons of most neuronal cells allowing saltatory conduction and increasing the motor nerve conduction velocity.

Myoclonus: a quick jerk of a body part produced by a brief muscle contraction typically originating from activity in the central nervous system (spinal, segmental, brainstem or cortical).

Myokymia: undulating movement of the skin overlying a muscle associated with spontaneous repetitive discharge of motor unit action potentials.

Myokymic discharge: burst of motor unit action potentials firing recurring for a short period of time.

Myotome: group of muscles innervated by a single spinal nerve root.

Myotonia: delayed relaxation of a muscle after voluntary contraction or percussion.

Myotonic discharge: repetitive discharge of a single muscle fibre which wax and wane, occurring following needle electrode insertion, muscle contraction or after muscle percussion.

M-wave: compound muscle action potential evoked from a muscle following electrical stimulation of the motor nerve that innervates it.

Nerve conduction velocity: speed at which electrical impulses propagate down a nerve, reported in meters per second.

Neurapraxia: mildest form of traumatic peripheral nerve injury, with focal demyelination at the site of injury, without disruption of the axon and surrounding connective tissues (endoneurium). This results in a transient conduction block.

Neuromyotonia: continuous muscle fibre activity manifested as continuous muscle rippling and stiffness.

Neuromyotonic discharge: motor unit action potentials firing at high rates (150-300Hz) and often starting or stopping abruptly.

Neurotmesis: Partial or complete nerve injury that includes the axons and endoneurium.

Near-field potential: potential recorded close to its source (i.e. compound muscle action potential, sensory nerve action potential, motor unit action potential...)

Orthodromic: propagation of a nerve impulse in the same direction as physiologic conduction.

Periodic: repetition of a pattern with relatively similar morphology and duration at regular intervals (inter-discharge interval). In practice, this corresponds to a less than 50% variation in the period length in the majority of the cycles. It is called pseudo periodic if the period is not exact.

Peripheral nervous system: part of the nervous system made of nerve roots of cranial and spinal motor and sensory nerves, peripheral nerves, neuromuscular junctions and muscles.

Phase: that portion of a waveform between the departure from and the return to the baseline.

Phase cancellation: with increase in latency of some fibres, positive peaks may arrive at the level of the recording site concomitantly with negative peaks, leading to cancellation of the peak on the recording display and therefore no recorded amplitude.

Polyphasic action potential: action potential with more than four baseline crossings.

Projected pattern: abnormal EEG activity believed to result from disturbance in a remote region of the brain generally in frontal region, of high amplitude and slow frequency

Recording electrode: to record an electrical potential difference, two electrodes are necessary (e.g. usually a pair of monopolar electrodes): the electrode close to the source of the signal is the 'active' electrode also called 'exploring' electrode (this is the cathode) and the other electrode is the anode.

Resting membrane potential: voltage across the membrane of an excitable cell in the absence of a stimulus.

Rhythmic: repetition of a waveform with relatively similar morphology and duration without an interval between consecutive waveforms (no inter-discharge interval). In practice, to be called rhythmic, the duration of one waveform of a rhythmic pattern should vary by less than 50% of the duration of the next waveform for the majority of the waveform pairs.

Sensory nerve: nerve containing only afferent nerve fibres.

Single-fibre electromyography (sfEMG): The recording of single muscle fibre action potentials using a needle electrode.

Spinal nerve: mixed nerve carrying sensory, motor and autonomic signals between the spinal cord and the body.

Stimulating electrode: to deliver a current for stimulation, two electrodes are necessary (e.g. a pair of monopolar electrodes): the negative terminal (cathode) and the positive terminal (anode); the stimulating electrode is the negative terminal placed near the structure to stimulate (e.g. a nerve for study of motor conduction velocity).

Temporal dispersion: desynchronisation of components of a compound potential due to different rates of conduction of each synchronously evoked component from the stimulation point to the recording electrode.

Threshold: voltage level at which an action potential is initiated in an axon or muscle fibre.

Voltage: potential difference between two recording sites (expressed in volts).

Volume conduction: spread of current from a potential source through a conducting medium (from the intracellular space through extracellular fluid and body tissues).

Wallerian degeneration: degeneration of the segment of an axon located distal to the site of injury.

APPENDIX II

List of abbreviations

Ach: acetylcholine

AchE: acetylcholinesterase

AchR: acetylcholine receptor

A: ampere

ASSR: auditory steady-state responses

BAER: brainstem auditory evoked responses

BIRD: Brief potentially ictal rhythmic discharges

CHAT: choline acetyltransferase

CK: creatine kinase

CMAP: compound muscle action potential

ColQ: collagen-like tail subunit of asymmetric acetylcholinesterase

ECG: electrocardiography/electrocardiogram

ED: epileptiform discharge

EEG: electroencephalography

EMG: electromyography

EOG: electrooculogram

ERG: electroretinography

G: gauge

GABA: Gamma-aminobutyric acid

GPDTW: Generalized periodic discharges with triphasic wave morphology

Hz: hertz

Ω: ohm

LGI1: Leucine-rech, glioma inactivated 1

LPD lateral periodic discharge

NMDA: N-methyl-D-aspartate receptor

MEPP: miniature end-plate potential

MiNAP: mixed nerve action potential

MNCV: motor nerve conduction velocity

m: meter

MUAP: motor unit action potential

OAE: otoacoustic emissions

POSTS: Positive occipital sharp transient of sleep

qEEG: quantitative electroencephalography

REM sleep: rapid eye movement sleep

s: second

SARDS: sudden acquired retinal degeneration syndrome

SE: status epilepticus

SED: sporadic epileptiform discharges

SNAP: sensory nerve action potential

SSEP: somatosensory evoked potential

SWC: spike-wave complex

THC: tetrahydrocannabinol

VGKC: voltage-gated potassium channel

VEP: visual evoked potential

V: volt

APPENDIX III

Reference range for common nerve conduction velocities and compound muscle action potentials in dogs and cats

Note that these are obtained from specific laboratories, as referenced, but values may vary from one clinic / laboratory to another.
Malik R, Ho S. Motor nerve conduction parameters in the cat. J Small Anim Pract. 1989; 30: 396–400

Canine - mean motor nerve conduction velocity (m/s +/- standard deviation)	Based on Lee and Bowen, 1970 (*) and Walker *et al.*, 1979 (**)
Peroneal	77 +/- 3.8 (*)
Tibial	60 +/- 1.7 (*)
Ulnar	60 +/- 1.1 (*)
Radial	72 +/- 1.9 (**)

Canine - mean compound muscle action potential amplitude (mV +/- standard deviation)	Based on Walker *et al.*, 1979	
	Proximal stimulation	Distal stimulation
Peroneal	19.8 +/- 1.4	19.5 +/- 1.5
Tibial	20.1 +/- 1.6	23.3 +/- 2.3
Ulnar	22.9 +/- 1.6	25.8 +/- 1.8
Radial	23.4 +/-1.5	21.6+/-1.6

Feline - median motor nerve conduction velocity [m/s (range)]	Based on Malik and Ho, 1989
Peroneal	115.1 (100.3-142.1)
Tibial (proximal-distal)	98.8 (90.5-107.9)
Ulnar	82.3 (76.9-100.0)

Feline - median compound muscle action potential amplitude range [mV (range)]	Based on Malik and Ho, 1989	
	Proximal stimulation	Distal stimulation
Peroneal	28.7 (24.1-33.1)	30.3 (26.7-36.4)
Tibial	16.2 (12.4-18.6)	20.5 (18.8-23.4)
Ulnar	14.7 (11.0-20.8)	17.9 (14.9-22.4)

Canine - mean sensory nerve conduction velocity (m/s +/- standard deviation)	Based on Redding *et al.*, 1984
Peroneal	64.4 +/- 5.25
Tibial	63.4 +/- 5.3
Ulnar	69.4 +/- 6.9
Radial	65.1 +/- 6.2

Feline - mean sensory nerve conduction velocity (m/s +/- standard deviation)	Based on Redding and Ingram, 1984
Peroneal	85.3 +/- 6.8
Tibial	80.2 +/- 7.9
Ulnar	89.2 +/- 10.3
Radial	83.6 +/- 8.3

Author Biographies

Lead Authors

Dr. Hélène Vandenberghe DVM, Dip ECVN, MRCVS

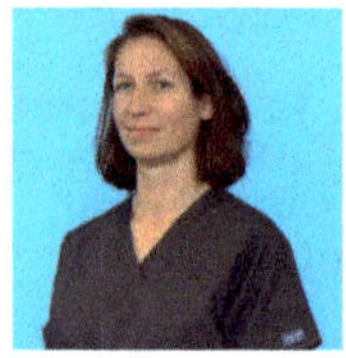

Hélène is a veterinary surgeon who graduated from the Nantes-Atlantic National College of Veterinary Medicine, France, in 2014 and subsequently completed an internship and a European College of Veterinary Neurology residency at the National Veterinary School of Alfort (Paris). She then moved to the United Kingdom in 2018 to join Highcroft Veterinary Referrals, which became Bristol Vet Specialists in 2023. By training, she has a strong interest in medical neurology and electrophysiology and has published and reviewed papers around those disciplines. Hélène takes an active part in teaching and lecturing in England and France.

Dr. Edward Ives MA, VetMB, Dip ECVN, MRCVS

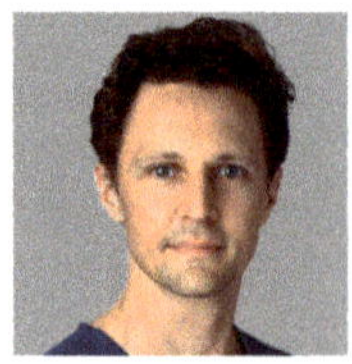

Edward is a veterinary surgeon who graduated from the University of Cambridge, UK, in 2007 before working in first-opinion small animal practice. He returned to the University of Cambridge in 2012 to complete a three-year Senior Clinical Training Scholarship in Veterinary Neurology and Neurosurgery, before joining Anderson Moores Veterinary Specialists, UK, where he is now Head of Service. Edward is a Diplomate of the European College of Veterinary Neurologists and RCVS-recognised specialist in Veterinary Neurology and Neurosurgery. He has lectured nationally and internationally on many aspects of veterinary neurology and co-authored a textbook aimed at veterinary students and general practitioners. He has a passion for teaching and trying to demystify subjects, such as electrodiagnostics, so that they are approachable to all.

Dr. Nicolas Granger DVM, PhD, FHEA, Dip ECVN, FRCVS

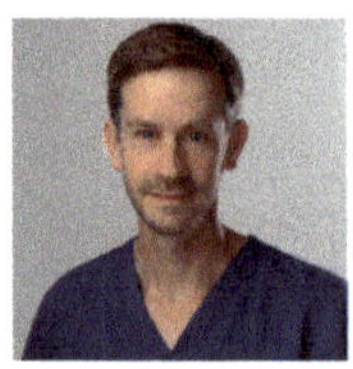

Nicolas is a veterinary surgeon. He is Head of the neurology and neurosurgery service at Bristol Veterinary Specialists (part of CVS referrals), RCVS-recognised specialist in Veterinary Neurology and Neurosurgery, Fellow of the Royal College of Veterinary Surgeons and visiting Fellow of the University of Bath. Nicolas graduated from the National Veterinary School of Alfort (Paris), in 2002, where he completed an internship and neurology residency to become a Diplomate of the European College of Veterinary Neurology in 2006. He led the neurology and neurosurgery service at the Queen's Veterinary School Hospital, University of Cambridge, UK, between 2006 and 2008 and worked there on a Medical Research Council funded PhD in neuroscience in 2012. He continued his research and teaching as Senior Lecturer at the University of Bristol until 2016. Nicolas' research focuses on treatments for spinal cord injury in dogs, in particular cell transplantation and neuromodulation for incontinence control. Nicolas' clinical activities and research have led him to study and exploit functional testing such as urodynamic and electrophysiology for companion animals.

Contributing Authors

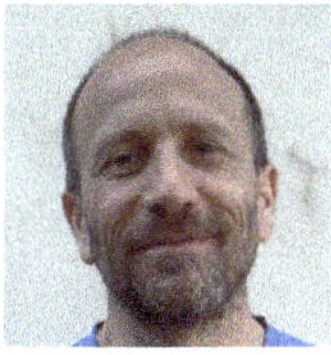

Dr. Ezio Bianchi DVM, Dip ECVN
Associate Professor, EBVS® European Specialist in Veterinary Neurology
Department of Veterinary Science, University of Parma,
Parma, Italy

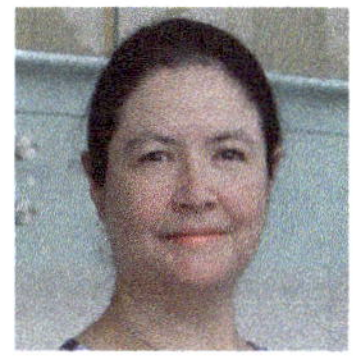

Dr. Fiona M.K. James, DVM, MSc, DVSc, Dip ACVIM (Neurology)
Professor & Chief Neurology and Neurosurgery Service
Graduate Program Coordinator
Department of Clinical Studies, Ontario Veterinary College, University of Guelph
Guelph, Canada

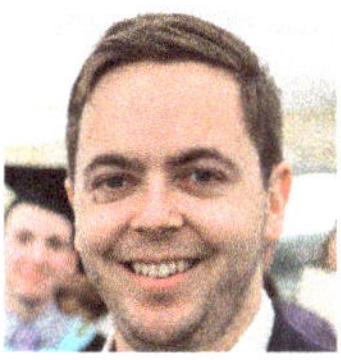

Dr. Benjamin Metcalfe FRSA, FIPEM, FHEA, CEng MIET, MEng (Hons)
Head of Department of Electronic & Electrical Engineering
Deputy Director of the Bath Institute for the Augmented Human
University of Bath
Bath, UK

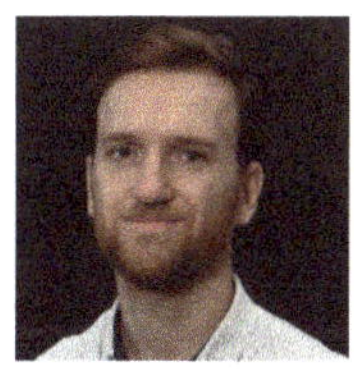

Dr. Thomas Parmentier, DMV, PhD, Dip ACVIM (Neurology)
Assistant Professor of Neurology and Neurosurgery
Département de sciences cliniques, Faculté de médecine vétérinaire, Université de Montréal
Centre Interdisciplinaire de Recherche sur le Cerveau et l'Apprentissage, Université de Montréal
Montréal, Canada

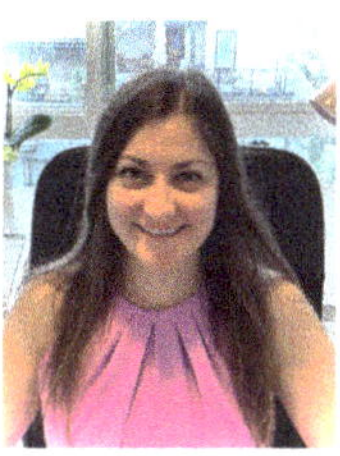

Dr. Francesca Samarani, DVM, Dip ECVN, MRCVS
Adjunct Professor Neurology and Neurosurgery
EBVS® Specialist in Veterinary Neurology
Department of Neurology Canada West Veterinary Specialists and Critical Care Hospital
Vancouver, British Columbia, Canada
Department of Clinical Studies,Ontario Veterinary College, University of Guelph
Guelph, Canada

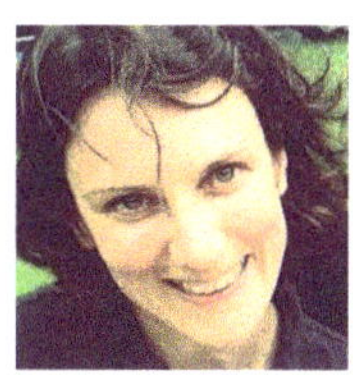

Dr. An Vanhaesebrouck DVM, CEAV (Int Med), Dip ECVN, DPhil, FHEA, MRCVS
Clinical Neurologist & Associate Teaching Professor
Department of Veterinary Medicine, Cambridge University
Cambridge, UK

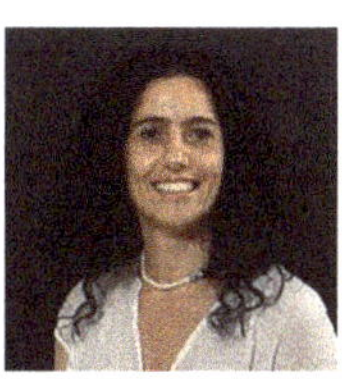

Dr. Maria Vanore, DMV, MSc, Dip ECVO
Assistant Professor in ophthalmology
Département de Sciences cliniques,
Faculté de médecine vétérinaire,
Université de Montréal, Canada

Acknowledgements

We would like to thank Professor Stéphane Blot – National Veterinary School of Alfort (Paris) – for initiating us to the world of electrophysiology and teaching us a discipline he masters.

We are also extremely grateful to An, Ben, Ezio, Fiona, Francesca, Maria, Nick and Thomas who have agreed to share their knowledge; without their expert contribution, the book would have been grossly incomplete.

Finally, this kind of work would not be possible without the support we receive daily from colleagues and family, in various forms, adding, layer after layer, confidence and understanding to what we do in our profession. We hope this will, in turn, help them too.

E.I. – To my father, for all the sacrifices he made to give me the opportunities I have had, and to Gemma, Gilbert and Taggie for their daily love, laughter and support. I'm forever grateful.

Index

Note: Page numbers in *italics* refer to figures and/or tables.

C

N

U

www.ingramcontent.com/pod-product-compliance
Lightning Source LLC
LaVergne TN
LVHW050907210926
848482LV00012B/368
* 9 7 8 1 9 1 1 4 5 0 9 3 1 *